Bottom Line's
ULTIMATE
Antiaging
SECRETS

Everything You Need to Know to Stay Healthier Longer

With Recipes by
Linda Gassenheimer

Bottom Line
Books

www.BottomLineSecrets.com

Table of Contents

A Lifestyle of Longevity

Explore simple changes you can make to ensure you live a long, healthy life. From maintaining a proper weight to increasing your fiber intake, follow these helpful guidelines to improve the quality of your life and increase your longevity.

Crucial Answers for a Longer Life

Find answers to many common questions about potential hazards to your health. Understanding certain risk factors—such as smoking, genetics and sun exposure—is an easy way to start incorporating important changes that will enhance your health.

Don't Let It Happen Again

Whether you have had a heart attack, stroke, or been diagnosed with cancer, disease strikes many people at some point in life. Examine the factors that cause these serious diseases, and find ways to live healthier and prevent a recurrence.

Low-Fat Eating: A Powerful Way to Preserve Good Health

Americans love fat. In fact, we love it so much that, on average, we eat the fat equivalent of six sticks of butter each week. Yes, you read it right—six! But eating that much fat month after month, year after year, takes its toll on our health. In fact, many doctors are convinced that eating excessive amounts of fat is second only to smoking as a health threat.

Fortunately, cutting back on fat can diminish its negative impact. According to Michael Klaper, M.D., director of the Institute of Nutrition Education and Research in Manhattan Beach, California, a growing arsenal of powerful evidence suggests that lowering dietary fat—at any age—can prevent or reverse heart disease, short-circuit strokes, and stifle the growth of many cancers.

Just How Bad Can Fat Be for Your Cardiovascular System?

Of the estimated 13.5 million Americans alive today with a history of heart attack, angina, or both, about 50 percent are age 60 and older. Eighty-three percent of the people who die of heart attacks are age 65 or older. Overall, heart disease and strokes annually kill more than 40 percent of all people who die in the United States.

Hans Diehl, Dr.H.Sc., director of the Coronary Health Improvement Project based in Loma Linda, California, says that five of the eight controllable risk factors for heart disease and stroke have been linked to high-fat diets:

- *elevated cholesterol*
- *elevated triglycerides*
- *high blood pressure*
- *diabetes*
- *excessive weight*

Dr. Diehl's lifestyle intervention program, which includes controlling the amount of fat in the diet, has helped more than 15,000 people worldwide reduce their risk of heart disease.

Heart disease, particularly the type caused by atherosclerosis (hardening of the arteries caused by fatty buildups in the circulatory system) can at least double your risk of stroke, says Ralph L. Sacco, M.D., director of the North Manhattan Stroke Study, which enrolled 260,000 people, and was conducted at Columbia-Presbyterian Medical Center in New York City.

The risk of ischemic stroke—the most common type of stroke, caused by blood clots that block arteries supplying blood to the brain—may be even higher if you also have heart disease. French researchers who examined 250 men and women in their sixties and seventies found that those who had deposits of fatty plaque narrowing their aortic arches (the main artery leading out of the heart) were up to nine times more likely to have ischemic strokes than those who didn't have such buildups.

Dr. Sacco agrees. "If you have plaque there, more than likely you're going to have it in the arteries leading to or inside the brain, too," he says.

And Then There's Cancer

Dietary fat may play a role in up to 40 percent of cancers in men and 60 percent of cancers in women, says Moshe Shike, M.D., director of clinical nutrition at Memorial Sloan-Kettering Cancer Center in New York City and co-author of *Cancer Free*.

Research shows that men in their sixties and seventies who eat lots of red meat have a risk up to three times greater for colon cancer. They also are more likely to develop rectal cancer and 2.6 times more likely to have prostate cancer than men who limit dietary animal fats. Women older than age 60 who load up on red meat are 2.5 times more likely to develop colon cancer.

Scientists are learning more about the role of fat in the development of breast cancer. Researchers at the University of Hawaii compared the eating habits of 272 postmenopausal women who were being treated for breast cancer with 296 women who lived in the same area but who were cancer-free. They found that overweight women who ate a lot of foods high in saturated fat, such as sausage, processed cold cuts, beef, lamb, and whole-milk dairy food, were at greater risk for breast cancer.

"We know that saturated fats have an impact on hormone levels in the body, and we think that has a role in promoting breast cancer," says Cheryl Ritenbaugh, Ph.D., head of nutrition research at the Arizona Cancer Center in Tucson.

Eating a high-fat diet might increase your risk of lung cancer, even if you don't smoke, says Michael Alavanja, Ph.D., senior scientist at the National Cancer Institute in Rockville, Maryland. In his study of 429 female nonsmokers ranging up to age 84, Dr. Alavanja concluded that those who ate the most saturated fat were six times more likely to have lung cancer than those who consumed the least amount of that fat.

"At least seven studies worldwide have shown an effect of saturated fat on lung cancer," Dr. Alavanja says. "The evidence is pointing toward the fact that fat increases the risk of lung cancer among smokers and nonsmokers."

None of these things need to happen to you. You could help prevent and possibly subdue almost every one of these diseases if you did just one thing: Slash the fat.

"It's very clear that our diet is totally devastating us," Dr. Diehl says. "We know that if we cut the fat content and eat a more plant food–centered diet, we could drastically cut our risk for most cancers, heart disease, and stroke."

So Why Do We Still Eat Fat?

A surprising number of people—particularly among those of us over age 60—haven't gotten the word yet.

In fact, one-third of 4,480 people who cook household meals told University of Nebraska researchers that they had never heard that fat was a problem.

"I was very surprised by that finding," says Nancy Betts, R.D., Ph.D., associate professor of nutritional science at the university in Lincoln, who conducted the survey. "The information about fat has been around for a long time. You'd think everyone would be aware of it, especially the people who are taking care of food preparation for an entire household."

Why are we so perplexed?

Well, first, many of us think, and rightly so, that dietary fat exists for a reason. Eating it can provide us with essential fatty acids that we need to regulate body temperature, maintain healthy skin and hair, and insulate and protect nerves and vital organs like the heart and kidneys.

The problem is, all fats are not created equal. There are three main types of fat in foods you eat, each with its own health consequences:

Monounsaturated fats, like olive and canola oils, and *polyunsaturated fats*, like corn and safflower oils, are considered relatively healthy—in moderation.

Saturated fats, which are found mainly in meats, eggs, and dairy products, can cause major health problems, especially if consumed in large quantities.

Trans-fatty acids, another type of harmful fat, are unsaturated fats that have been artificially solidified by food manufacturers to make products like margarines and vegetable shortenings. They have little dietary value.

Unfortunately, many foods don't contain purely unsaturated or saturated fats. When you eat a typical American meal, you're likely to consume a mixture of good and bad fats. That's how it's possible to unwittingly load up on bad fats, even if you cut obvious problem fats—like butter—out of your life.

Why Cut Back Now?

The average American eats about 34 percent of calories from fat—which is down from 43 percent just a few years ago. But many people in their sixties, seventies, and eighties continue to consume 40 to 50 percent of their calories from fat, says Cheryl Pingleton, R.D., a dietitian at the Grand Court Lifestyles, a retirement community in Phoenix. And they're mostly eating the harmful fats.

"Many of the people I see are eating a lot of fried foods, creamy salad dressings, and rich desserts," Pingleton says. "They feel as if they've worked their whole lives and now literally want to enjoy the fat of the land."

But if you enjoy the harmful fats too much, it can lead to serious health problems. If, however, you switch to a low-fat lifestyle, eating mostly unsaturated fats, you may quickly feel rejuvenated, particularly if you have a chronic ailment.

"You can lose weight, feel more energetic, have fewer digestive problems, and just feel better about yourself," Pingleton says. "No matter what your age or medical condition—diabetes, gout, high cholesterol, heart disease—low-fat eating is the way to go."

In 2002, the Institute of Medicine (IOM) said that up to 35 percent of total calories in your diet could come from fat—as long as most of it is the healthful unsaturated variety. Many researchers recommend that fat should fill an even smaller portion of your dinner plate—down to 20 percent or possibly as low as 10 percent of total calories. The American Heart Association urges you to limit saturated fat to less than 10 percent of your daily calories, and the IOM warns against trans-fatty acids as well.

The Skinny on Fat

This table lists the percentage of saturated fat and unsaturated fat in common cooking oils and fats. (Please note that the percentages do not add up to 100 percent because these fats have small amounts of other fatty substances.)

Oil/Fat	Saturated (%)	Monounsaturated (%)	Polyunsaturated (%)
11 superb choices...			
Canola oil	7	60	30
Safflower oil	9	13	76
Walnut oil	9	23	65
Sunflower oil	11	20	67
Corn oil	13	25	59
Olive oil	14	76	9
Soybean oil	15	24	59
Peanut oil	17	47	32
Rice oil	19	42	38
Wheat-germ oil	19	15	63
Margarine	20	48	32
...and 7 ugly ones			
Coconut oil	89	6	2
Butter	64	29	4
Palm oil	50	36	9
Lard	39	45	11
Chicken fat	30	45	20
Cottonseed oil	26	18	53
Vegetable shortening	25	45	20

"Cutting back on fat will help, and the more drastically you can cut back, the better off you'll be, with the lower limit being around 7 percent of calories from fat for nutritional adequacy," says Lee Lipsenthal, M.D., medical director of Preventive Medicine Research Institute in Sausalito, California, where Dean Ornish, M.D., is conducting his pioneering research on reversing heart disease. "You'll certainly have less

angina. You'll also have less risk of stroke, heart attack, and cancer."

It's Not Too Late

The good news is that you can benefit from a change to low-fat eating at any age. Dr. Lipsenthal says, "Every study that I've ever looked at says it's never too late to make these important changes in your diet."

Sorting Out Light, Lean, and Everything in Between

For some of us, telling the difference between Minnesota Fats and monounsaturated fats is a challenge. (A hint: Monos don't play pool.) Here are some of the key words and phrases that you should look for on food labels and what they really mean.

Saturated fats are loaded (saturated) with hydrogen atoms. Saturated fats are found primarily in animal foods like meat, poultry, and dairy products such as butter. These fats tend to raise levels of the "bad" low-density lipoprotein (LDL) cholesterol in the blood and increase the risk of heart disease and stroke. Saturated fat has also been linked to several cancers including colon, prostate, lung, and breast.

Monounsaturated fats, such as olive and canola oils, lower levels of LDL cholesterol in the blood and may reduce the risk of heart disease, stroke, and cancer. They are called monounsaturated because they are missing one pair of hydrogen atoms and, therefore, are unsaturated.

Polyunsaturated fats, such as corn, safflower, sesame, and sunflower oils, are missing more than one pair of hydrogen atoms. Although they aren't as harmful as saturated fats, polyunsaturated fats should be used cautiously because they do lower both LDL and "good" high-density lipoprotein (HDL) cholesterol levels and may increase your risk of cardiovascular disease. Polyunsaturated fats also promote cell division, and that can increase your cancer risk.

Hydrogenated fats are created when food manufacturers add hydrogen atoms to unsaturated fats so that they solidify and transform into saturated fats like vegetable shortenings and margarine.

Trans-fatty acids are solidified polyunsaturated fats created during hydrogenation. They raise LDL cholesterol levels about as much as saturated fat. To be safe, avoid foods with ingredient lists that include hydrogenated or partially hydrogenated fat.

Cholesterol, a fatty chemical compound manufactured by the body, also is found in many meats, dairy products, and other animal foods. It helps make important hormones and cell membranes. Excessive amounts of LDL cholesterol narrow artery walls. HDL cholesterol helps sweep LDL out of the body.

What Fat-Content Labels Mean:

Fat-free. A product carrying this label has less than 0.5 gram of fat in each serving.

Low-fat. This food has 3 grams of fat or less per serving.

Lean. Less than 10 grams of total fat, 4 grams of saturated fat, and 95 milligrams of cholesterol are in each serving of this food.

Light. It contains one-third fewer calories or no more than half the fat of the regular product.

Cholesterol-free. Fewer than 2 milligrams of cholesterol and 2 grams or less of saturated fat are in this product.

Switching to a low-fat lifestyle, even in your later years, can help quash all of the big three killers—heart disease, stroke, and cancer.

How Fatty Foods Damage Your Heart

Within five hours of eating a fatty meal like a slice of pepperoni pizza or a bologna sandwich (both of which are loaded with saturated fat), radical and dangerous changes occur in your body's chemistry, Dr. Klaper says.

Here are some of the ways dietary fat harms your heart:

- First, a tide of fat oozes into the bloodstream and coats red blood cells with a sticky film. "Under normal conditions, blood serum is clear. But after you eat a fatty meal, it is thick, white, and greasy. It looks like household glue," Dr. Klaper says.

- Because they're so sticky, these cells begin to clump together. It is this clumping that eventually forms the blood clots in the arteries, which lead to stroke or heart attack.

- At the same time, saturated fat raises the harmful LDL cholesterol levels in the blood by suppressing the production of enzymes in the liver that would normally help destroy these compounds.

- Adding to your woes, as the body processes the fat, it produces free radicals, the same oxidizing molecules that cause metal to rust and food to spoil. Inside your body, these free radicals cause cholesterol to cling to artery walls and clog them up.

Years of eating like that virtually guarantees that a person over age 60 will have at least some atherosclerosis, the underlying disease that can lead to stroke and heart attack. In addition, this arterial rust makes it more difficult to deliver oxygenated blood, says Dr. Diehl. This starves the tissues and leads to changes that can cause impotence, hearing loss, degenerative disk disease, memory loss, and vision problems.

Reversing Heart Damage

Atherosclerosis is totally unnecessary," Dr. Diehl says. "It is reversible, even after age 60. All you have to do is take better care of yourself, particularly how you eat. The simpler your diet, the better your chances of reversing the narrowing of arteries and increasing blood flow to more adequate levels once again."

According to Dr. Diehl, it won't take long for the effects to kick in. "In as little as three weeks, most people can eat themselves out of angina symptoms just by switching to a simpler diet that includes very low fat foods." Several exciting studies have shown that eating a very low-fat and low-cholesterol diet in conjunction with other lifestyle changes like exercise, smoking cessation, and stress reduction can, as Dr. Diehl explains, actually reverse heart disease.

Here are three diet plans based on these studies of how to restore the heart to good health:

- **The Pritikin Research:** "Our experience has shown that within days of starting a low-fat diet, patients with angina can show an immediate and dramatic decrease in their symptoms," says Monroe Rosenthal, M.D., medical director of the Pritikin Longevity Center in Santa Monica, California. In addition, studies have shown that coronary artery blockages can actually be reversed over a one- to two-year period, he says.

Researchers at Pritikin, for example, studied a group of 4,587 people that included men and women in their eighties and nineties. After three weeks, those who ate a diet that had less than 10 percent of calories from fat and consisted mostly of fruits, vegetables, and whole grains lowered their total cholesterol levels by 23 percent. This reduction sliced their heart attack risk in half.

Fat-Busting Starts Here

Before you can break away from high-fat living, you need some information about your dietary requirements. First, you should calculate roughly how many calories you need to eat daily based on your age, says Moshe Shike, M.D., director of clinical nutrition at Memorial Sloan-Kettering Cancer Center in New York City and co-author of *Cancer Free.*

To do that, multiply your body weight by 13. (The average person needs to eat 13 calories per pound to do normal daily activities.) Next, subtract 2 percent of that total for each decade after age 30.

For example, if you are 80 years old and weigh 160 pounds, multiply 160 by 13. That's 2,080 calories. Now deduct 10 percent to account for your age—that leaves you with 1,872 calories. That's your basic caloric need. Now you can use the following chart to figure out the maximum number of fat grams you want to eat per day based on 30, 25, 20, 15, or 10 percent of calories from fat. Tallying your fat grams each day will help you make better decisions when you're reading food labels and preparing meals.

If You Eat (in Calories)	Calories from Fat				
	30%	25%	20%	15%	10%
1,200	40 g.	33 g.	27 g.	20 g.	13 g.
1,400	47 g.	39 g.	31 g.	23 g.	16 g.
1,600	53 g.	44 g.	36 g.	27 g.	18 g.
1,800	60 g.	50 g.	40 g.	30 g.	20 g.
2,000	67 g.	56 g.	44 g.	33 g.	22 g.
2,200	73 g.	61 g.	49 g.	37 g.	24 g.
2,400	80 g.	67 g.	53 g.	40 g.	27 g.
2,600	87 g.	72 g.	58 g.	43 g.	29 g.
2,800	93 g.	78 g.	62 g.	47 g.	31 g.

"There was little difference in the drop in cholesterol levels between the young people and the older people. This is clear proof that it's never too late to change your lifestyle and improve your health," says R. James Barnard, Ph.D., author of the study and professor of physiology in the Department of Physiological Science at the University of California, Los Angeles.

■ **The Ornish Research:** Even more dramatic results come from Dr. Dean Ornish's landmark work in Sausalito. Dr. Ornish divided 43 men and five women who had severe ather-osclerosis—many in their fifties, sixties and seventies—into two groups. The "treatment" group was instructed to go on a strict vegetarian diet deriving fewer than 10 percent of calories from fat. No meat, poultry, fish, or cheese. No nuts or seeds. No chocolate, no coffee, no cooking oils. In addition, they walked for at least one hour, three times a week; practiced meditation and yoga daily; and if they smoked, they quit.

Meanwhile, the other group was advised to follow the standard American Heart Association lifestyle program. That is, reduce their fat intake

Minor Menu Fixes Create Major Health Benefits

Small changes can make a big difference in percentage of calories from fat in your meals without sacrificing taste. Here is an example. The daily menu on the left is similar to the typical American diet—2,400 calories, 34 percent of calories from total fat and 12 percent of calories from saturated fat. The healthier menu on the right provides 2,300 calories, but only 26 percent of calories from total fat and 7 percent of calories from saturated fat. The subtle changes make a huge dent in the amount of fat. Both were prepared by Nelda Mercer, R.D., of the University of Michigan Medical Center and co-author of *The M-Fit Grocery Shopping Guide: Your Guide to Healthier Choices.*

Typical American Diet	The Healthy Alternative

Breakfast

8 oz. orange juice	8 oz. orange juice
12 oz. coffee	12 oz. coffee
1 Tbsp. half-and-half creamer	1 Tbsp. half-and-half creamer
1 cup puffed rice cereal	1¼ cups ready-to-eat oat cereal
¾ cup 2% milk	1 cup skim milk
	¾ cup strawberries

Midmorning Snack

12 oz. coffee	12 oz. coffee
1 tsp. nondairy powdered creamer	1 tsp. fat-free creamer
1 plain doughnut	1 blueberry muffin

Lunch

12 oz. cola	12 oz. instant tea (unsweetened)
1 cup carrot sticks	1 cup carrot sticks
1 oz. potato chips	—
Ham-and-cheese sandwich made with:	Grilled chicken sandwich made with:
1 oz. regular ham	4 oz. grilled chicken breast
1 oz. cheddar cheese	1 oz. Swiss cheese
1 Tbsp. mayonnaise	2 lettuce leaves
2 slices white bread	1 tomato slice
	1 Tbsp. mayonnaise
	1 wheat bun

Afternoon Snack

1 chocolate bar	1 oz. pretzels
	1 medium apple
	12 oz. diet cola

Minor Menu Fixes...continued

Typical American Diet	The Healthy Alternative
Dinner	
5 oz. chicken breast (fried)	1½ cups cooked spaghetti
¾ cup mashed potatoes	¾ cup tomato and mushroom sauce
¾ cup canned peas and carrots	1 oz. meatballs
Salad made with:	Salad made with:
1 cup iceberg lettuce, tomatoes, and carrots	1 cup romaine lettuce, tomatoes, and carrots
2 Tbsp. ranch salad dressing	2 Tbsp. light ranch dressing
1 brown-and-serve roll	1 whole-wheat roll
1 tsp. corn oil margarine	1 tsp. corn oil margarine
Evening Snack	
1 cup vanilla ice cream	1 cup low-fat vanilla ice cream

to less than 30 percent of calories, stop smoking, and exercise moderately.

After one year, 82 percent of those in the treatment group had shown reversal of coronary blockage. The average amount of reduction was about 5 percent. But even that modest regression can mean a 100 percent improvement in blood flow, Dr. Lipsenthal says. Those on the AHA diet didn't experience these striking results, although, the progress of their heart disease appeared to slow down.

"It's a world of difference. I'm doing things that I never imagined I could do again," said Victor K., a retired nuclear engineer from California. When he began the Ornish program, he had one artery almost completely blocked, had suffered from persistent angina, and could walk less than a block.

While Victor followed the Ornish plan, his total cholesterol dropped from 290 to 150 milligrams per deciliter, he lost 30 pounds, his angina disappeared, and he began regularly hiking in the hills around his home. He also climbed the equivalent of 130 floors on his stair-climber in

a half-hour and backpacked in the High Sierras at 8,000 feet with 40 pounds on his back.

"The diet is really the foundation of the whole program," he said. "I feel so much better now physically and mentally because of it. And it's a diet that really isn't hard to stick to—when you consider the benefits."

■ **A More Gradual Way:** Even if you can't see yourself curbing your fat consumption by as much as Dr. Ornish suggests, just shaving a modest amount of fat from the obvious sources can produce positive effects.

In the St. Thomas' Atherosclerosis Regression Study in London, for instance, 26 men up to age 66 were put on a diet that limited fat intake to 27 percent of calories and lowered saturated fat to 8 percent of calories. In a similar group, 24 men were allowed to eat their usual English diets, which typically consist of about 40 percent of calories from fat. Three years later, the group on the limited-fat diet reported better control of angina and had three times fewer deaths and coronary surgeries and two times fewer heart attacks.

"Anything that you can do to lower your fat intake is better than doing nothing at all," Dr. Barnard says. "It's like a game of Russian roulette. It just depends on how many bullets you want to stick in that revolver. If it holds six bullets and you eat the typical American diet, then you have five bullets in it. If you can eat 20 percent, you're down to four. If you go to 15 percent, you're down to three. And if you can manage to get down to less than 10 percent, you may only have one bullet in that pistol, and your risk of these diseases is dramatically reduced."

The Risk of Cancer Grows

Fat doesn't directly cause cancer. Instead, Dr. Klaper says, the consumption of excess fat promotes cancer—much like listening to high-decibel sounds on a regular basis increases the chance you will develop hearing loss.

Although researchers aren't certain how this happens, they do have plenty of theories:

■ Some suspect that free radicals, produced as the body metabolizes fat, damage a cell's genetic codes and hype cancer growth.

■ Others believe that fat may interfere with the body's ability to shut down cell growth or that it disrupts the immune system, which may have a protective role against cancer.

■ High-fat meals also may stimulate production of sex hormones, like estrogen and testosterone, that can promote cancer, particularly in the breast and prostate.

Whatever the reason, it is becoming increasingly clear that the longer you stick to a high-fat lifestyle, the less likely it is that you will remain cancer-free in what should be the best years of your life. "Eating high-fat foods is like throwing gasoline on a fire," Dr. Klaper says. "You're just fanning the flames of the cancer and helping it spread."

Derailing Tumors

As with heart disease and stroke, prevention works to reduce the risk of cancer. Even in your sixties, seventies, and eighties, slashing dietary fat might help you to halt the progression of certain tumors before they become cancerous and prevent recurrences, Dr. Ritenbaugh explains. It may be too late, for instance, for dietary changes to stop a tumor from developing in the next couple of years, but "tumors that would have gotten you four, five, or ten years from now, you can still do something about," he says.

Here are some conditions that excess dietary fat may facilitate:

■ **Skin Cancer:** Cutting back to 20 percent of calories from fat, for example, may reduce your risk of developing precancerous skin growths and prevent skin cancer in your sixties and beyond, according to researchers at Baylor College of Medicine in Houston. In their study, researchers found that people who continued eating the typical American diet developed three times more precancerous skin lesions, called actinic keratosis, than those who ate a low-fat diet.

■ **Prostate Cancer:** Men over the age of 60 who have been cancer-free all of their lives run a 21 percent risk of being diagnosed with prostate cancer, the second leading lethal cancer among American men. But switching to low-fat eating may help stop the growth of microscopic prostate cancers before they have a chance to cause major problems, says William R. Fair, M.D., chief of urologic surgery and chairman of urologic oncology at Memorial Sloan-Kettering Cancer Center in New York City.

In his animal studies, Dr. Fair is finding that decreasing fat consumption to less than 20 percent of calories can halt the progression of these tiny tumors. "I really don't think a low-fat diet

Slash More Than 100 Fat Grams Painlessly

If You Eat:	Grams of Fat	Switch to:	Grams of Fat	Fat Savings
Blueberry muffin	6	A toasted (unbuttered) English muffin with jam	1	5
1 oz. bag of potato chips	10	1 oz. bag of pretzels	1	9
3½ oz. fried chicken with skin	17	3½ oz. roasted light meat chicken without skin	5	12
2 Tbsp. regular French dressing	13	2 Tbsp. reduced-calorie French dressing	2	11
3 store-bought chocolate chip cookies	7	3 fig bars	3	4
½ cup rich chocolate ice cream	15	½ cup peach frozen yogurt	4	11
3 oz. corned beef	16	3 oz. lean roast beef (eye of round)	4	12
1 cup cream of mushroom soup	19	1 cup minestrone soup	3	16
3-in. square fudge brownie	6	2-in. square angel food cake with fresh strawberries	0	6
1 Tbsp. margarine	11	1 Tbsp. whipped margarine	7	4
1 Tbsp. half-and-half in 2 cups of coffee = 2 Tbsp. daily	4	2 Tbsp. evaporated skim milk in 2 cups of coffee = 4 Tbsp. daily	0	4
2 oz. whole-milk American cheese	18	2 oz. light cheese	8	10
TOTAL:	142		38	104

could cure a sizable tumor, but if it can halt the progression of a microscopic tumor, then that would be tantamount to a cure," Dr. Fair says.

■ **Colon Cancer:** Cutting back on fat may also stave off colon cancer, according to Harvard University researchers who followed nearly 52,000 male health professionals for two years. Those who ate about 24 percent of their calories in fat were half as likely to develop precancerous colon polyps as the men who consumed more fat.

"These studies suggest that eating a healthy diet that includes lower amounts of animal fat and higher amounts of fruits and vegetables that have lots of fiber and micronutrients is an important part of what we can do to prevent colon cancer," says Eric Rimm, Sc.D., an assistant professor of epidemiology and nutrition at the Harvard School of Public Health. (See Chapter 2 for more about fiber.)

■ **Breast Cancer:** Women can dramatically reduce their risk of other common types of

11

cancer—particularly breast cancer—if they significantly ease up on fat, Dr. Klaper says.

Researchers put 13 postmenopausal women at the Pritikin Longevity Center in Santa Monica, California, on an eating plan that included less than 10 percent of calories from fat. In three weeks, their blood levels of estradiol, a form of the hormone estrogen linked to breast cancer, fell nearly 50 percent. As a result, Dr. Barnard estimated at the end of the study, the women were far less likely to develop breast cancer.

Even if a woman age 60 or older does get breast cancer, reducing fats may be a good move. Women who have breast cancer might substantially improve their chances of surviving by eating low-fat diets, according to researchers at the University of Minnesota in Minneapolis who polled 42,000 women between the ages of 55 and 69 on their eating habits. Of the 698 women who developed breast cancer in the next five years, those who reported eating 56 grams of fat a day (almost 2 ounces) had twice the risk of death as women who ate less fat, says Aaron Folsom, M.D., professor of epidemiology at the university and co-author of the study.

"High-fat diets raise the levels of sex hormones like estrogen in the bloodstream, and many breast cancers depend on estrogen to grow," Dr. Klaper says. He believes that low-fat diets can be effective in both the treatment and prevention of breast cancer.

■ **Ovarian Cancer:** Cutting down on fat also may help women slash their risk of ovarian cancer, a disease that becomes more common as women reach their early sixties, says Harvey A. Risch, M.D., Ph.D., associate professor of epidemiology and public health at Yale University School of Medicine.

Dr. Risch and his colleagues evaluated the eating habits of women up to age 79, 450 with ovarian cancer and 564 without the disease.

They concluded that cutting 10 grams of saturated fat a day (about the same amount as in one cheeseburger with all the fixings) could trim the risk of ovarian cancer by 20 percent. And adding 10 grams of vegetable fiber a day—what you would get in about 1 cup of cooked lentils—may take the risk down by another 37 percent.

"It appears possible to cut your risk of ovarian cancer in half by assertive modification of the diet," Dr. Risch says.

How to Start Lowering Fat

Cutting back on total fat intake and sorting out the best low-fat foods from the worst high-fat offenders may take some adjustments, but these changes don't have to be time-consuming or costly—or sap flavor from your favorite meals. Sheah Rarback, R.D., an American Dietetic Association spokesperson in Miami, says, "Changing a lifetime of eating habits, particularly for people age 60-plus, can be challenging. But I don't think it's as hard to do as many people perceive. It doesn't have to be all or nothing. Over time, even small changes in your eating habits can improve your health."

Here's a step-by-step outline incorporating some of the basics that can get you started gradually:

1. Keep score. For the next couple of days, jot down on a piece of paper or 3" x 5" cards all the foods and beverages that you eat and drink. Note the amount and type of fat listed on the nutrition labels. If you're eating in a restaurant, estimate your intake of food, Dr. Shike suggests. This will give you an idea about how much fat you're eating now and how much you'll need to cut back. Every three months or so, do this all over again so that you can see your progress.

2. Set a goal. Give yourself something to strive for, but make it practical, Pingleton says.

Most doctors and dietitians recommend that no more than 30 percent of your calories come from fat. But it seems that the more you slash the fat you eat, the more dramatic the impact on your health. So be adventurous in your planning, Dr. Klaper suggests. While revising a lifetime of eating habits in a week probably isn't realistic, getting your total fat intake under 25 percent of calories during the next six months is a reasonable goal.

3. Experiment. Cravings for fat won't disappear immediately. But don't despair. "You can retrain yourself at any age by making shifts gradually away from high-fat foods," says John Foreyt, Ph.D., director of the Nutrition Research Clinic at Baylor College of Medicine in Houston. Here are several ways you can develop a taste for lower levels of fat in your meals:

a. Pick a day of the week. On that day, make a bean dish, or pasta, or a salad the centerpiece of your meals. If you are dining out on the day of the week you are cutting fat, try low-fat ethnic foods or vegetarian dishes. Then, gradually increase the number of days of the week you eat low-fat meals all day. Over a month or two, your taste buds will adapt to eating less fat. (Check Chapter 5 for some low-fat recipes you might enjoy.)

b. Make one small overall change a week. For instance, if you use whole milk in your coffee or on cereal, try a 50/50 mixture of whole milk and 2 percent milk for a week. Then switch to 2 percent for seven days. Next, use a mixture that is half 2 percent and half 1 percent, and so on until you are using skim milk. If skim milk alone doesn't satisfy your taste buds, you can stir in some nonfat powdered milk to improve its texture and flavor, Dr. Foreyt says. You can use the same strategy to wean yourself off cheeses, shortenings and oils, ice cream, and other high-fat foods.

c. Reinvent your favorites. The worst thing that you can do is give up your favorite dishes, because you'll feel deprived and may develop cravings that make it harder to stick to a low-fat lifestyle, Dr. Foreyt says. Instead, experiment with low-fat ingredients. "Take your 10 favorite recipes and go into the supermarket and buy low-fat substitutes for the ingredients that you would normally use," says Dr. Castelli. (If you prefer not to modify your recipes, Dr. Foreyt suggests that you serve the original versions less often—only on holidays and special occasions, for instance—and take only half of the portion that you would normally eat.)

4. Eat with friends. Make your transition to low-fat living a social celebration, Rarback says. Ask a few friends to join you in a lunch or dinner club. On a rotating basis, one of you makes a low-fat main entrée while the others bring the bread, salad, fruit, or dessert. "It will help all of you experiment with new low-fat recipes, and it is fun to eat together," she says.

5. Splurge now and then. High-fat foods like country-fried steak should be a once-a-month treat rather than daily fare, says Michele Tuttle, R.D., director of consumer affairs for the Food Marketing Institute in Washington, D.C. "I've never met anybody who can eat perfectly. In fact, that's probably the best recipe for failure, because the thought that you can never have chocolate fudge cake again in your life will drive you crazy," Tuttle says. "So go ahead and have a little bit with some friends. One dessert split four ways is not a big deal."

6. Make up for lapses later. Any one food or any one meal can have some extra fat as long as you compensate for it, Dr. Foreyt says. "Over a week you want your fat consumption to be certainly less than 30 percent of calories and closer to 20 percent of calories if you can get

Count Grams for Fats—and Saturated Fats—on Food Labels

You may find it easiest to control fat consumption by counting grams, because that's how total fat and saturated fat are measured on nutrition labels, says William Castelli, M.D., epidemiologist, medical director of the Framingham Cardiovascular Institute and former director of the Framingham Heart Study in Massachusetts.

Here's how you can figure out how to limit your fat intake to 20 percent:

1. If you eat 2,000 calories a day, multiply 2,000 by 20 percent. That's 400 calories.

2. Now divide 400 by 9—which is the number of fat calories in 1 gram. That means you want to limit yourself to about 44 grams of fat from the foods you eat each day.

Beware of your high-fat favorites. For instance, a beef bologna sandwich made with two pieces of meat and a 1-ounce slice of regular cheddar cheese has about 36 grams of fat—nearly an entire day's fat allowance in one meal. So try to use those fat grams more thoughtfully, Dr. Castelli says.

Castelli also recommends that you cut your consumption of saturated fat—the really bad fat—to under 20 grams a day (10 grams if you have already suffered a heart attack). Again, read the food labels carefully.

What can you eat and stay under 20 grams of saturated fat? "You could have rolled oats, fruit, and low-fat yogurt for breakfast; a chicken, tuna, or turkey sandwich for lunch; and shrimp cocktail, a 3-ounce filet mignon, vegetables, salad, and fat-free dressing for dinner—and you'd still be under 20 grams of saturated fat for the day," Dr. Castelli says. "Now does that sound like such a miserable experience?"

---

there," Dr. Foreyt says. "So if you eat a hamburger or cheesecake on a Monday, that's fine. But you should adjust your eating plans so that you eat less fat during the rest of the week."

Low-Fat Living Starts in the Pantry

Filling your pantry with high-fat foods is like asking a compulsive gambler to live next door to a casino. It's too much of a temptation.

"If you don't have the right things in your pantry, you're going to prepare the foods you do have in the same old way, or you're going to be tempted to say 'the heck with it' and go out to eat at a high-fat restaurant," Tuttle says. "So it only makes sense to stock your pantry well."

Here are a few suggestions for how to follow a low-fat living plan:

■ **Abide by the 75/25 rule.** "Whenever you open the refrigerator, a kitchen cabinet, or the bread box, 75 percent of what you see should be plant-derived foods—pastas, breads, beans, cereals, grains, and fresh, frozen, or canned fruits and vegetables. Then the remaining 25 percent can be made up of small amounts of lean meats and low-fat dairy products like milk and cheese. If the bulk of your pantry is like that, then your plate will probably look that way, too," says Elizabeth Somer, R.D., author of *Nutrition for Women.*

■ **Consider pasta.** Pastas, such as spaghetti, linguine, and fettucine, have earned a bizarre reputation for being fattening. But in reality, these grain foods are almost devoid of fat and are a great source of complex carbohydrates—your body's best fuel. "If you fill up on pasta, you'll be more inclined to eat less meat, and that will mean that you're eating even less fat," Rarback says. So keep several boxes of your favorite pastas within reach. Whole-wheat pastas are especially healthy.

■ **Be wary of the sauces you put on the pasta.** What fattens up most pastas is what we put on it, says Rarback. A typical white sauce, for instance, has 71 percent of its calories from fat. And many bottled spaghetti sauces have up to 9 grams of fat in a ½-cup serving. Instead of those, always keep in your refrigerator a jar of spaghetti sauce that has 5 grams of fat or less to pour over pasta, spread on pizza crust or even on baked potatoes, says Elaine Moquette-Magee, R.D., author of the book series *Fight Fat and Win: How to Eat a Low-Fat Diet Without Changing Your Life.*

■ **Count on beans and rice.** Dried beans like pinto, navy, lima, and black beans, and grains like brown rice are virtually fat-free and are terrific sources of protein that can reduce or eliminate the need for fat-laden meats in stews, chili, salads, and other traditional dishes, Rarback says. Instead of using 10 ounces of beef in a stew recipe, for example, use 5 ounces and round out the dish with lentils.

■ **Look for cracker meal.** Unlike packaged bread crumbs, which contain a bit of fat, cracker meal is fat-free, Moquette-Magee says. Cracker meal can be used for coating oven-roasted chicken or fish, as a topping for low-fat fruit crisps and casseroles, or as a filler for meat loaf.

■ **Stock up on low-fat cream soups.** Be sure to have in your pantry plenty of low-fat condensed cream soups, like 99 percent fat-free cream of broccoli or cream of chicken, says Evelyn Tribole, R.D., author of *Healthy Homestyle Cooking.* They're great in casseroles and as sauces on meats, poultry, and fish.

■ **Stay away from solid cooking oils.** If you use cooking oils, stock up on liquid olive or canola oils that are loaded with monounsaturated fat. These oils and tub margarines are better for you than solid oils and fats like shortenings that contain lots of saturated fat, says Edith Howard Hogan, R.D., a spokesperson for the American Dietetic Association in Washington, D.C. Better yet, coat your cookware with a vegetable oil cooking spray.

■ **Brown foods in broth.** Keep defatted chicken broth in your cupboard instead of vegetable oil, Moquette-Magee suggests. "I use chicken broth all the time to sauté vegetables, pan-simmer meats or boil and flavor rice. All it does is keep the food moist and transfer heat. Those are the same things the oil would be doing, except the broth doesn't have all that fat."

■ **Slash fat with a splash.** Alcohol is another good substitute to have on hand, says Moquette-Magee. You can use beer and wine to stir-fry meats and simmer mushrooms, green peppers, onions, and other vegetables.

■ **Juice up your salads.** White grape, apple, orange, and pineapple juices are all light-flavored alternatives to oil in homemade salad dressings or marinades, Tribole says.

■ **Find substitutes for fats in baking.** Pureed prunes are one of the best fat substitutes in baked chocolate favorites like brownies and cakes, Tribole says. They're chewy and contribute a naturally sweet flavor to the dessert. A ½ cup of prunes can save you more than 800 calories and almost 100 grams of fat compared to a ½ cup of butter. (For convenience, Tribole suggests buying baby-food jars of prunes that have already been pureed.)

"Applesauce is another great substitute," Tribole says. "You can use it in place of cooking oils or butter in brownies, muffins, and cakes. For every ½ cup of applesauce you use, you'll save about 109 grams of fat and 900 calories."

Eat Like a Peasant, Live Like a King

It's cheap, it's easy, and it's quick. A hamburger and fries at a drive-through? Wrong. It's the traditional Mediterranean diet that—from Spain to Sicily, Corsica to Crete, and Athens to the Alps—has been the peasant's staple for centuries. Ranging up to 40 percent of calories from fat, the Mediterranean diet would also seem to be a sure killer. Yet people in this vast region live longer than Americans do, and heart disease and cancer are far less common. "It's one of the healthiest diets that human beings have developed in the past 2,000 years," says R. Curtis Ellison, M.D., chief of preventive medicine and epidemiology at Boston University School of Medicine.

Researchers aren't absolutely certain why the Mediterranean diet works. But it may have a lot to do with the type of fat that Mediterraneans eat. Nearly 75 percent of the fat that is consumed is from heart-healthy olive oil, which is loaded with monounsaturates. And most of the foods are low-fat—fresh fruits, vegetables, and grains, including oranges, apples, tomatoes, eggplant, spinach, onions, peppers and lots of bread. Red meat, a prime source of worrisome saturated fat, isn't daily fare in the traditional Mediterranean diet. In fact, it is usually only eaten once or twice a month. Poultry and fish are also eaten less often than in the United States.

French researchers have shown that people in their sixties who begin living this lifestyle can have a 70 percent drop in heart attack risk. Preliminary evidence also suggests that monounsaturated fats may reduce your risk of breast and endometrial cancer, and perhaps lung cancer, too, says Dimitrios Trichopoulos, M.D., director of the Harvard Center for Cancer Prevention at the Harvard School of Public Health.

But is the Mediterranean diet better than eating the diet with much lower fat that scientists are recommending? "I think both are excellent alternatives to the traditional American fare of meat and potatoes," Dr. Ellison says. "But low-fat is a huge change that is less acceptable to many Americans. Mediterranean eating is a less radical change, and more Americans are trying it and liking it."

■ **Bake with cocoa instead of chocolate.** If you bake, keep your pantry well-stocked with unsweetened cocoa powder. It provides rich chocolate taste without the fat of unsweetened baking chocolate, Tribole says. For each ounce of unsweetened chocolate called for in a recipe, substitute 3 tablespoons of unsweetened cocoa powder, she advises.

■ **Use lower-fat milk products.** Evaporated skim milk is terrific for sauces and soups because it has the texture and flavor of cream but without the fat, Tribole says. Each cup contains 80 grams less of fat and 600 fewer calories than heavy cream. Plain nonfat or low-fat yogurt is also a versatile addition to any refrigerator, says

Moquette-Magee. It can be used to replace sour cream and make salad dressings, and it is a good, quick add-on to breakfast cereals and desserts.

■ **Try butter substitutes.** There are butter-flavored sprinkles like Molly McButter or Butter Buds that add taste to foods without the extra fat or calories, Rarback says.

■ **Pour on the spice.** Low-fat foods may seems less flavorful when you first try them, because fat adds flavor to some foods—flavor that you're used to. Also, as we age, our taste buds become less acute. To add zip to meals, keep plenty of herbs and spices like basil, garlic, ginger, onion powder, tarragon, and oregano in your pantry. "By using different spices and herbs

Low Fat? High Fiber? What Do the Labels Mean?

Kathy Pompliano, R.D., manager of the M-Fit Supermarket Program at the University of Michigan in Ann Arbor, explains it for you: If an item contains 5 percent or less of the Daily Value for a particular nutrient, it is considered "low." On the other hand, if an item contains 20 percent or more of the Daily Value for a particular nutrient, it is considered "high." Look for foods that are low in total fat, saturated fat, and sodium, and foods that are high in fiber, vitamin A, vitamin C, and calcium.

in your food, you're going to bring back flavor and zest to the meal and make it more enjoyable, while still eliminating fat," says Rarback.

■ **Invigorate with vinegar.** "Using a flavorful vinegar like raspberry, tarragon, or rice wine vinegar allows you to decrease the oil in homemade salad dressings. Keep them in your kitchen and experiment with them," Rarback says.

■ **Remake your mayo.** Regular mayonnaise is 98 percent fat. "It's just egg yolks and oil," Moquette-Magee says. "I can't think of anything worse for you." Try the light, low-fat or fat-free varieties, or create your own mayo: Either mix ½ cup of light or low-fat mayonnaise with ½ cup of plain yogurt, or whip ½ cup of low-fat cottage cheese in a food processor or blender. (If you don't like how a mayo substitute tastes on sandwiches, opt for mustard, salsa, cranberry sauce, barbecue sauce, or plain yogurt instead.)

■ **Keep a "bite" box.** Put a variety of low-fat snacks like grapes, dates, celery, rice cakes, and other crunchy, chewy things into a container in your kitchen so that you can quickly satisfy yourself without being tempted to dash out for high-fat goodies between meals.

Shopping for Low-Fat Food

If you're the cook in the family, your first line of defense against high-fat living is at the grocery store," Pingleton says. Most supermarkets have a tremendous variety of nonfat and low-fat options. But they are also filled with prominently displayed, high-fat enticements.

Here are some ways to get through the grocery store without loading up on fat:

■ **Make a list.** This may seem like obvious advice, but some people in their sixties, seventies, and eighties still don't do it, Somer says. Before you go to the store, sit down and plan out what you would like to eat that week. In the long run, a list will save time and reduce the risk that you'll impulsively throw a high-fat food into your cart, advises Somer.

■ **Never shop on an empty stomach.** "You want your mind working, not your stomach, as you stroll the grocery store aisles," Somer says. "If you're hungry, you're going to be reaching for all the high-fat stuff that you shouldn't be eating." Go grocery shopping after a meal or a snack like low-fat cheese and crackers, she says.

■ **Shop from the outside in.** Generally, the fresher, lower-fat foods like fruits and vegetables are on the perimeter of the store. So shop on the outside aisles first. That way, you'll load your cart with healthier foods and be less tempted to fill it with the more processed, higher-fat products on the inner aisles, says Jayne Newmark, R.D., a nutrition consultant in Phoenix.

■ **Read those labels.** The Nutrition Facts labels on packaged foods can be your best weapon in the war against high-fat eating. Among other

The Gas Factor

Beans can cause gas. To prevent this unwanted side effect, soak your dried beans overnight in a bowl of water, then drain them and use fresh water to cook them. Or try taking over-the-counter products containing enzymes such as alpha-galactosidase (Beano) that can prevent gas by breaking down sugars in the digestive system.

things, each label is now required by law to list the amount of total calories, total fat, saturated fat, and sodium per listed serving size.

■ **Read the ingredients list, too.** Compare products and choose the one with fewer fat sources listed. Common fat sources include vegetable oil, meat fat, whole milk, butter, cream, and eggs. Check breads and cereals for fiber-rich whole grains, such as whole or rolled oats, or whole, cracked, or stone-ground wheat.

■ **Take it slow.** Of course, reading every label on every food every time you shop would be tedious and time-consuming. Instead, each time you shop pick out a couple of foods and read those labels very carefully, recommends Mona Sutnick, R.D., Ed.D., a nutrition consultant in Philadelphia and a spokesperson for the American Dietetic Association. "Today, for example, you could read salad dressing labels and pick one that has little or no fat," she says. "If you like it, you don't have to read salad dressing labels anymore, because you've found one that suits you. That approach will work for virtually every food in the store."

■ **Skip hydrogenated foods.** Foods like baked goods or margarines may list hydrogenated or partially hydrogenated oils as ingredients. This means hydrogen has been added to unsaturated liquid oils to make them solidify. But adding hydrogen does two things. First, it transforms unsaturated fat into saturated fat,

says George Seperich, Ph.D., a food scientist and associate professor of agribusiness at Arizona State University in Tempe. Second, it creates trans-fatty acids, molecules that raise LDL cholesterol as much as saturated fat does. "When I'm shopping and I see the word 'hydrogenated' on the label, that food goes right back on the shelf because I know it is loaded with things that I don't want in my body," Dr. Klaper says.

■ **Watch the margarine.** Pick a margarine that lists water as its first ingredient. It will almost certainly be low-fat, Dr. Castelli says. Whipped margarines also are a good choice because they have more air, and that reduces the fat content, says Gerry Bates, R.D., nutritional program manager for the Florida Department of Elder Affairs in Tallahassee.

■ **Pick frozen veggies.** "For many people in this age group who live alone, buying fresh fruits and vegetables is often a problem because they rot before they're eaten," Rarback says. "Frozen vegetables packed without sauces are a very good alternative. Then a person living alone or a couple doesn't have to worry about spoilage; a fresh-tasting vegetable is readily available that they can take out of the freezer and microwave quickly, or use as a base in soups or stews."

■ **Become a cereal fan.** "There didn't used to be a lot of low-fat, low-sodium breakfast cereals, but now there is a multitude of very good ones," says Jeanne Jones, cookbook author and "Cook It Light" syndicated columnist in La

Reduced Fat Products May Not Always Be Healthier

Holly McCord, author of *Prevention's The Peanut Butter Diet* and nutrition editor of *Prevention* magazine, says reduced-fat peanut butter can be worse for you than ordinary peanut butter. The reduced-fat version replaces monounsaturated fat (the kind that's good for your heart) with sugar, which can add calories.

Bottom Line Personal

Jolla, California. Good choices include shredded wheat, oatmeal, and puffed rice, corn, or wheat.

■ **Look for low-fat cheese.** Most regular cheeses have about 9 grams of fat per ounce, according to Moquette-Magee. Instead, look for low-fat cheeses that have 6 grams of fat or less per ounce, or part-skim varieties of ricotta and mozzarella that have 5 grams or less. (Nonfat cheeses taste fine in sandwiches but don't cook well.) Reach for nonfat cream cheese, too, since regular varieties are high in fat and saturated fat. Look for whipped products that contain more air.

■ **Avoid most foods labeled "nonfat."** Many nonfat processed products—particularly sweets like cakes and cookies—are packed with gums and sugars that cause the formation of free radicals and drive up your triglycerides—the type of fat that increases your risk of heart disease. People also tend to eat larger amounts of high-calorie nonfat foods because they don't get the feeling of fullness that fat gives them. Dutch researchers also have found that fat substitutes can reduce your body's ability to absorb vitamin E and health-promoting antioxidants like carotenoids. *Exceptions:* Nonfat products such as fat-free sour cream, cream cheese, yogurt, and mayonnaise are fine if used sparingly on sandwiches or to make other foods like vegetable dips and salad dressings, Dr. Seperich says.

■ **Try something new.** Every time you go shopping, purchase a new low-fat food: a fruit, vegetable, grain, bean, or pasta that you've never tried before, like kiwifruit, bok choy, couscous, Anasazi beans, or whole wheat ziti, Pingleton suggests. It will wake up your taste buds.

■ **Get the right ground meat.** Ground turkey breast or ground chicken breast are among the leanest meats you can buy, Pingleton says. Be wary, though, if the label doesn't indicate 100 percent breast meat; otherwise, the package may include skin and other poultry fat. If ground turkey breast or chicken breast isn't available, consider 15 percent–fat ground beef. It is leaner than plain ground turkey, Pingleton says.

■ **Buy the "select" meats.** Marbling in meat is pure fat. The U.S. Department of Agriculture grades meat by the amount of marbling it has, and lists the grade on the package, as follows:

Select grade meats have the least amount of marbling (and may be cheaper than other meats, too). Choose "select" cuts for the lowest fat content.

Choice is the next highest grade. Get "choice" meats if "select" meats are not available.

Prime grades have the most marbling, so avoid buying them except for special occasions.

Also, packs of leaner cuts of beef contain the words "round" or "loin," as in "top round" or "sirloin." Lean cuts of pork usually are loins or legs. For ham, Pingleton recommends lower-fat varieties or Canadian bacon.

■ **Go for fish.** Most varieties of seafood are low in fat, and those that are high-fat contain a

Macaroni Makeover

To lower the fat content of packaged macaroni and cheese, add vegetables like broccoli, carrots, or cauliflower, and use low-fat or skim milk in the preparation. Try 1½ tablespoons of margarine or butter and 2 tablespoons of light sour cream instead of the 4 tablespoons of butter the package recommends.

polyunsaturated type that is heart-healthy. "From all we know, fish is better for you than red meat," says Walter Willett, M.D., Dr. P.H., professor of epidemiology and nutrition, chairman of the Department of Nutrition at the Harvard School of Public Health in Boston, and author of several classic studies on fish consumption.

■ **Be wary in the deli.** While it is true that many deli meats and salads are loaded with fat and sodium, there are healthier varieties at supermarkets today, says Pompliano. Look for chicken breast, turkey breast, or other lean and extra-lean meats for a low-fat protein source. (To reduce the amount of sodium in them, Pompliano suggests rinsing the meat gently under cool water and patting it dry before making a sandwich.) Ask the deli clerk about lower-fat options in the salad department. Some delis have fat-free or low-fat macaroni salads, potato salads and chicken salads, he says.

■ **Avoid oil packs.** Tuna and other seafoods packed in oil add unwanted fat to your meal. Pick water-packed tuna, or seafood like clams canned in their own juices, Jones suggests.

■ **Dump the doughnuts and muffins.** Because half of the calories in a doughnut comes from fat and a third of the calories in a muffin comes from fat, neither makes a healthful breakfast bread. A bagel is your best choice— it's nearly fat-free. "A bagel is a great breakfast food. It is fast, convenient and readily available in most areas," Pompliano says.

■ **Don't go nuts for the nuts.** Eating nuts —excellent sources of monounsaturated and polyunsaturated fats—may protect you from heart disease, according to researchers at Loma Linda University in California. They studied the eating habits of 31,000 Seventh-Day Adventists in their fifties, sixties, and seventies and found that those who ate nuts four or more times a week had half the risk of fatal heart attacks than people who munched on them less than once a week. But the fats in nuts still count toward your daily fat total, and most nuts are chock-full of calories. A cup of peanuts, for example, has about 800 calories. "For the average person, nuts can be dangerous because they're like potato chips. It's hard to just have one," Newmark says. Instead of eating them by the handful, use five or six nuts to add flavor or texture to foods like oatmeal, pasta, salads or frozen desserts.

Low-Fat Cooking with a Personal Touch

By age 70, the average person who cooks for a family has made about 49,000 meals. Unfortunately, most household cooks also have a limited repertoire of about 14 main dishes, so they're likely to feed their families the same high-fat meals that they've always made, day after day.

For a low-fat entrée to replace one of those 14 dishes, consider these changes:

■ **Stick with no-stick pans.** Buying no-stick cookware is worth the investment because its special coating allows you to cook or bake without greasing it with fat, Rarback says. "I know a

Get Out of the Frying Pan

Gerry B. has an easy time recalling her late husband's favorite dishes: fried chicken, fried catfish, fried eggs...

"My husband didn't think something was cooked unless it was fried," says Gerry, who happens to be a registered dietitian. She says that his eating habits contributed to his death of heart disease at age 59.

But times are changing. A growing number of people in their sixties, seventies, and eighties are adopting low-fat cooking methods in hopes of avoiding a similar fate or simply to add variety to their meals, Gerry says. "It is surprising to a lot of them that they can get away from the frying pan and cook something in a different way and still have it taste good."

Here's a glimpse at some of the lean ways Gerry suggests for creating delicious meals without added grease, butter, or oil:

Steaming and microwaving allow you to quickly cook rice, vegetables, and other foods without added fat. These methods also help retain the nutrients, flavor, and moisture in the food. To steam vegetables, for instance, bring about 1 inch of water to a boil in a large saucepan. Place the veggies in a steamer basket and set the basket in the saucepan so that it sits above the water. Cover the saucepan with a tight-fitting lid and cook until the vegetables are crisp-tender. When microwaving vegetables, you need to add only a small amount of water before cooking.

Poaching means cooking food in a simmering liquid, often stock, broth, or water. This healthful alternative to frying works well with boned poultry and firm-fleshed fish like salmon.

Baking and roasting are excellent ways to cook meats, poultry, fish, squash, potatoes, and many other foods. To keep foods moist, you can cover them for at least part of the cooking time. Bake meats by setting them on a roasting rack or meat-loaf pan to keep them from soaking in fat drippings.

Braising, also known as stewing, means slowly cooking food in a small amount of boiling water or other liquid. The longer you braise the meat, the more fat leaches into the cooking liquid. When the meat is done, strain the broth into a container and refrigerate it overnight. The next day, skim off and dispose of the fat that has congealed on top and reserve the remaining broth for soup stock. This works well for combination meat dishes such as chicken and rice, chicken and dumplings, meat stews, or soups made with meat.

woman in her sixties who has been using the same cooking pots and pans since her wedding years ago, and there have been a few innovations since then," Rarback says.

■ **Don't drown your pans.** If you still want to use some oil or butter to grease your pans, try dabbing a small spot— about the size of a quarter—onto a paper towel and swabbing the pan with it, Hogan advises. Better yet, use fruit juice or defatted chicken broth instead.

■ **Throw out your frying pan.** Bake, roast, grill, microwave, or sauté foods that you would normally fry, Dr. Foreyt says. These cooking methods allow fats to run off the meats so they can be discarded.

■ **Be a poacher.** Poaching fish in white wine rather than frying it trims fat and helps keep the fish flavorful and moist, Rarback says.

■ **Shrink the meat portions.** Use a serving of 2 to 3 ounces (after cooking) to complement a

How I Did It: A Weatherman Alters His Forecast

Fred P., a retired journalist, thought he had been doing all he could to protect himself from heart disease when he was young. He was wrong.

Although he ran 5 miles a day and didn't smoke, Fred drank whole milk by the gallon, ate eggs by the dozen, and eagerly sopped up every bit of fat on his dinner plate.

"When I was pre-40, my diet was absolutely atrocious. I overindulged in fats, heavy creams, cheeses, and meats...the works. Now when I think about what I ate, I just want to pass out. I really was a walking time bomb," says Fred.

Fortunately for Fred, doctors defused the bomb in his arteries before it killed him— although it did take quadruple heart bypass surgery to do it. That was when Fred was in his fifties, but he still remembers the lesson he learned.

"After the surgery, I knew what I had to do. Throw the fat out," Fred says. And he did. Now he briskly walks 2 miles a day and doggedly sticks to a low-fat diet.

"I just know that I wouldn't be here if I had continued eating and drinking the junk that I used to," he says.

The first food that he abandoned was whole milk.

"When you make the switch, the message you need to put into your brain is simply this: Skim milk is a clean, cold, delicious drink that doesn't have any fat," he says. "I wouldn't be caught dead drinking anything else now."

He eats lots of fruits and vegetables, prefers poultry with all the visible fat trimmed, rarely eats red meat, uses the lowest-fat margarine he can find, and dresses his salads with oil and vinegar only.

"The funny thing is, once you get yourself off all that high-fat junk, you wonder how you ever managed to eat it," Fred says. "I don't miss it one bit. I enjoy the good low-fat foods I eat now more than ever, and I feel like a million."

low-fat meal instead of letting it crowd fruits and vegetables off the plate, Pingleton says. Tuttle suggests limiting your total meat consumption per day to no more than 6 ounces. "Many people of this generation, especially men in their sixties and seventies, are used to eating 16-ounce steaks," Somer says. "If you eat a 16-ounce steak, you're eating about three days' worth of meat in one serving."

■ **Pile on the vegetables.** For every bite of meat, take four bites of fruits, vegetables, beans, and grains, Somer says. It will help you develop a sense of proportion that leads to a low-fat lifestyle.

■ **Forget frozen dinners.** Many frozen meals are loaded with fat and sodium, and in some cases take just as much time to prepare as fresh foods, Jones says. In the same 10 minutes that it takes to make fat-laden boil-in-the-bag Swedish meatballs, for instance, you could brown ground turkey breast in a skillet, add some low-fat spaghetti sauce, and pour it over cooked pasta.

■ **Lighten puddings.** Evaporated skim milk gives body and richness to puddings, but unlike whole milk, it doesn't add any fat, according to Tribole.

■ **Throw away the yokes.** If your recipe calls for whole eggs, use fat-free egg substitute instead (1/4 cup substitute equals one whole egg). Since fat content of the substitutes varies,

What About Those "Fatty" Fish?

Fish such as salmon and tuna are rich in a polyunsaturated fat called omega-3 fatty acids. Researchers have found that eating one or two servings of these fatty fish each week is healthy for your heart. However, they are backing away from earlier claims that eating five or six servings a week is any more beneficial.

check the label before buying. For baking, however, using two egg whites in place of each whole egg is a better choice, because it reduces the fat, yet maintains the flavor and texture of the original recipe, Rarback says.

■ **Soak your food.** Marinades add flavor to roasted or grilled meats, but instead of using oil-based marinades, try plain nonfat yogurt, Rarback says. Allow meat or skinless poultry to soak for several hours or overnight. Marinate fish for only an hour or so because of its delicate texture.

■ **Shred the cheese.** Instead of putting a full slice of cheese on a sandwich, grate it or shred it. You'll use less cheese, Rarback says, yet get the same flavor while cutting the fat in half.

■ **Cook now, eat later.** Once or twice a month make large quantities of low-fat soups, stews, waffles, and other favorites. Then divide them into one- or two-serving packets and store them in the freezer, Pingleton says. Then when you don't feel like cooking, you'll have a ready-made low-fat meal that you can reheat in minutes.

■ **Give up the grease bucket.** "A lot of people like to save the grease from bacon and other fatty foods in a bucket for use in cooking later. Get rid of it," Pingleton urges. Grease-bucket fat is mainly saturated and causes the most havoc in your body. (If you insist on using it, discard the oils that harden on top and use the liquid oil underneath, because it is less saturated.)

■ **Lighten vinaigrette.** Traditional vinaigrette is made with two parts oil to one part vinegar. Switch that around: Double the vinegar and halve the oil, and you've created an exciting lower-fat salad dressing and marinade. Try this formula with a balsamic or Japanese rice wine vinegar and a tasty olive oil. Throw in a crushed garlic clove and dash of dry mustard. If you like it sweet, add a sprinkle of brown sugar. Whip the combination in a blender and keep it in your refrigerator.

■ **If you insist on butter:** Don't use it in cooking, but add a small amount—about the size of a postage stamp—when the dish is done,

For No-Fry Fried Food...

Instead of frying chicken, remove the skin, coat the pieces with a dusting of flour and egg white, dip in bread or cornflake crumbs, and bake.

If you crave french-fried potatoes, cut 4 medium potatoes into strips, coat them with 1 tablespoon of oil by stirring them in a bowl, and bake on a baking sheet in a 450°F oven for 30 to 40 minutes, turning frequently. Sprinkle with paprika or (lightly) with salt or salt substitute.

for flavoring only. On bread or toast, spread butter thinly, so that you can still see the bread fiber. If you're making a sandwich, only butter one slice of bread. Better yet, Pingleton suggests using an all-fruit spread, low-fat mayonnaise, or margarine instead. "A lot of foods will surprise you by how good they taste without butter," Tribole says. "You really won't miss it in most cases."

Dining Out: Dodging High-Fat Temptations

The same rules you use for eating at home apply when you eat out. You just have to be more vigilant, and you can't assume anything," Somer says. "You still want to minimize the amount of meat that you eat and focus on fruits, vegetables, and grains."

Here are some ways to cut the fat when you're eating out:

■ **Call first.** Most high-quality restaurants will accommodate your needs if you give them sufficient notice, Dr. Lipsenthal says. Call a day or so beforehand, explain that you're eating low-fat foods, and ask if they can fulfill your specific requests for lowering fat. Ask for food to be prepared any way but fried.

■ **Get a menu for homework.** If you eat at a restaurant frequently, ask for a copy of the menu to take home with you, Dr. Shike advises. That way you can study your food choices without feeling pressured to order immediately.

■ **Go slow at fast-food restaurants.** Many of the foods are 40 to 55 percent fat, so order salads, plain hamburgers, or grilled chicken, or ask for a copy of the restaurant's nutritional information so that you can make wise selections, suggests Shike.

■ **Ease back on the appetizers.** Many appetizers, like buffalo wings, fried zucchini, and creamed soups, are high in fat. If you want something to munch on while you wait for your entrée, ask for bread sticks, grain breads, crackers, pretzels, or fresh vegetables like carrots and celery with honey-mustard dressing (not ranch), and salads with dressings on the side, Pingleton says. Or look for a soup with broth as its base.

■ **Get feisty.** Ask the waiter lots of questions and don't stop until you're satisfied, Somer says. How is the fish grilled? If it is in butter, ask for it dry. If a fried entrée is offered on the menu, Shike suggests asking if the chef can bake it, broil it, grill it, or steam it to cut down on the fat. Then see that they follow up. "It's your meal, you're paying for it, and within reason you should be able to get it the way you want it," Somer says. "If they say they can do something and they don't, send it back. You need to hold them to their promise."

■ **Start with a take-home portion.** Ask your server to bring a doggie bag when your meal is served. That way you can cut the meal in half and put part of it in the bag for later—before you take your first bite, Somer says. You'll not only have a meal for the next day, you'll slash the amount of fat and calories in each serving. "Don't start eating until you do that," Somer says, "because once you start eating you'll be likely to finish it."

■ **Carry a restaurant survival kit.** In a small sandwich bag, carry packets of low-fat dressings, herbal teas, spices, hot-pepper sauce, and other essentials that may not be readily available at the restaurant, Newmark suggests.

■ **Split a meal with a friend.** Order soup or salad à la carte with one entrée and ask the waiter for an extra plate. It will save you money and reduce the fat in each meal, Somer says.

■ **Get dressings on the side.** Many restaurants put more than 3 tablespoons of dressing on their salads, which can add more than 16 grams of fat to those veggies, Somer says. Always order salad dressings on the side so that you can

If You Love Your Gravy...

Pingleton suggests some ways to create lower-fat gravies:

Put meat drippings in the freezer for a few minutes. Then discard the crust of saturated fat that hardens on the top and use the flavorful broth underneath to make your gravy. Be sure to use skim or low-fat milk, as well.

For last-minute low-fat gravy or sauce, mix a can of condensed low-fat cream soup, such as cream of chicken or mushroom, with a half-can of water. Then pour the mixture over cooked meat, fish, or poultry and let it simmer for 5 to 10 minutes.

control the portion, and try to stick with oil and vinegar. It spreads more evenly than cream dressings, so you'll use less of it, she says.

■ **Omit the extras.** Cheese, bacon, olives, eggs, and croutons add unnecessary fat to a salad. Ask your server not to use them, Bates says.

■ **Cut back on rich sauces.** The sauce for fettuccine Alfredo is often referred to as "heart attack on a plate," Dr. Foreyt says. Avoid rich sauces on pasta, meats, or fish, or ask for the sauce on the side.

■ **Slow down on desserts.** If you want dessert, ask if you can get a child's portion, Somer says. That will cut some of the fat and still satisfy your sweet tooth. Or share one full-sized dessert with your dining companions.

■ **Turn down meat toppings on pizza.** Choose a pizza parlor that has a salad bar so that you can fill up on fresh fruits and vegetables while you're waiting for your pizza to cook, Somer says.

Steer clear of pies that are made with fatty meats like sausage or pepperoni. Try a vegetarian pizza—ask for extra veggies and skimp on the cheese—and limit yourself to one or two pieces.

■ **Hold the mayo.** Many delis use regular mayonnaise on their sandwiches. Instead, ask for a low-fat substitute or leave it off altogether. If mayo is a must, Moquette-Magee suggests asking the clerk to just barely wet the bread rather than slathering it on.

■ **Skip the tartar sauce.** Tartar sauce, which is served with many fish entrées, gets 96 percent of its calories from fat, Moquette-Magee says. Use it sparingly, if at all. "If you order a fish fillet sandwich at a fast-food restaurant and scrape the tartar sauce off the bun, or ask that it not be put on in the first place, you're cutting the fat in that sandwich by 50 percent," she says.

■ **Take a no-thank-you portion.** "Years ago, if a child told his mother that he didn't want

Nonfat "Cream Cheese"

Put a cheesecloth into a hand sieve and scoop in a tub of plain nonfat yogurt. Put a plate on top of the sieve and set it over a bowl in the refrigerator so that the whey can drip out. After 12 hours, the yogurt should look like thick, creamy, loosely packed cream cheese. If it tastes too sour, stir in a few drops of maple syrup to sweeten it.

a particular food, she'd put a little on his plate anyway. It was called a no-thank-you helping. If you are tempted by a high-fat food, ask for a no-thank-you helping—a tablespoon of it—so that you still get a taste and won't feel deprived," Hogan says.

▪ **Wash the sauce away.** In restaurants, ask for your vegetables steamed without added oils, butter, margarine, or creamed sauces. If the waiter tells you that the vegetables are already prepared with one of those ingredients, ask if your portion can be put in a colander and rinsed with boiling water to wash away the unwanted add-ons, says Francine Grabowski, R.D., at Cooper Hospital in Camden, New Jersey, and co-author of *Low-Fat Living for Real People.*

▪ **Make bacon a special treat.** "Just one slice of cooked bacon has approximately 3 to 5 grams of fat, and it's about 80 percent calories from fat. I tell people not to even buy it or keep it at home," Pingleton says. "If you must have it, get it at a restaurant where you're only going to be served one to two slices instead of the 10 that you would be tempted to eat at home." (When shopping, look for turkey bacon, which is lower in fat.)

If You Crave Fatty Foods...

If you're berating yourself because you simply can't seem to cut back on potato chips, ice cream or some other tempting food—stop. Your problem may not be a lack of willpower. Food cravings are linked to low levels of critical nutrients and/or an imbalance of brain chemicals that affect appetite as well as mood, says Elizabeth Somer, R.D., a nutritionist in Salem, Oregon, who appears regularly on NBC's *Today* show and is a contributing editor to *Shape* magazine. She is the author of *Food & Mood* and *The Origin Diet.*

Somer says the craving for fat is driven, in part, by a brain chemical called galanin. Galanin levels are lowest in the morning, rise during the day and peak in the afternoon. Eating fatty foods keeps galanin circulating in the body, which stimulates the craving for more fat later in the day. This physiological response makes sense in evolutionary terms. Fat was once scarce, so people had to eat as much as possible—whenever it was available—in order to survive.

Today, with rich food all around, fat cravings can be controlled if you:

Substitute fat-free creamy foods. The texture of foods such as fruit-and-yogurt smoothies or pureed squash soup is similar to high-fat foods, and helps reduce cravings.

Eat half a small avocado or one ounce of nuts daily. Such foods contain mono- or polyunsaturated fats, which usually satisfy fat cravings in a more healthful way than the saturated fat found in meat and rich desserts.

Bottom Line Health

Prescription for Low-Fat Eating

Eating foods loaded with fat on a regular basis can clog arteries and lead to heart disease and stroke. Excessive dietary fat also can promote the growth of some types of cancer. Lowering the amount of fat you eat, even after age 60, can prevent or even reverse these diseases.

DO:

▶ **Count grams.** Multiply the average number of calories you eat each day by 20 percent. Then divide the resulting number by 9 (the number of fat calories in a gram). The result is a moderate number of fat calories that you might eat daily.

▶ **Read labels.** Almost all foods list fat grams per serving. Study nutrition labels carefully before buying.

▶ **Make a grocery list.** It will discourage you from impulsively buying high-fat foods.

▶ **Leave foods that contain hydrogenated or partially hydrogenated oils** on the grocery shelf.

▶ **Buy ground turkey or chicken breast that has been processed without the skin.** These are among the leanest meats that you can get.

▶ **Fill your pantry and refrigerator with plant foods**—pastas, breads, beans, cereals, grains, and fresh, frozen, or canned fruits and vegetables. Only one in four items should be a lean meat or low-fat dairy product.

▶ **Keep low-fat snacks** like grapes, dates, celery, and rice cakes handy.

▶ **Experiment with low-fat ingredients** in your favorite recipes.

DON'T:

▶ **Use solid oils** like shortening for cooking. Instead, reach for liquid canola or olive oils.

▶ **Shop on an empty stomach.**

▶ **Automatically reach for nonfat foods.** They may contain substances that drive up triglycerides, a type of fat that increases your risk of heart disease. A low-fat alternative may be a better choice.

▶ **Grease your cooking pans.** Use fruit juice or defatted chicken broth instead.

▶ **Eat fried foods.** They're loaded with fat. Grill, bake, broil, or steam food instead.

▶ **Order appetizers** in restaurants. Many are high in fat.

2

How Fiber Helps Fight Disease

If your body had a yard sale, fiber would be in the bin marked "Free—take it away." Fiber is the last vestige of the food you eat, the waste that remains after your body has wrung out all the goodness it can. But fiber is far from being an expendable part of your diet. As it passes through your system, this throwaway stuff actually acts as an important fighter against cancer, heart disease, and stroke.

Unfortunately, if you're like most older Americans, you probably get no more than 14.8 grams of fiber a day. You need 25 to 35 grams for disease protection.

Luckily, you can make up the difference easily. Researchers note that people who do nothing more than increase fiber and cut fat see cholesterol levels plummet from over 300 milligrams per deciliter (mg/dL) to under 200 mg/dL. That 33 percent drop in cholesterol translates into a whopping 60 percent lower risk of heart disease and stroke.

Some forms of cancer can be prevented with a high-fiber diet. On its way through your body, fiber keeps cancer-causing substances from combining forces to make trouble and helps to eliminate them faster. Fiber also contains perillyl alcohol, one of the valuable compounds now being tested as an experimental treatment for people with advanced cancer. "These compounds, called isoprenoids, actually slow down the growth of tumors or stop their growth entirely," says Charles Elson, Ph.D., a researcher at the University of Wisconsin at Madison.

Most foods contain a combination of two types of fiber—insoluble and soluble. Each type fights disease differently.

Keep Cancer at Bay with Insoluble Fiber

What is insoluble fiber, anyway? Much of it comes from substances that form in the cell walls of plants. It's called insoluble because your body can't easily break it down during the digestive process. It gives your stool its bulk, which helps it move more quickly through your system. (That is why foods high in insoluble fiber—bran, for instance—are known as nature's own laxatives.)

Get Rid of the Gas

How can high-fiber eating be, well, socially acceptable? You know that old song about beans. Along with all the benefits, fiber has two side effects that you would rather do without. It might give you that bloated feeling that makes you need to loosen your belt. And, of course, there is always gas.

Here's how to get the fiber you need without the unpleasantness:

Increase your intake gradually. Each week, increase your daily intake by no more than 5 grams. That is the amount of fiber that you would get in 2 cups of sliced, unpeeled apples, says Belinda Smith, R.D., research dietitian at the Veterans Affairs Medical Center in Lexington, Kentucky. If you add fiber gradually but experience discomfort, keep your fiber intake constant for a few days until symptoms clear up. If they still persist, cut back a few grams and wait several days before trying to make another addition. Also, introduce high-fiber cereals or fiber supplements even more slowly and take them with low-fiber foods.

Drink more water. "You need to increase the amount of water as you increase the fiber you take in, because fiber actually draws water into the bowel," says Alan Adelman, M.D., associate professor in the Department of Family and Community Medicine at the Milton S. Hershey Medical Center of Pennsylvania State University in Hershey. Nutritionists recommend 8 to 12 (8-ounce) glasses per day to reduce the buildup of gas that leads to bloating.

Soak the beans. "Before you cook them, soak dried beans," says Dr. Adelman. Replace the soaking water with fresh water when it is time to cook. This will help get rid of the sugars that cause gas.

Take a gas preventer. To reduce gas, try an over-the-counter product that contains enzymes, such as alpha-galactosidase (Beano), suggests Dr. Adelman.

Grain products and vegetables boast lots of insoluble fiber.

How could that stuff fight cancer, you might ask? At first glance, it looks more like lawn mulch than food. But studies show that insoluble fiber protects you from colon cancer, and researchers believe it wards off breast, prostate, and pancreatic cancer as well.

In Finland, diets rich in cereals go along with low rates of breast and colon cancer. In some parts of Africa, where people eat lots of high-fiber foods, there is virtually no intestinal disease—and that includes colon cancer. In laboratory studies, one component of insoluble fiber, phytic acid, actually prevents the beginning of colon cancer.

Here's how insoluble fiber works to protect you:

■ **Diluting problem elements.** Insoluble fiber soaks up water like a sponge. This makes stools bulkier. The extra bulk means that cancer-causing agents get spread out over a larger area. They can't join forces to do as much damage.

■ **Giving a speed boost.** In the intestinal highway, bulk translates into speed. Insoluble fiber gets things moving fast, so there is less time for interaction between the cells that line the colon and cancerous agents.

■ **Creating a cancer-unfriendly environment.** Fiber tinkers with the acid levels in

A Fibrous Bonus: Weight Loss

Fiber aids weight loss by absorbing water in the stomach, says Om P. Ganda, M.D., associate professor of medicine at Harvard Medical School and director of the lipid clinic at Harvard's Joslin Diabetes Center (both in Boston). As the water is absorbed, it makes you feel full faster and decreases your appetite.

Bottom Line Personal

your intestines. This changes the way bacteria do their jobs. The end result: more fermentation. While that may give you gas (see the box at the top of page 31), it also makes it harder for carcinogens to get into your system. Fiber also helps control levels of the intestinal bile acids that play a part in the start-up of colon cancer.

■ **Tying up carcinogens.** Substances that lead to cancer of the breast, prostate, and pancreas tend to latch onto fiber. This means that when fiber exits the body, it carries away any carcinogens that have become attached.

■ **Lowering estrogen levels.** Insoluble fiber may help reduce levels of the harmful estrogen that contributes to the beginnings of breast cancer. In addition, when you eat a lot of fiber, you generally eat less fat. Researchers believe that dietary fat is a big player in postmenopausal breast cancer. Laboratory experiments suggest that doubling your fiber intake and lowering the amount of fat you eat can decrease the tumor rate by 50 percent. In an Australian study,

women who ate 28 grams of fiber a day had half the breast cancer risk of women who ate less than 14 grams a day.

Foods Rich in Insoluble Fiber

If you're eating fiber-rich foods, you're likely to be getting an ample amount of the insoluble type. That's because virtually all fiber-rich foods contain more insoluble fiber than soluble fiber. Eat plenty of the following foods to make sure that you're getting enough:

■ **Beans.** You get as much fiber benefit from canned beans as dried beans that you soak and cook yourself. Belinda Smith, R.D., research dietitian at the Veterans Affairs Medical Center in Lexington, Kentucky, suggests adding a can of beans to vegetable and other soups, and putting them in lasagna, casseroles, and salads.

■ **Oat bran.** Add it to cereals that you normally prepare, such as oatmeal. Also use oat bran instead of white bread as a filler in meat loaf.

Limit Your Wheat Intake

Andrew Rubman, N.D., associate professor of clinical medicine at the College of Naturopathic Medicine, University of Bridgeport, and director, Southbury Clinic for Traditional Medicines (both in Connecticut), suggests that you limit your servings of wheat products to two times a week. Wheat has a high-gluten content that can set off a condition called gluten enteropathy, which damages the intestinal lining, causing headaches, allergies and autoimmune diseases, such as lupus. Many people aren't even aware that they have the condition, he says.

Bottom Line Personal

Maximize the Bean Benefit

Maybe you bring packages of beans home from the store in little plastic bags, plop them into the cupboard and forget about them. Well, here's how to bring beans out into the open and get the most out of them, according to James W. Anderson, M.D., professor of medicine and clinical nutrition at the Veterans Affairs Medical Center in Lexington, Kentucky.

Put beans on plain view. Store beans in airtight containers (glass jars let you keep them in sight) at room temperature. They'll keep for up to a year, and you'll be more likely to use them if you see them every time you're in the kitchen.

Prepare beans carefully. Get rid of pebbles and other debris that may be in the package along with the beans. Then soak dried beans overnight, or boil them and then soak them for two hours before cooking. Always use fresh water for cooking.

■ **Brown rice.** Try instant brown rice instead of instant white rice, says Alan Adelman, M.D., associate professor in the Department of Family and Community Medicine at the Milton S. Hershey Medical Center of Pennsylvania State University in Hershey. Brown rice supplies 3.32 grams of fiber per cup—white rice weighs in with only 0.74 grams per cup.

■ **Whole-grain bread products.** Choose whole-grain bread products, which can provide 3 or more grams of fiber per slice. That means you can get 6 grams from one sandwich. Refined wheat loses fiber in the milling process. "Refined, processed foods not only lose the fiber, but refining takes out a lot of the trace minerals and possibly the beneficial phytochemicals," notes Rosemary

Fiber Fights Cholesterol and Cancer

Imagine substances in your food that can stop or slow the growth of tumors. Substances that researchers are using—right now—to treat advanced cancers. And imagine that these same substances block the synthesis of cholesterol in your body.

You would eat such a substance morning, noon, and night, yes? Well, that's exactly what you get when you eat foods that are rich in fiber. That's because tocotrienols, components of a protective group of compounds called isoprenoids, are bound to the fiber in many foods. You eat them in cereal products like oats, rice, and barley, as well as olive oil. And you get similar substances in fruits and vegetables.

Tocotrienols are structurally similar to vitamin E. "They're closer in structure than a golden retriever is to a Labrador retriever," says Charles Elson, Ph.D., a researcher at the University of Wisconsin at Madison. He notes that plants produce some of these substances to protect themselves from fungus or insect attacks.

In the laboratory, combinations of isoprenoids offer more protection against disease than individual isoprenoids. "This suggests that you're better off eating a variety of the foods rich in isoprenoids, especially tocotrienols," Dr. Elson says.

How One Researcher Personally Discovered the Cholesterol-Busting Power of Oat Bran

James W. Anderson, M.D., world-renowned professor of medicine and clinical nutrition at the Veterans Affairs Medical Center, recalls that he began eating oat bran in 1977. A pioneer in oat bran research, he couldn't even get the stuff from food suppliers then. Oat bran's main use at the time? Face powder.

But Anderson found that just a bowl of cereal and three to four oat bran muffins a day lowered his cholesterol from 285 to 175 in five weeks. He also lost 8 pounds in that same time. He has continued researching (and eating) oat bran ever since.

Newman, R.D., Ph.D., professor of food and nutrition at Montana State University in Bozeman. These chemicals guard against a wide number of diseases, including heart disease, cancer, and stroke.

How to Bulk Up Your Diet

When you go grocery shopping, read the fine print on the nutrition labels. They tell you the amount of fiber per serving in a food. For instance, "In a bread, the first listed ingredient should be a whole grain," says Dr. Newman. "Better yet, the first three or four listed should be whole grains. That means there are more grains than anything else in the product." If you get tired of picking up and checking every loaf, concentrate on those with labels that make high-fiber claims, such as "good source of fiber."

Here are some simple techniques for adding fiber to your diet:

■ **Balance the benefits of fiber versus other ingredients.** For instance, even if the granola bar of your dreams has 1 or more grams of fiber, it's a good deal only if the fat and calorie content are low. "A snack bar with something like 100 calories, 2 grams of fat, and a gram of fiber is fine. But some have around 300 calories and a lot more fat. That's too much," says Dr. Newman.

■ **Increase fiber in your diet gradually.** Set small, realistic goals that you can meet, suggests Smith. Once you have accomplished those goals, set new ones. To keep yourself on track, keep a diary of what you eat.

■ **Store easy-to-prepare items in your pantry.** Even if you're an avid cook, says Smith, there will be days when you don't feel like getting busy in the kitchen. Stock up on items like baking potatoes, low-fat canned soup, canned beans, and cereals that are easy to prepare. Keep the freezer well-stocked with vegetables that you can quickly cook in a steamer or a microwave oven.

■ **Look for company in increasing the fiber content of your diet.** Get on the phone and flesh out your social calendar. When there are friends and family around, fixing a high-fiber meal can seem like no effort at all, Smith notes. Other avenues for social eating: Join community groups or start your own luncheon club.

Soluble Fiber: The Heart Protector

Soluble fiber shows up mostly in fruits, barley, oats, and beans. Study after study shows that soluble fiber lowers cholesterol, cutting your risk of heart disease and stroke. It may also help clear out your arteries, dropping your risk of high blood pressure. You get soluble fiber in the

Soluble Fiber: A Plan for 10 Grams

Here's how to get 10 grams of soluble fiber each day, which is the amount researchers recommend for lowering your cholesterol, says Belinda Smith, R.D., research dietitian at the Veterans Affairs Medical Center in Lexington, Kentucky.

For breakfast, eat a bowl of high-soluble-fiber cereal (for instance, $2/3$ cup cooked oatmeal) and fruit (say, an orange) for approximately 3.4 grams.

With lunch or dinner, have a serving of cooked legumes for another 2.5 grams. You will get what you need from any of the following choices:

$3/4$ cup bean soup made with navy beans

$3/4$ cup vegetarian chili made with pinto beans

1 cup of three-bean salad made with kidney beans, chickpeas, and green beans

$1 1/4$ cups lentil soup

$1 1/2$ cups split pea soup

$3/4$ cup minestrone soup made with kidney beans

During the course of the day, eat two more fruits or vegetables that are high in soluble fiber for an additional 2 grams of soluble fiber. (See "Play the Numbers for Protection" on pages 34–35 for a list of the best choices.) Chances are, you will get 3 grams of soluble fiber from the rest of the foods you eat.

So without breaking a sweat, you'll make it to 10 grams. But remember, you still need to consume a total of 25 to 35 grams of fiber a day, the rest made up from insoluble fiber.

outer part of certain grains, the white rind in citrus fruits, and the membranes that contain each little section of grapefruit pulp. But in some plants, such as beans or barley, you find soluble fiber throughout.

In your body, soluble fiber combines with water, swelling up to create a gelatinous substance that does wonders to shield you from heart attacks and strokes.

Here's how soluble fiber works to protect your heart:

■ **Cutting cholesterol.** The higher your cholesterol levels, the greater your risk of heart disease and stroke. "The total amount of fat in the diet is probably the major factor in cholesterol control," says Dr. Newman. Researchers believe that once soluble fiber reaches the small intestine, it interferes with absorption of fat. In addition, soluble fiber may trap bile, which must

be replaced. The replacement material is cholesterol, which is drawn out of the blood and tissues." That cholesterol-laden bile heads on down the intestinal highway and out of the body.

But the benefits don't stop there. Elsewhere on the digestive route, bacteria break down soluble fiber to create short-chain fatty acids. When these are absorbed back into the body, they restrict the body's ability to synthesize cholesterol, reducing your blood's cholesterol levels still more.

Researchers note that some people can lower cholesterol much more cheaply and just as effectively with fiber than with cholesterol-lowering medication. At the University of Minnesota, researchers looked at 10 studies of oat bran and found that eating just 3 grams of soluble fiber a day (what you would get in one cup of ready-to-eat oat bran cereal) can drop cholesterol levels by 2 to 3 percent. In people whose levels were over

Play the Numbers for Protection:
Foods That Are Tops in Soluble Fiber

Food	Portion	Soluble Fiber (g.)
Vegetables		
Artichoke, cooked	1 medium	2.2
Celery root, fresh, chopped	½ cup	1.9
Sweet potato, cooked	½ cup	1.8
Parsnip, cooked	½ cup	1.8
Turnip, cooked	½ cup	1.7
Acorn squash, baked	½ cup	1.6
Potato with skin, baked	1 medium	1.6
Brussels sprouts, cooked	½ cup	1.4
Cabbage, fresh	1 cup	1.3
Green peas, cooked	½ cup	1.3
Broccoli, cooked, chopped	½ cup	1.2
Carrots, cooked, chopped	½ cup	1.1
Carrot, raw	7½" long	1.1
Cabbage, cooked	½ cup	1.1
French-style green beans, cooked	½ cup	1.1
Cauliflower florets, cooked	¾ cup	1.0
Asparagus, cooked	¾ cup	1.0
Fruits		
Mango, sliced	1 cup	2.9
Strawberries, whole, capped	1 cup	2.0
Figs	2	1.7
Kiwifruits	2	1.4
Orange	1	1.4
Plums	2	1.4
Pear	1 small	1.1
Grapefruit	½ medium	1.1
Blackberries	¾ cup	1.1
Apricot halves, dried	7	1.1
Apple with skin	1 small	1.0
Prunes	3	1.0
Peach	1 medium	1.0

Play the Numbers for Protection...continued

Food	Portion	Soluble Fiber (g.)
Cereals		
Quaker Oat Bran	1 cup cooked (1/2 cup dry)	3.0
Quaker Oat Bran Cereal, ready-to-eat	1 1/4 cups	3.0
SmartBeat High Fiber Oatmeal	1 packet, instant	3.0
H-O Super Bran High Fiber Cereal	3/4 cup	3.0
Kellogg's Bran Buds	1/3 cup	3.0
Quaker Oatmeal, cooked	1 cup	2.0
Health Valley Healthy Crunch	1/2 cup	1.4
Raisin Bran	1 cup	1.2
Quaker Instant Oatmeal	1 packet	1.0
Nabisco 100% Bran	1/3 cup	1.0
Kellogg's All-Bran	1/2 cup	1.0
Post Oat Flakes	2/3 cup	1.0
Kellogg's Common Sense Oat Bran	3/4 cup	1.0
Cheerios	1 1/4 cups	1.0
Nabisco Shredded Wheat 'N Bran	2/3 cup	1.0
Post Bran Flakes	1/2 cup	1.0
Grains		
Pearl barley	3/4 cup cooked	1.8
Oat flour	1/4 cup	1.6
Rye flour	1/4 cup	1.3
Wheat germ	4 1/2 tablespoons	1.0
Legumes		
Large lima beans, canned	1/2 cup	5.7
Kidney beans, cooked	1/2 cup	2.8
Cranberry beans, cooked	1/2 cup	2.7
Butter beans, cooked	1/2 cup	2.7
Baked beans, canned, cooked	1/2 cup	2.6
Black beans, cooked	1/2 cup	2.4
Navy beans, cooked	1/2 cup	2.2
Lentils, cooked	1/2 cup	2.0
Pinto beans, cooked	1/2 cup	1.9
Great Northern beans, cooked	1/2 cup	1.4
Chickpeas, cooked	1/2 cup	1.3
Split peas, cooked	1/2 cup	1.1

Reduce Cholesterol in Three Easy Steps

Soluble fiber is a mighty cholesterol-buster. James W. Anderson, M.D., professor of medicine and clinical nutrition at the Veterans Affairs Medical Center in Lexington, Kentucky, recommends this three-stage program using soluble fiber to cut your blood cholesterol. Stay at each level for four to six weeks.

Level I: Adjust your diet so that you take in 10 grams of soluble fiber a day. You will probably get a 5 to 10 percent drop in your cholesterol levels. Generally, the higher the levels you start with, the bigger the drop.

Level II: Consume 15 grams of soluble fiber per day for a total 10 to 15 percent cholesterol reduction.

Level III: Combine 15 grams of soluble fiber with a psyllium supplement (under your doctor's supervision). This will give you a total 15 to 20 percent cholesterol reduction.

230 mg/dL, cholesterol declined more steeply, an average of 6 to 7 percent. And it seems that the more oat bran people eat, the more their cholesterol goes down. In one study, consuming 6 to 9 grams of soluble fiber reduced cholesterol levels of over 260 by 23 percent.

■ **Clearing out your arteries.** Researchers theorize that soluble fiber may also be an arterial housecleaner, helping to reduce the risk of plaque buildup in your arteries that can lead to heart attack and stroke. By lowering the levels of cholesterol that circulate in your body, soluble fiber automatically drops your risk of an artery-clogging buildup.

■ **Controlling blood sugar.** Soluble fiber improves the body's ability to maintain normal blood sugar by slowing absorption of starchy foods. This helps forestall the plaque buildup in arteries, which can lead to a heart attack or stroke.

■ **Fighting high blood pressure.** Researchers studied 850 Yi people, members of an ethnic minority in southwest China. They found that the Yi diet, high in oats and buckwheat, resulted in lower blood pressures and lower levels of the harmful low-density lipoprotein (LDL) cholesterol.

■ **Slashing cancer risk.** In one laboratory study, researchers studied a modified form of pectin, a soluble fiber. They found that this special kind of pectin helped prevent cancer from spreading. It kept cancer cells from sticking to the walls of the lungs, keeping lung tumors from getting a start.

In Search of the Soluble

One-fourth of the fiber that you take in should be soluble, according to Dr. Newman. The problem is that most people who eat fiber don't get enough of the soluble type. Many foods that are gold mines of insoluble fiber contain almost no soluble materials. For example, you'll get 3 grams of fiber from 3 cups of popcorn. But a mere 0.1 gram will be soluble fiber.

The valuable soluble fiber shows up mostly in fruits, barley, oats, and beans (these foods generally contain plenty of insoluble fiber as well). Although most foods contain much more insoluble fiber than soluble, you can increase your intake of soluble fiber by making small changes in how you handle foods you're probably already eating.

Here are some suggestions for increasing the soluble fiber in your diet:

More Benefits of Fiber

Fiber can do more for you than just help to forestall heart problems, cancer, and stroke. It can prevent other unpleasant side effects of aging as well:

Fiber stops constipation.

Fiber alleviates diverticulosis, the formation of little pockets in the colon that can trap bacteria, bleed, and become inflamed. (This malady affects more than half of all people over age 70.)

Fiber reduces hemorrhoid flare-ups.

Fiber improves the appearance of your hair and fingernails, when it's eaten as part of a balanced diet.

■ **Don't throw out the liquid from beans.** The liquid that comes with canned beans contains a lot of dissolved soluble fiber (the reason why it is soupy instead of watery). Unless you have salt-sensitive high blood pressure or congestive heart failure, the salt in the liquid should not bother you. Save the liquid and combine it with soups. Or, for a low-salt or no-salt substitute, cook your own beans and save the leftover liquid, says Dr. Anderson.

■ **Don't peel fruits or vegetables.** The peels of many of them—apples, pears, peaches, or potatoes, to name a few—are rich in soluble fiber. Eat the white inner rind of oranges, which is high in pectin. For grapefruit sections, spoon out the membrane with the pulp for extra soluble fiber, says Dr. Anderson.

■ **Eat fruits and vegetables whole.** While you get concentrated nutrients from many juices, you lose the fiber in the fruit. An 8-ounce glass of extracted carrot juice, for instance, contains just 2 grams of fiber, compared with the 14 grams you would get from the six carrots (1 pound) that went into the juicer, says Dr. Adelman.

■ **Take a soluble fiber supplement.** "A lot of people find that it's easier to take a soluble fiber supplement than to adjust their diets," says Dr. Adelman. The main ingredient in fiber supplements like Metamucil is psyllium, which comes from the ground-up seed husks of a plant grown in India. It has been used as a laxative for more than 60 years. You get the most benefit if you take psyllium with a meal. But taking a supplement may not be the best way to reward your taste buds. "My patients who use a supplement tell me that they make it palatable by mixing it with orange juice or apple juice," says Dr. Adelman.

Psyllium is also available in some cereals. In one study, people with mildly high cholesterol levels ate Bran Buds, a cereal high in psyllium, for two weeks. Their cholesterol levels dropped by 8 percent.

Warning: Don't use a psyllium supplement without your doctor's okay, since it can interfere with other medicines that you may be taking.

■ **Look for food products rich in soluble fiber.** TrimChoice, formerly known as Oatrim, is a fat substitute made from oat flour, which is rich in soluble fiber. Produced by Mountain Lake Manufacturing, it may appear as an ingredient called "hydrolyzed oat flour" in cheese, baked goods, confections, and meat, as well as a variety of other low-fat products. While

TrimChoice is touted for its low-fat benefits, it also cuts cholesterol. In a U.S. Department of Agriculture study, 24 people with high levels of cholesterol who ate products containing Trim-Choice experienced a 16 percent drop in total cholesterol in five weeks. Their levels of protective high-density lipoprotein cholesterol were unchanged. Other benefits: Their blood pressures went down and their blood sugar levels became more stable.

Two Quick and Tasty High-Fiber Recipes

Belinda Smith, R.D., a research dietitian at the Veterans Affairs Medical Center in Lexington, Kentucky, recommends this quick-and-easy two-in-one recipe developed by Constance Pittman Lindner for the *Tufts University Diet and Nutrition Letter* to add fiber to your diet. Store individual servings in the freezer and have a home-cooked meal whenever the mood strikes.

Chili and Spaghetti Sauce: Two Recipes in One

Basic Meat Mixture

2 tablespoons olive oil
2 onions, chopped
2 cloves garlic, minced
1 pound ground turkey or chicken

2 cans (28 ounces each) chopped
    tomatoes or tomato purée
1 can (12 ounces) tomato paste
1 1/2 cups water

In a large saucepan, add the onions and garlic to the heated oil. Sauté over medium heat for 5 minutes, or until the onions are tender. Crumble the turkey or chicken into the pan. Break up the meat with a wooden spoon and cook for five minutes, or until it is browned. Drain off any fat that has accumulated in the pan. Add the tomatoes or tomato purée, tomato paste, and water to the meat mixture. Simmer for 20 minutes. Divide the meat mixture into two portions: Use two-thirds of the meat and one-third of the sauce for the chili, and the rest for the spaghetti sauce.

Chili

Portion of the Basic Meat Mixture
2 cans (16 ounces) kidney beans,
    rinsed and drained
1/2 green pepper, seeded and chopped

1 1/2–2 teaspoons chili powder
1 1/2 teaspoons ground cumin
1 cup shredded low-fat sharp Cheddar
    cheese

Mix the beans, green peppers, chili powder, and cumin with the basic meat mixture. Simmer for 5 minutes. Serve sprinkled with the Cheddar.
Makes 8 (1 cup) servings. Per serving: 276 calories, 7.1 g. fat (23% of calories), 7 g. dietary fiber, 38 mg. cholesterol, 911 mg. sodium.

Spaghetti Sauce

Portion of the Basic Meat Mixture
2 tablespoons honey
1 teaspoon dried basil

1 teaspoon dried oregano
1/2 teaspoon ground black pepper

Add the honey, basil, oregano, and pepper to the basic meat mixture. Simmer for 5 minutes.
Makes 5 (1 cup) servings. Per serving: 325 calories, 8.4 g. fat (23% of calories), 6.6 g. dietary fiber, 53 mg. cholesterol, 1,110 mg. sodium.

Prescription for Increasing Fiber

Eating more fiber can substantially lower your cholesterol levels, greatly reducing your risk of heart disease and stroke. High-fiber diets also slash your risk of some forms of cancer, including breast, colon, pancreatic, and prostate cancer.

DO:

▶ **Eat wheat products and vegetables** for insoluble fiber.

▶ **Get soluble fiber from fruits, oats, and beans.**

▶ **Increase your fiber intake** by adding beans to soups, lasagna, casseroles, and salads.

▶ **Eat brown rice** instead of white rice and replace refined flour with whole-wheat flour.

▶ **Choose whole-grain bread products.**

▶ **Drink 8 to 12 (8-ounce) glasses of water** each day. Fiber draws liquids out of your system.

DON'T:

▶ **Peel apples, pears, peaches, or potatoes.**

▶ **Add a high-fiber psyllium supplement** if you're on other medications without first checking with your doctor.

3

Plant Power:
Vital Weapons for Healthy Aging

Imagine an array of well-armed forces battling heart disease, cancer, and stroke, catching cancerous invaders and throwing them out of your system before they destroy healthy cells. Shrinking any tumors that get started. Sending blood pressure tumbling down. Cleaning out the fat in your arteries. Keeping your arteries clear of the blood clots that lead to strokes. Protecting cells against DNA damage. Even slowing down the aging process.

Sounds like the antics of superheroes in your grandchildren's video games? It's also what goes on in your body when you eat fruits, vegetables, and grains.

Scientists have discovered that when you eat food made from plants, you get the benefits of powerful defenses. They come from *phytochemicals,* a term that refers to certain chemicals in plants. They are separate substances from the the vitamins that plants contain, and they may be even more valuable.

For a long time, scientists thought that phytochemicals were just plain useless. But the picture is changing as experts sift through the thousands of different phytochemicals in plants. No one knows exactly what each one does, but they appear to help ward off cancer, heart disease, and stroke. In fact, more than 200 studies have shown that diets high in fruits and vegetables cut cancer risk. That protection becomes increasingly important as you get older and your risk of disease increases.

How Do These Mysterious Chemicals Work?

Sometimes protective phytochemicals make their presence known: You can see their calling cards in the bright orange color of carrots or sweet potatoes. Or you get a whiff of phytochemicals when you come nose-to-clove with garlic. You taste them in the sharp bite of freshly cut watercress. But many others are undetectable.

"These chemicals are there to protect the plants," says James Duke, Ph.D., an ethnobotanist who was formerly with the U.S. Department of Agriculture Research Service in Beltsville, Maryland. Researchers theorize that some antioxidant phytochemicals evolved to protect plants from oxygen (since plants feed on carbon dioxide, with oxygen as waste), as well as wind, weather, and insects. "These

Bonus from Eating Plants:
Vegetarians Have Less Arthritis Pain

A few days on a vegetarian diet may soothe your aching joints. John McDougall, M.D., medical director of the McDougall Program (a diet and exercise program in Santa Rosa, California), says patients who ate a diet with no animal products or added fats or oils for four weeks experienced a significant reduction in arthritis symptoms, including pain and joint tenderness. Their diet, which included corn, beans, fruits, and vegetables, reduced the blood levels of antibodies that attack joint tissue.

Bottom Line Health

substances keep plants from oxidizing under the hot sun's ultraviolet radiation. They protect bulb plants that grow underground from an onslaught of microbial and insect hazards," says Suzanne Paxton Pierson, a pharmacy doctor and president of Preventive Nutrition Consults in Woodinville, Washington. "But you can borrow the protective benefits," says Dr. Duke.

Plant Foods Can Slash Cancer Risk

Up to 33 percent of potential cancers might be prevented just by eating a diet rich in fruits and vegetables, according to scientists at the National Cancer Institute.

"We can save more than 150,000 lives a year, right now, with no treatments, no medical costs, no long-term recovery—if people would just eat the foods that protect them," says Edward Miller, Ph.D., professor of biomedical sciences in the Department of Biomedical Sciences at Baylor College of Dentistry in Houston, who researches oral cancer.

"Studies worldwide show that phytochemicals protect against cancer," says Paul Lachance, Ph.D., chairman of the food science department at Rutgers University in New Brunswick, New Jersey, and an internationally known researcher in the field. But, he cautions, "There is no panacea phytochemical, no one thing you can take or eat for protection."

If you eat lots of plant foods (which provide plenty of phytochemicals), you have a lower risk for cancers that attack the lungs, bladder, cervix, mouth, larynx, throat, esophagus, stomach, pancreas, colon, and rectum. In the laboratory, phytochemicals keep cancer-forming substances and defective cells—which can turn into cancers—from getting a foothold or spreading.

Scientists also believe plant foods may help protect you from breast and prostate cancer. Some phytochemicals in plants contain hormones that disrupt the growth of breast cancer and prostate cancer cells.

Plant Foods Can Cure Cardiovascular Problems

Phytochemicals in plants keep your heart healthy, too. "The 60-to-80 age group has a much greater risk of heart disease than younger people do. If your diet is rich in fruits and vegetables, you can reduce risk," notes Dexter Morris, M.D., vice chairman of the Department of Emergency Medicine and a heart researcher at the University of North Carolina at Chapel Hill School of Medicine.

Certain plant chemicals may help your cardiovascular system by neutralizing harmful low-density lipoprotein (LDL) cholesterol that, if left unchecked, can lead to hardening of the arteries. Others act on the walls of your blood vessels and, in the process, lower blood pressure or make blood platelets less sticky and less likely to clot so that you're not as vulnerable to strokes.

In a study begun in 1973, researchers kept track of 1,883 men ages 35 to 59 who had high cholesterol levels. Over the next 20 years, the men who had the highest levels of carotenoids (a phytochemical) in their blood had 60 percent fewer heart attacks and deaths.

Plant Foods Can Combat Free Radicals

Many phytochemicals in plants do double-duty as antioxidants, neutralizing free radicals in the body—unstable molecules that damage or destroy your healthy cells. Your body produces these harmful free radicals routinely. You also get them from a variety of exterior sources, including cigarette smoke, pollutants, medications, pesticides, and household cleaners.

Free radicals have been linked to more than 60 diseases and medical problems. Beyond heart disease, cancer, and stroke, these include premature aging, stiff joints, wrinkled skin, arthritis, diabetes, and liver cirrhosis.

"Antioxidants are particularly important for people aged 60 to 80 because they reduce the effects of aging system-wide," says Joanne Slavin, Ph.D., professor in the Department of Food Science and Nutrition at the University of Minnesota in St. Paul.

Protective Phytochemicals in Plants

In this relatively new field, research is ongoing. Scientists are still finding out exactly how phytochemicals work.

Here is a list of phytochemicals that appear to provide the most protection:

ORGANOSULFUR COMPOUNDS

The aromatic scent and pungent flavor that you get from plants belonging to the allium family—such as garlic, onions, leeks, chives, and shallots —are actually signs that protective phytochemicals are at work. These particular phytochemicals are called organosulfur compounds. You can also get these compounds in cruciferous vegetables, such as broccoli, cabbage, and cauliflower.

■ **Fighting Cancer**—Foods rich in organosulfur compounds could be called dietary anti-carcinogens, according to John Potter, M.D., Ph.D., head of the Cancer Prevention Research Program at the Fred Hutchinson Cancer Research Center in Seattle. Studies have shown that some of the powerful organosulfur compounds in these plants, such as diallyl disulfide, block or suppress carcinogens. Plus, they help the body intercept and eject cancer-causing agents before they can do any damage.

Another important organosulfur compound, alliin, works as a powerful antioxidant, disposing of free radicals that damage healthy cells and promote both cancer and atherosclerosis. In animals, alliin interferes with tumor growth and prevents the molecular changes that lead to cancer.

Some of these chemicals also help your immune system stay strong by increasing the number of infection-fighting T cells. Researchers at the University of Minnesota School of Public Health looked at the eating habits of more than 41,830 Iowa women aged 55 to 69. Those who ate garlic, a particularly rich source of organosulfur compounds, had a one-third reduction in their risk of colon cancer.

In other studies, researchers note that the bacteria-fighting organosulfur compounds may also fight off cancer. They disarm *Helicobacter pylori*, a bacteria found in the stomach that can lead to stomach cancer.

Danish scientists have discovered that chemicals in garlic not only block the growth of cancer cells but also delay the normal aging process of healthy cells.

■ **Fighting Heart Disease**—Organosulfur compounds found in onions, garlic, and other members of the allium family also defend your heart. "When you eat a hearty meal, you get an influx of fats into the bloodstream. This makes your blood more likely to clot. The alliums, particularly onions, will help your body manufacture substances to get rid of the fat quickly," says Isabella Lipinska, Ph.D., a nutritional counselor for the Cardiac Rehabilitation Program at St. Elizabeth's Medical Center in Boston. This lowers your risk for heart disease and stroke.

Organosulfur compounds help to lower blood pressure without the common side effects, such as headaches and impotence, that some people get from prescription medication. Experts theorize that these compounds dilate the muscle cells in the arteries, opening up the blood vessels. They may also help the blood circulate to the smaller vessels more efficiently, lowering blood pressure even more.

They also decrease levels of harmful LDL cholesterol that can narrow artery walls. And they increase levels of the beneficial high-density lipoprotein (HDL) cholesterol that keeps your arteries free of plaque and protects against heart disease and stroke.

Scientists in Australia examined the results of eight trials with a total of 415 people. Those who consumed a commercial dried garlic powder for one to three months lowered their blood pressure. Project researchers speculate that if, in long-term studies, garlic eaters sustain this lowered blood pressure, the studies might also show 30 to 40 percent fewer strokes and 20 to 25 percent less coronary heart disease.

Another study measured cholesterol levels, revealing an 11 percent drop in harmful LDL cholesterol and a 6 percent drop in total cholesterol in people who took 900 milligrams a day of garlic powder tablets (the equivalent of about three cloves) over a 12-week period. That's important because researchers estimate that every 1 percent drop in total cholesterol could translate into a decreased heart attack risk of 2 percent.

■ **Fighting Stroke**—You get protection against stroke from organosulfur compounds, too. At Brown University, men aged 30 to 70 who had cholesterol levels of 230 to 290 consumed 700 milligrams of garlic a day. Their total cholesterol and LDL cholesterol levels declined by 8 percent. Their levels of beneficial HDL cholesterol did not change.

Here are some ways to get the most benefit from organosulfur compounds:

■ **Purée veggies in soup.** As you get older, your body doesn't absorb food as easily, a problem compounded if you have dentures and don't chew your food properly. Dr. Lipinska advises using a blender to purée vegetables into vegetable soups, complete with onion and garlic.

■ **Eat garlic every day.** "For health benefits, based on retrospective epidemiologic studies, eat two to three cloves of garlic a day," advises Dr. Paxton Pierson.

Yu-Yan Yeh, Ph.D., professor of nutrition science at Pennsylvania State University in University Park, conducted a study of men aged 35 to 55 with high LDL ("bad" cholesterol) levels. They received supplements equal to two to three cloves, and their LDL cholesterol levels dropped. Still, Dr. Yeh says, "It's better to incorporate fresh garlic into daily cooking and to eat healthy foods instead of taking a supplement. You get extra benefits from vegetables you eat with garlic."

■ **Pass up rich food.** Adding garlic or other foods rich in phytochemicals may tempt you toward the wrong kinds of food. A garlicky sauce, for instance, is hardly a wise choice if it's also full of butter or other animal fats, advises

How I Did It:
Now She Knows Beans—and Carrots

Diagnosed with breast cancer at age 49, Grace M. recalls, "I knew I would beat it. I just put one foot in front of the other mentally. But I didn't really make any big changes in my life then, with one exception—I stopped smoking."

When the New York resident reached menopause, she did change her diet. "I always loved meat and fruit but hated cooked vegetables. With menopause, I noticed that I put on another 10 pounds. That wasn't healthy, so I knew that I had to change."

Grace says that her downfall wasn't a sweet tooth. It was cheese and other high-fat foods. "It was a real sacrifice to give those foods up," she sighs, recalling a special treat—cheese and pâté.

"I can't say that it made my life better right away, but switching to more fruits and vegetables made my life a lot easier. I've always hated cooked vegetables. In fact, I cook them for my husband, but I can't stand to eat them. So I tried them raw. I discovered that I liked raw carrots and fresh string beans."

Each week, Grace bought bunches of carrots and a pound or so of beans. She peeled and sliced the carrots, pulled the strings and the ends off the beans, and stored them in separate, sealed containers in the refrigerator to keep them fresh. "I realized that the string beans, in particular, are delicious, with a crunchy, fresh taste. I would bring things like that to work with me."

She added tomatoes to her assortment and stocked up on fruit. "I've always loved fruit, and it was wonderful to have an excuse to buy more," Grace says. She started buying watermelons, cutting them up and storing them in the refrigerator, along with her vegetable assortment. "I'd just nosh on that when I wanted a snack." Pretty soon, eating fruits and vegetables got to be routine for her.

"But I haven't given up everything," she says. "I have my wine with dinner every night. My husband, Robert, and I eat out twice a week. We try to order sensibly, but I figure that because I eat carefully almost all the time, I'm entitled to an occasional treat. The other day at a French restaurant, I even had pâté."

Around the time she turned 60, Grace started to worry about other ailments. "I was scared of debilitating things like strokes," she says. "Several friends died." Still, she didn't act until her gynecologist remarked about her borderline high blood pressure.

"Hypertension runs in my family. I worried about that. My internist told me to limit my salt intake, which worked a little. She also put me on a very low dose of medication."

That's when Grace made more lifestyle changes to keep her heart healthy. "I'm doing a lot of bicycle riding, just for flexibility. I have arthritis of the spine, and I've found that movement also helps my arthritis. Plus, I do weight-bearing exercises. And I started playing tennis an hour a day on the handball wall. "

The effort has paid off. Now she has more stamina. "I didn't behave myself when I was young, and it's nice not to have to pay too much for your past sins when you get older," Grace says. "It has been a sacrifice, but I'm glad for the result—I don't think that I look my age, and I feel great."

Do You Chew?

The stomach can't break down food into usable forms unless it has been thoroughly mixed with saliva. If you don't chew your food thoroughly, nutritional deficiencies may result, warns Andrew Rubman, N.D., associate professor of clinical medicine, College of Naturopathic Medicine, University of Bridgeport, and director, Southbury Clinic for Traditional Medicines (both in Connecticut). Not only will you lose access to your food's protection against cancer, heart attack, and stroke, but you can also develop chronic colds, fatigue, and even memory loss.

Bottom Line Personal

Dr. Yeh. "The benefits won't offset the health hazards of rich food."

■ **Sauté the garlic.** Avoid eating raw garlic because, like other bulb vegetables, it grows underground in close contact with bacteria that may be harmful to you. So don't mix raw garlic in oil, for instance, and store it in the refrigerator. Raw garlic also gives some people intestinal irritation, says Dr. Yeh. "You'll get the most benefit out of alliums (garlic and its relatives) by chopping them up and then sautéing them in a little oil," he says. "Use olive oil or canola oil, because they're high in monounsaturated fat and don't seem to contribute to higher LDL cholesterol levels the way other oils do." He adds that chopping activates some phytochemicals while heat gets others going.

■ **Use garlic powder for flavor only.** Condiments such as onion or garlic powder may add flavor to your food, but processing techniques have probably cost them much of their protective benefits. Your taste buds are the only part of you that are likely to benefit from them.

■ **Use the vegetable immediately.** The enzymes that activate protective phytochemicals dissipate within 12 to 24 hours. So you'll get more benefit when your garlic and onion are freshly chopped, according to Dr. Lachance. If you cut up the vegetable and save it for another day, all you'll get from it is the taste.

Warning: Check with your doctor before increasing your intake of organosulfur compounds if you are on anticlotting medicine or aspirin.

ISOTHIOCYANATES

You find plant chemicals called isothiocyanates in leafy green vegetables, such as watercress, arugula, cabbage, Chinese cabbage, and brussels sprouts, as well as broccoli and cauliflower.

■ **Fighting Cancer**—These beneficial compounds help the body get rid of cancer-causing substances. "They take the trash out, to put it in the simplest terms. Fewer carcinogens reach their cellular targets," says Stephen Hecht, Ph.D., professor of cancer prevention at the University of Minnesota Cancer Center in Minneapolis.

Isothiocyanates make it difficult for cancer-causing substances to zero in on the DNA (genetic material) of healthy cells. In the laboratory, they have kept tumors from forming and have detoxified carcinogens. In one experiment, rats that ate a diet containing an isothiocyanate from watercress and a carcinogen from tobacco were 50 percent less likely to develop lung tumors than those exposed only to the carcinogen.

Here's how you can get the most benefit from the isothiocyanates in your food:

■ **Eat some of the vegetables raw.** "Isothiocyanates are released when you chew the raw vegetable or chop it up," says Dr. Hecht.

"You know it's happening because of the sharp taste. Cooking reduces some of the compounds, but the vegetables still contain a lot of beneficial chemicals."

■ **Eat the vegetables as soon as possible.** While the phytochemicals in these vegetables are fairly stable, you'll get more if you eat vegetables while they are fresh, adds Dr. Hecht. If, for example, you chop up watercress or broccoli and use it the next day, the taste will be subdued—and the benefits will be slightly less, according to Dr. Duke.

■ **Eat plenty of them.** "The National Cancer Institute recommends at least five helpings a day of fruits and vegetables. While you won't be immune to cancer if you eat a lot of cruciferous vegetables, they do contain a large number of compounds that we strongly suspect to be anticarcinogens," says Dr. Potter.

■ **Eat the leaves.** "Phytochemicals are most concentrated in the broad leaves of many vegetables to protect the plant, although we also see some concentration in seeds," says Dr. Duke.

INDOLES

Like Laurel and Hardy, indoles and isothiocyanates go together. When you eat the leafy greens of cruciferous vegetables like broccoli, cauliflower, and cabbage, you get the benefits of both.

■ **Fighting Cancer**—Indoles protect against breast cancer because they alter the body's estrogen metabolism. But it's not for women only—it has the potential for use as a possible preventive treatment for prostate cancer in men.

"In humans, indoles stop the growth of small virus-caused tumors. In animals, these vegetables prevent breast cancer," says Leon Bradlow, Ph.D., director of the Murray Rayburn Laboratory of Biochemical Endocrinology at Strang

Cancer Research Laboratory in New York City. "This makes us optimistic that we'll see similar results in humans. We already know that people in China and Korea, who eat cabbage all their lives, have much lower breast cancer rates than people in the West."

You get added benefits from broccoli, a rich source of indoles. It also contains sulforaphane, a phytochemical that prevents mammary tumors in rats.

■ **Fighting Heart Disease and Stroke**—Because indoles are estrogen-like substances, they may help lower the risk of heart disease and stroke. Estrogen has been linked to lower levels of harmful LDL cholesterol and may even help control high blood pressure and reduce the blood's tendency to clot.

Here's how to benefit the most from indoles:

■ **Eat a quarter a day.** For maximum protection, Dr. Bradlow suggests that you eat the equivalent of a quarter head of cabbage a day or an equal amount of broccoli (about half a bunch), brussels sprouts, or cauliflower. "We have found that the highest levels of indoles are in savoy cabbage—the crinkly looking type—and in purple broccoli," he says.

ISOFLAVONES

Isoflavones are a group of plant estrogens found in soy products.

■ **Fighting Cancer**—"In countries where people consume a lot of soy, the rate of breast and prostate cancer is very low," says Clare Hasler, Ph.D., director of the Functional Foods for Health Program at University of Illinois at Urbana–Champaign. The powerhouse isoflavones in soy are *genistein, daidzein,* and *equol.* In laboratory tests, they keep cancerous cells from growing. Some studies on animals show genistein

Eat Right to Fight Disease

Ever think that you could protect yourself from disease every time you put food in your mouth? You can, if you eat foods rich in protective phytochemicals. Here is how to get more of the foods that defend you from cancer, heart disease, and stroke.

Minimize meats. Gradually decrease the amount of meat and other high-fat items on your plate and increase the amount of vegetables. Slowly cut back until your meat serving is the size of a deck of cards or smaller, and the rest of the space is filled with vegetables, pasta, or rice, says John Potter, M.D., Ph.D., head of the Cancer Prevention Research Program at the Fred Hutchinson Cancer Research Center in Seattle. Try meatless meals using recipes from the Mediterranean region as well as India, Japan, China, Indonesia, Southeast Asia, and North Africa. If you make changes gradually, the shift will be easier to tolerate.

Open a cookbook. Get ideas for new foods by checking out cookbooks from the library or buying a few. Look for books that promote the consumption of fruits and vegetables and other plant foods, suggests Dr. Potter.

Ask for support. Tell your family and friends that you're trying new foods for health and enlist their psychological support. "Learning new styles of cooking takes time, and you will screw up," says Dr. Potter. "It's easier if your friends and family are tolerant of your failures. I sometimes think that cooking is a skill that has gone the way of the horse and buggy. I would like to see people get it back."

Throw a party. "Work on your own or enroll in cooking classes," suggests Dr. Potter. "You get to meet new people and eat more healthy foods." Get together with friends for "moving dinners," perhaps held once a week at a different person's home. That way, you can all learn together, Dr. Potter says.

Prepare balanced meals. Whether you pop a clove or a pill, you'll get maximum benefit if you consume phytochemicals with a meal of plant foods, because the intake of protein, fat, and carbohydrate helps your body absorb and use the phytochemicals more effectively, says Paul Lachance, Ph.D., chairman of the food science department at Rutgers University in New Brunswick, New Jersey, and an internationally known researcher in the field.

Eat what you like. "If you don't like something, you probably won't eat it," says Dexter Morris, M.D., vice chairman of the Department of Emergency Medicine and a heart researcher at the University of North Carolina at Chapel Hill School of Medicine. If you only like tomatoes and hate other vegetables, just eat more tomatoes. "There are probably enough different kinds of phytochemicals in every vegetable to do you some good," he says. "It's not like there is only one kind in a tomato and another kind in a carrot. There are mixtures in all. It's more important to eat vegetables than to worry about which ones."

also keeps tumors from getting the blood supplies they need. In fact, when leukemia cells divide, genistein helps them to return to their original healthy state.

In laboratory studies, the phytoestrogens in soy reduce the number of mammary tumors in rats and prevent the growth of human breast cancer cells. Researchers also think that phytochemicals such as isoflavonoids may slow the growth of prostate cancer.

In a Japanese study, the diets of 142,875 women were followed for 17 years. Breast cancer

Soy Helps When You Have a Cold

Eat soy at least once a day when you have a cold, says Andrew Rubman. The saponins it contains destroy infectious organisms, but do not contribute to the increase in antibiotic-resistant diseases.

Bottom Line Personal

risk was lowest in women whose diets included miso soup, made from soybean paste. Researchers theorize that the isoflavones do the job. Studies also show that soy consumption is tied to a lower rate of colon and rectal cancers.

Soy is a good source of another group of phytochemicals called saponins. In the laboratory, saponins fight cervical, pancreatic, gastric, colon, breast, and prostate cancers.

■ **Fighting Heart Disease and Stroke—** "Studies have shown that soy can bring cholesterol from the high-risk to moderate- or low-risk range," says Dr. Hasler.

"Soy contains a variety of chemicals that probably interact. Even independently, some of them do lower levels of harmful cholesterol," says Susan Potter, R.D., Ph.D., associate professor of nutrition at the University of Illinois at Urbana–Champaign.

Scientists believe that plant estrogens found in soy lead to the low levels of heart disease in Asian countries. Scientists speculate that those phytoestrogens also slow down atherosclerosis, protecting the arteries.

Soy is unique among plants. The important protectors, genistein and daidzein, are only found to any significant extent in soybeans and the foods that come from them. They may keep LDL cholesterol from oxidizing so that it can't easily attach to artery walls. Genistein may also keep artery walls from thickening and keep platelets from clumping together, reducing the risk of heart disease and stroke.

Researchers at the University of Kentucky reviewed 38 previous studies to show that soy protein lowers LDL cholesterol and triglyceride levels but does not affect levels of the beneficial HDL cholesterol. In some experiments, soy-rich diets have reduced total cholesterol by 10 percent and LDL levels by 13 percent. Cardiologists estimate that a cholesterol reduction of 10 percent lowers risk of death by 30 percent.

Dr. Potter studied the blood cholesterol and bone density of women aged 50 to 70. Findings showed that the women who consumed 40 grams a day of soy protein isolate, the powerful stuff in soy foods, ended up with a drop in LDL and an increase in HDL cholesterol levels.

"We also found that bone density improved in those women taking a soy protein isolate with slightly higher levels of isoflavones," adds Dr. Susan Potter. "Soy consumption may possibly be an alternative to estrogen therapy." Unfortunately, the typical American diet is virtually soyless.

Try these methods to increase your soy consumption:

■ **Try tofu.** It may be bland by itself, but it absorbs the taste of spices and other foods with which it is cooked. This means that you may easily transform the bland into the sublime.

■ **Look for Asian recipes.** For grilling and sautéing, use extra-firm tofu—it won't crumble. Add small cubes of tofu to salads. Under a light dressing or with a topping of nuts or seeds, you won't even know it's there, says Dr. Hasler.

Don't Take Too Much Soy

High levels of phytoestrogens found in soy may increase breast cancer risk. Excessive soy consumption can also interfere with thyroid function. Andrew Weil, M.D., director, Foundation for Integrative Medicine in Tucson, Arizona, says most people can get enough benefits to lower their cholesterol levels and reduce breast cancer risk from moderate soy consumption—one serving a day, providing up to 50 milligrams of isoflavones, is a safe and healthful amount. That's 1/2 cup tofu or cooked soy protein, 1 cup soy milk, or 1 ounce roasted soy nuts.

■ **Experiment with tempeh.** Fermented soy products such as tempeh are available in dense, firm blocks. Researchers theorize that fermented soy products are easier for your body to use. Tempeh, which is firmer than tofu, is perfect for grilling or stir-frying.

■ **Stick to low-fat products.** Buy low-fat (1 percent) tofu, tempeh, and soy milk products. Avoid the high-fat varieties, advises Dr. Hasler.

■ **Drink soy milk.** "I drink soy milk," says Dr. Hasler. "The beany flavor is great on whole-grain cereals or granola." Soy milk comes in many different flavors like vanilla and carob, and you can find it in most grocery stores. Powdered soy protein can also be found as a supplement in health food stores.

■ **Eat a veggie burger.** Some vegetarian hamburger substitutes are made with soy products. Check the label, says Barbara P. Klein, Ph.D., professor of foods and nutrition at the University of Illinois at Urbana–Champaign. Look at the fat content as well: Some veggie burgers contain more than their fair share. If you just can't do without meat, use half meat and half soy substitute in recipes.

■ **Lay off the soy sauce.** It contains very little soy, says Dr. Lachance. It also tends to be loaded with salt, which can raise your blood pressure. Other condiments, such as Bac-Os, contain soy, but in such small amounts that they won't do you any good.

■ **Make a substitution.** When you bake, trade 25 percent of your regular flour for soy flour. You'll get those soy benefits, and most recipes will come out the same, says Mark Messina, Ph.D., a nutritionist and soy expert in Port Townsend, Washington, and author of *The Simple Soybean and Your Health*.

LIGNANS

"This is a new area for research, and we don't know that much about it yet," cautions Dr. Hasler. Lignans appear to protect the body from cancer, heart disease, and stroke. These powerful plant estrogens are most plentiful in flaxseed (also known as linseed), something that you probably don't normally include in your diet. You do get small amounts in cereals and vegetables.

■ **Fighting Cancer**—Lignans seems to prevent breast cancer, at least in the laboratory. In addition to working as phytoestrogens, which means they provide the body with estrogen, lignans are antioxidants, helping to prevent cell damage and stop cancers before they start.

■ **Fighting Heart Disease and Stroke**—As antioxidants, lignans may help prevent damage from dangerous LDL cholesterol, which can lay the groundwork for heart disease.

In a study at the University of Western Ontario, rats ate flax and flaxseed oil (which contain lignans)—and their blood pressures held stable, while blood pressures rose in the rats that got no flax in their diets. In another study, people ate three slices of bread containing flaxseed as well as 15 grams of ground flaxseed a day and saw drops in their LDL cholesterol levels and in the clotting action of their blood.

Here's how you can get lignans into your diet:

■ **Search for flax.** "Some baking companies add small amounts of flax or linseed to give breads and other baked goods a nutty flavor," Dr. Hasler says. "You can get products made with flaxseed in health food stores, too." She suggests that if you want to add flaxseed to your diet, do so very slowly, perhaps sprinkling a little fortified flax (no more than a teaspoon) on your breakfast cereal. Adding flax to your diet too quickly can cause intestinal distress.

CAROTENOIDS

You see evidence of protective carotenoids in the bright red, orange, and yellow pigments of some plants. You'll find them in carrots, tomatoes, sweet potatoes, cantaloupe, winter squash, parsley, green peas, pink grapefruit, Swiss chard, spinach, beet greens, pumpkin, watermelon, broccoli, mangoes, oranges, papaya, and tangerines. They're also in okra, red peppers, leafy green vegetables, and fish liver oil.

■ **Fighting Cancer**—"Study after study shows that diets rich in carotenoids fight disease," says Dr. Lachance. In one study, a high-carotenoid diet helped reduce the risk of lung cancer in nonsmokers. Researchers studied the diets of 1,197 people in Hawaii. Those who ate a variety of fruits and vegetables and consumed high amounts of three carotenoids had less lung cancer. The European Institute of Oncology in Milan looked at rates of oral cancer in Beijing, China, and found that carotenoid consumption reduced risk.

A particularly powerful carotenoid, lycopene, comes in tomatoes and everything made from them, including pizza sauce and ketchup. Lycopene also shows up in watermelon, guava, and pink grapefruit.

In a survey of 3,000 northern Italians, people who ate seven or more servings of raw tomatoes a week ended up with a 50 to 60 percent lower risk for cancers of the mouth, esophagus, stomach, colon, and rectum. Researchers also think that carotenoids reduce the risk of cancers of the cervix and pancreas.

In the laboratory, tomato juice extract has been shown to prevent the formation of cancer-causing compounds. An Israeli study showed that lycopene knocks out human endometrial, breast, and lung cancer cells. It also affects the systems that allow the cells to grow into tumors. Researchers at Harvard Medical School found that people who ate tomatoes, tomato sauce, tomato juice, and pizza had lower rates of prostate cancer.

Beta-carotene is another carotenoid that is a potent disease preventer. You get it in sweet potatoes, carrots, apricots, spinach, collard greens, cooking pumpkins, and cantaloupe.

Your body converts beta-carotene into both vitamin A and retinoic acid, which thwarts precancerous and cancerous cells while it enhances T cells, a key part of your body's immune system. As antioxidants, beta-carotene and lycopene root out the dangerous free radicals that can turn cells cancerous.

Researchers note that beta-carotene seems to help reduce the risk of cancers that affect organ linings, including colon cancer. Researchers think that precancerous colon polyp tissue that contains beta-carotene may be less likely to turn malignant. In a combined Swiss and Italian study,

Travel to an Exotic Aisle

As you work on adjusting your diet for disease prevention, it is likely that you will want to change your shopping habits as well. So grab a grocery cart and be prepared to take a few turns off the beaten path.

Fill 'er up with produce. When you shop at the supermarket, head straight for the fruits and vegetables section and fill up your cart there. That way, says Isabella Lipinska, Ph.D., a nutritional counselor for the Cardiac Rehabilitation Program at St. Elizabeth's Medical Center in Boston, you'll be less likely to head for the more familiar aisles of the store that are filled with less nutritious foods.

Find strength in numbers. Lots of cities have co-op food stores, where members buy food in bulk and split up the distribution chores. Usually, you get top-quality fruits and vegetables at a lower price. If you and your friends organize a combined "buying and cooking" club, you'll reap benefits in taste, health, and finances, notes John Potter, M.D., Ph.D., head of the Cancer Prevention Research Program at the Fred Hutchinson Cancer Research Center in Seattle.

Buy it off the truck. Make your shopping more fun by frequenting farmers' markets, where local produce often has more taste than the prepackaged stuff in the big stores, suggests Dexter Morris, M.D., vice chairman of the Department of Emergency Medicine and a heart researcher at the University of North Carolina at Chapel Hill School of Medicine. With some extra charm in your shopping expedition and a tastier time in the dining room, you'll be more likely to stick to the fruits-and-vegetables habit.

beta-carotene in the diet protected against endometrial cancer.

The carotenoids work together, too. In a study conducted by the University of Hawaii, diets rich in beta-carotene, alpha-carotene, and lutein resulted in lower risks of lung cancer in a study of more than 1,200 people. You get lutein in broccoli, green peas, celery, spinach, kale, collard greens, Swiss chard, mustard greens, red peppers, okra, and romaine lettuce.

■ **Fighting Heart Disease and Stroke—** Researchers agree that the more carotenoids you eat, the lower your risk will be for chronic heart disease. "They work as antioxidants and prevent the formation of LDL cholesterol," says Dr. Morris.

Use these methods to get the biggest boost from carotenoids:

■ **Add a little fat.** "Since most of the carotenoids are fat soluble, eat them with other foods that contain a hint of fat," says Dr. Morris.

■ **Cook them.** Most carotenoids are not damaged by cooking, says Dr. John Potter.

■ **Look for color.** Reds, oranges, and deep greens tell you that carotenoids are present, even in fruits and vegetables where you might not expect them. For instance, red-leaf lettuce has more carotenoids than iceberg lettuce, and you get more carotenoid benefit from pink grapefruit than from white grapefruit. If you're a meat-and-potatoes sort of person, put some yams or sweet potatoes on your plate for an extra carotenoid boost. (Not that there is anything wrong with white potatoes—they are a good source of potassium, an important mineral, says Dr. Lipinska.) If your lunch features a piece

How We Did It: Supermarket Savvy

Manhattanites Claire and Stanley M. were struck by the double whammy of cancer and heart disease several years ago. Claire, then age 68, was diagnosed with breast cancer, while an electrocardiogram revealed that her husband had previously suffered a silent heart attack.

"I realized that we could do more to control our health, especially by adding fiber and decreasing fat to help reduce the risk of heart problems and cancer," says Claire. "So I started to read labels carefully. I stayed away from processed foods, especially ones that contain a lot of chemicals. I spend much more time in the supermarket now because I read the labels. I look for high fiber, low fat, and serving size. For instance, one brand will call three crackers a serving and another will call six a serving. It often makes a big difference when you add up the total in fiber, fat, and calories."

Before label reading became part of her shopping routine, Claire says, "I used to buy foods that contained chemicals and preservatives. Now I'm more careful. We really emphasize fresh fruits and vegetables. We make it a point to get broccoli, apples, and oranges for fiber and other nutrients."

Stanley wasn't as careful about his diet before his heart attack. "We've both come to enjoy the high-fiber, low-fat diet," Claire says. "I never had any problems with constipation, but Stanley really knows the difference when he doesn't take in enough fiber."

The healthy diet has become a habit. "These days, we maybe eat meat twice a month. When we first tried to change our diet, we used to say to each other, 'What is there to eat?' It was just hard to figure out what we could eat. We bought low-fat cookbooks and concocted recipes of our own using a lot of pasta, vegetables, and beans. Now, if we go off our diet, both of us feel guilty."

Claire had just retired from her job as a controller at an advertising agency when her cancer was diagnosed. "One of my best survival tactics centered on making attitude changes. After my illness, I was very tense and anxious. I learned to meditate, using breathing exercises to relax."

Exercise helps, too. "I always walk a lot, mostly because my husband and I like to go to museums, movies, theaters, and concerts. I started doing floor exercises for my back. I must be in better shape now, because when I started, I'd get so exhausted that I'd almost be nauseated. Now I can do them with ease."

Claire does volunteer work with SHARE, an organization that helps women fight breast and ovarian cancers. She has found an important sense of community in helping others. "I lead discussion groups and work on the hotline. It's been very meaningful.

"Facing mortality has made us stronger—more appreciative of the time we have. It has underscored how precious life is, and that you can make changes in your life if you go step by step and do what you can."

of broiled chicken and potatoes, add a slice of red pepper or tomato, she suggests.

■ **Snack on vegetables and crackers.** Raw vegetables plus a high-fiber, low-fat cracker or two give you the most phytochemical benefit, says Dr. Lipinska. The small amount of fat contained in the cracker enables your body to take in the fat-soluble phytochemicals as well as water-soluble ones. Make your snack even more beneficial by choosing a bright orange or green vegetable, which is high in carotenoids.

If Garlic Gives You Heartburn...

According to Dr. Yeh, garlic and other alliums may not agree with everyone's digestive tract. If you get heartburn, try a deodorized garlic, such as aged garlic extract. People who participated in one study consumed the deodorized supplemental equivalent of three cloves a day. They got the benefits, and no one felt the burn.

■ **Concentration helps.** You'll get more carotenoids from some concentrated products, says Dr. Morris. Tomato paste, ounce for ounce, contains twice as many carotenoids as do fresh tomatoes, for instance. Tomato purée contains 20 percent more.

Warning: Carotenoids are more healthful if they come from food rather than supplements. They are fat soluble, which means that your body stores them until they are used. If you take a bit too much, the side effects will be obvious to everyone you see. "You can turn orange. This doesn't happen if you get carotenoids in food, because you'd have to eat an awful lot. But it's easy to take too many supplements," says Dr. Morris.

Another reason you're better off getting your carotenoids from food rather than from a bottle: It's hard to know the quality of supplements and how well your body can use the substances they contain. Besides, researchers haven't yet figured out whether it's the carotenoids themselves that help your body, or whether other substances linked with them in fruits and vegetables are providing the real benefit.

FLAVONOIDS

You're in luck. The valuable flavonoids can be found in just about every plant, from apples to onions to soy. Even black tea and green tea contain flavonoids that help ward off cancer.

■ **Fighting Cancer**—"Flavonoids help dissipate the substances that cause cancer. They prevent—they don't cure," says Dr. Lachance. Studies at Rutgers University have shown that, at least in laboratory mice, green tea blocks the development of cancer tumors by 90 percent. Black tea, says Dr. Lachance, performs only a little less impressively.

Many flavonoids are also powerful antioxidants. Researchers have found that the process used to make green tea leaves activates a key antioxidant, epigallocatechin gallate. In the lab, it prevents tumors of a broad range of cancers.

According to researchers, some flavonoids, such as quercetin in onions and kaempferol in leeks and garlic, fight off the earliest stages of cancer. In a Dutch study involving 58,279 men and 62,573 women aged 55 to 69, scientists found that onion eaters decreased their risk of developing stomach cancer.

■ **Fighting Heart Disease and Stroke**— In a Canadian laboratory study, a flavonoid called purpurogallin protected the heart against the injuries that occur during a heart attack.

Another Dutch study followed 805 men aged 65 to 84 over a 25-year period. Researchers found that those who ate a diet high in flavonoids (mostly from black tea, but also from onions and apples) had a 58 percent drop in risk of dying of a heart attack. The average daily tea consumption? About 3.4 cups.

The Dutch study was part of a larger, seven-country study which revealed that a high-flavonoid diet was the reason for a 25 percent variance in coronary heart disease among all the countries studied. Researchers in Israel discovered that red wine, which is high in flavonoids, lowers LDL cholesterol levels which, when raised, leads to hardening of the arteries. Laboratory research shows that flavonoids can reduce the tendency of blood platelets to stick together and cause clots.

To get the most from flavonoids, try these tips:

▪ **Sip wine.** Researchers are actively scrutinizing "the French paradox," where people who drink wine regularly seem to have lower rates of heart disease even when they dine on a rich cuisine like France's. "We think that the chemicals in wine are potent antioxidants, and they may keep blood from clotting," says Andrew Waterhouse, Ph.D., a researcher in the Department of Viticulture and Enology at the University of California, Davis. The people who benefit, studies show, drink just a little wine on a daily basis.

▪ **Drink tea.** Dr. Lachance says that tea will give you an effective dose of flavonoids—but you have to drink it regularly. "I drink a cup of coffee in the morning and then drink black tea the rest of the day," he says. "I drink around a half-dozen cups. It's safer than coffee, too, because it's not as stimulating." If you are sensitive to caffeine, you might want to try decaffinated black tea, which has the same benefits.

TRITERPENES AND MONOTERPENES

Triterpenes are a group of compounds that include limonoids, found in fruits with vitamin C, especially the seeds, fruit, and juice of citrus plants. Monoterpenes also are found in the skin or peel of citrus fruits. In addition, monoterpenes are present in caraway seeds in the form of D-carvone. Both these phytochemicals can help protect against major diseases.

▪ **Fighting Cancer**—"We're excited about these substances as possible anticancer agents because people consume them at high levels anyway," says Dr. Miller. "We used to think that vitamin C was the protective component in citrus, but studies suggest other agents." For this reason, it's better to eat an orange than to take a vitamin tablet. Epidemiological studies show that citrus consumption is linked to protection against a whole slew of cancers—oral, esophageal, and pancreatic, among others.

In laboratory rats, some of the phytochemicals in citrus reduce the number of tumors by up to 60 percent, but so far this has only been tested at very high dosages that have unwanted side effects. However, citrus does appear to help your body increase the production of enzymes that dispose of cancer-causing substances.

Dr. Miller is studying limonoids, a group of cancer-fighting phytochemicals that fend off oral cancer in animals. Two substances, limonin and limonin 17-beta-D-glucopyranoside, actually block and suppress tumors. In one study, researchers applied orange-peel oil directly to skin tumors and found that the tumors grew much more slowly.

▪ **Fighting Heart Disease and Stroke**—A University of Wisconsin at Madison study shows that monoterpenes can decrease the harmful LDL cholesterol that contributes to heart disease and stroke. You get a lot of other good things from citrus, too (such as vitamin C and fiber).

Here's how to obtain the most benefit from monoterpenes and triterpenes:

▪ **Add fruit to salads.** Combine fruits to make a fruit salad (avoid canned fruits—they lose vitamin C during storage). Buy a variety of fruits and, every day, serve them in different combinations—a slice of plum, apricot, peach, and apple, for example.

■ **Use citrus peel.** Orange or lemon peel, finely grated, can be a flavor enhancer in fruit drinks and carbonated beverages and on salads, vegetables and even meats. The peel is rich in protective d-limonene.

■ **Eat and drink the real thing.** To get limonoids, avoid watered-down citrus drinks or carbonated citrus drinks. Eat the actual fruit or drink the real juice, recommends Dr. Miller.

TANNINS

You might think of tannins as colorful concoctions used in dying, making inks, and tanning leather. One tannin, ellagic acid, is in the foods that stain your clothing—strawberries, raspberries, blackberries, and loganberries. And tannins can make a lasting impression on your body, too, by protecting you from disease.

■ **Fighting Cancer**—Research on tannins (and ellagic acid, in particular) is getting under way in laboratory studies. Researchers believe that ellagic acid may keep cancerous substances from altering the DNA of healthy cells. In the laboratory, it neutralizes cancer-causing substances and helps prevent cancers in tissues of the lung, liver, skin, and esophagus.

■ **Fighting Heart Disease and Stroke**— In the laboratory, ellagic acid works as an antioxidant, preventing oxidation of the fats that turn into LDL cholesterol.

Here's how to get more tannins into your system:

■ **Skip juices in favor of fruits.** For instance, grape juice may be a sweet refreshment, but you're better off eating the grape itself to get all the benefits of the phytochemicals clustered in the grape peel. (You'll also get more fiber from whole fruits.)

■ **Check jam labels.** If your tastes run to jellies and jams, take a close look at the contents listed on the labels. Pick products listing a higher content of real fruit, which is more likely to be the premium jams.

■ **Top off foods with berries.** Find inventive ways to work berries into your daily eating pattern. Sprinkle them over cereals, waffles, pancakes, and desserts like sherbet or a slice of melon.

Prescription for Tapping Into the Power of Plants

When you eat a diet rich in fruits, vegetables, and grains, you stoke up your defenses against heart disease, cancer, and stroke. You may cut your disease risk in half.

DO:

▶ **Eat at least five servings a day of fruits and vegetables.**

▶ **Choose bright orange or dark green vegetables.**

▶ **Add vegetables rich in organosulfur compounds to soups.** Choose garlic, onions, leeks, chives, shallots, broccoli, and cauliflower, for example.

▶ **Enjoy raw vegetables with a few crackers** to get the benefits of both water-soluble and fat-soluble phytochemicals.

▶ **Eat the leaves, seeds, and peel,** where many phytochemicals are concentrated.

▶ **Drink milk made from soybeans and try soy-based vegetarian meat substitutes.**

▶ **Drink tea,** which is rich in phytochemicals, instead of coffee.

DON'T:

▶ **Add more than just a teaspoon of flax** to your cereal.

▶ **Rely on canned fruits,** because they lose valuable nutrients during storage.

4

The Top 100 Foods for Healthy Aging

Good news: You can easily get cheap, good-tasting medicine that helps ward off cancer, heart disease, and stroke without ever going to the pharmacy. These powerful, disease-preventing substances can be found—thankfully—in the everyday, garden-variety foods available in any grocery store.

The secret lies in eating a wide variety of foods containing an assortment of these disease-fighting substances. That way, you create a protective mosaic of vitamins, minerals, and enzymes that help you stay disease free. Your body absorbs these nutrients more safely from food than from supplements. Besides, relying on supplements for nutrients may contribute to an overdose, which is never a problem when you get them from foods. So be sure you eat an extravagant abundance of fruits and vegetables, seafood and lean meats, grains and legumes—with a moderate amount of milk products and a small bit of fat. The five-plus servings of fruits and vegetables recommended by the National Cancer Institute and leading nutritionists are especially important. Most people, unfortunately, forget all about them.

How Can These Foods Work to Keep You Healthy?

To start, you have to eat the recommended number of servings to protect you from disease. But what is the proper size of a serving, you may well ask? The standard serving size for cooked vegetables or chopped raw vegetables is $1/2$ cup, and for raw leafy vegetables the serving size is 1 cup. For fruit a serving is one medium apple, banana, or orange or $1/2$ cup of chopped, cooked, or canned fruit. A serving of cooked cereal, rice, pasta, or cooked dried beans is $1/2$ cup. A serving of seafood or meat is 3 ounces. Eat five to six servings of grains—preferably whole grains—each day, and two servings of beans, seafood, or meat.

The "Daily Value" is another strange term related to the food you eat, and it's mentioned often in this chapter. The term refers to the amount of a given nutrient that scientists figure you need each day. This is based on eating a 2,000-calorie diet. If you eat more calories or less, the Daily Value you need will be higher or lower accordingly.

The following 100 foods stand out as top-notch disease fighters and are easily found in the supermarket:

ALMONDS

Not what you would expect to head up a list of healthy foods—almonds weigh in like sumo wrestlers in the amount of calories and fat they contain. Fortunately, most of the fat is monounsaturated, the kind that may actually reduce high blood pressure and cholesterol levels.

■ **Fighting Cancer**—Almonds deliver copper to power up your immune system, which needs more of a boost as you get older. One serving of almonds (the amount that fits in your hand, about an ounce, or 24 whole kernels) gives you 13.5 percent of the Daily Value for copper. Plus, they provide some fiber (1.9 milligrams per serving) and calcium to help lower your risk of colon cancer.

■ **Fighting Heart Disease and Stroke**— In one study, people eating 3½ ounces of almonds a day reduced cholesterol levels by 20 points. Almonds are a good source of riboflavin, which has been associated with lower heart disease rates. In addition, a handful of almonds is high in magnesium—it provides 21 percent of the Daily Value, which may help prevent blood clots and lower blood pressure.

APPLES

Whole, sliced, juiced, cooked, or sauced, apples deliver protection from disease.

■ **Fighting Cancer**—Take a bite and take in some glutathione (well, it does sound as if you're talking with your mouth full when you try to say it). This tongue twister protects your mouth because it cuts the risk of oral and throat cancer by up to 50 percent compared to the risk for people who don't eat apples. It also makes your immune system work as though it belongs to someone much

younger. The problem is that most people over age 60 have 17 percent lower blood levels of glutathione than people under 40. This antioxidant is available only from raw vegetables and fruits, so eat your apples raw. (You'll have to think of another excuse to eat apple pie.) Raw or cooked apples are a great source of another mouth-saver—vitamin C, which helps guard your mouth against cancer. Apples also provide you with flavonoids, antioxidants that help to halt cancer's start-up process. A medium-size apple, with peel, gives you a little more than 2.5 grams of total fiber, protection against both cancer and heart disease.

■ **Fighting Heart Disease and Stroke**— When researchers in the Netherlands studied 805 men aged 65 to 84, they found that the apple eaters had a 32 percent lower risk of dying from heart disease, in part because of flavonoids concentrated in the apple peel.

Researchers think that the vitamin C in apples also performs such feats as lowering your blood pressure, which could help protect your arteries and heart. Vitamin C also helps prevent oxidation of blood cholesterol and, therefore, slows clogging of the arteries. Apples are high in flavonoids, which have antioxidant properties, and one small apple with skin gives you 1 gram of soluble fiber, which can aid heart health.

APRICOTS

The taste is tart, but the benefits are sweet. This tiny, low-fat, low-cal, zero-cholesterol fruit packs a lot of protection in the form of beta-carotene, dietary fiber, and vitamin C. And remember that apricots in the dried form contain even greater concentrations of their beneficial nutrients.

■ **Fighting Cancer**—Eating a serving of three fresh apricots boosts your body's defenses as a source of more than half of the Daily Value of vitamin A. People who eat a lot of vitamin A/

beta-carotene have lower rates of breast, cervical, and uterine cancer. They may also get protection against cancer of the esophagus, stomach, colon, and mouth. Vitamin A also helps keep invaders out by strengthening the mucous membranes that line the digestive, respiratory, reproductive, and urinary tracts.

The vitamin C helps lower your risk of cancer of many vital organs. More than 1 gram of insoluble fiber is in a ½-cup serving of canned apricots, and there are 5 grams of total fiber in ¼ cup of dried apricots, which helps fend off colon and breast cancer.

■ **Fighting Heart Disease and Stroke—** Proof that good things come in small packages, seven dried apricot halves give you 1.1 grams of soluble fiber to help bring down high cholesterol and high blood pressure.

Apricots provide potassium, which helps to lower high blood pressure. One serving of three fresh apricots is the source for more than half the Daily Value of vitamin A, which may protect you from the harmful low-density lipoprotein (LDL) cholesterol buildup that can lead to hardening of the arteries. Stroke victims in Belgium fared better when their diets included lots of sources of vitamin A.

ARTICHOKES

Perhaps the citizens of ancient Rome were thinking about taste, not disease protection. Regardless, they paid more for artichokes than any other garden vegetable.

■ **Fighting Cancer—** A ½-cup serving of artichoke hearts gives you 4.5 grams of total dietary fiber for protection against colon cancer. Plus, you get 10 percent of the Daily Value of copper to boost your immune system. And 14 percent of the Daily Value of vitamin C helps protect you against a variety of cancers.

■ **Fighting Heart Disease and Stroke—** One medium cooked artichoke gives you 2.2 grams of soluble fiber for heart health. Vitamin C also defends your body against hazardous LDL cholesterol and other fats in the blood by keeping them from latching onto artery walls where they can build up and cause damage.

A serving provides almost 11 percent of your Daily Value for folate (the natural form of the supplement folic acid), which helps prevent homocysteine levels from rising. Elevated homocysteine may increase the risk of heart disease. Researchers estimate that if people took in more folate, between 13,500 and 50,000 deaths from coronary artery disease could be prevented every year. A ½-cup serving of artichoke hearts provides you with more than 12 percent of your Daily Value of magnesium, which may prevent the blood clotting that increases your risk of a heart attack or stroke. It also helps lower blood pressure.

ASPARAGUS

It's a stand-up kind of vegetable. Next time you see a bunch of asparagus upright in a pan of water at the grocery store, think about how these low-cal, cholesterol-free little green spears stand up to disease.

■ **Fighting Cancer—** According to research, asparagus could actually help block tumor development. Obviously, you wouldn't want to go on an all-asparagus diet, but these laboratory findings make it clear that your body will benefit from a regular helping of these great defenders. In the laboratory, compounds in asparagus keep cells from mutating and prevent tumors from forming.

Weighing in with 1.4 grams of insoluble fiber, a single serving of cooked fresh asparagus (about six spears) beefs up your defenses against colon cancer. Asparagus also provides vitamin C to protect you from a variety of cancers and copper to help strengthen your immune system.

Raw asparagus is a very good source of an antioxidant called glutathione, which has been found in animal studies to inhibit tumor growth. Asparagus gives you almost 33 percent of a day's requirement for folate, which keeps cells healthy. Studies show that people who eat a diet rich in folate have lower levels of cancer of the cervix, colon, and rectum, and folate may also help prevent cancer of the esophagus.

■ **Fighting Heart Disease and Stroke**— The ingredient list for asparagus reads like a Who's Who of heart protection: It's a source for nearly 10 percent of your Daily Value of vitamin A/beta-carotene, which helps prevent the buildup of harmful LDL cholesterol in your arteries. At the same time, people with high amounts of beta-carotene have higher levels of the protective high-density lipoprotein (HDL) cholesterol than people with low amounts of beta-carotene.

As you age, it becomes harder for your body to absorb the B vitamins, so you have to take in more than you used to. B vitamins are plentiful in asparagus: Folate and vitamin B_6 protect your heart, partly by lowering levels of the harmful amino acid homocysteine. Homocysteine is associated with high risk of heart attack and stroke. Riboflavin boosts the other B vitamins, and the soluble fiber in asparagus lowers the levels of LDL cholesterol and fats in your blood.

AVOCADOS

Avocados contain a lot of protective nutrients, but they're also high in fat. One avocado supplies you with almost 31 grams of fat. That's a bigger problem now that you're older and trying to slow the buildup of the body fat that increases your risk for heart disease, some cancers, and weight gain. But there's a silver lining: About two-thirds of the fat in avocados is monounsaturated, which may actually help lower cholesterol levels. Plus, you can use mashed avocados or guacamole as a healthy mayonnaise substitute.

■ **Fighting Cancer**—Heading up the protective roster are 5.3 grams of insoluble fiber— a lot of protection from colon cancer. You get as much insoluble fiber from one avocado as you do from 5 tablespoons of toasted wheat germ.

A standard serving, half of an avocado, gives you 14 percent of the Daily Value of vitamin B_6. If you're low on vitamin B_6, your immune system gets sluggish—a condition you can't afford as you get older. But studies show that increasing your intake of vitamin B_6 will reverse that slump. You also get 14 percent of the Daily Value of copper, which will help shift your immune system into high gear. The beta-carotene in avocados helps to disable cancer-causing agents before they strike. Avocados also provide vitamin C to guard against a variety of cancers and glutathione to help strengthen your immune system.

A serving of avocado contains more than 15 percent of the Daily Value of folate. Researchers think that this nutrient protects healthy cells from cancerous invasion. High levels of folate are also linked to low rates of cancer of the cervix, colon, rectum, lung, and possibly of the esophagus. In the laboratory, substances in avocados even keep tumors from getting started.

■ **Fighting Heart Disease and Stroke**— In one study, people who ate ½ to 1½ avocados each day reduced their cholesterol levels from an average of 236 milligrams per deciliter (mg/dL) of blood to 217. Even better, the levels of the beneficial HDL cholesterol, which lowers your risk of heart attack, didn't go down.

Go Light on Meat

Meat tends to be high in calories, fat, and iron—but some cuts fit easily into a healthy diet. Here are the top choices for meat dishes. All give you over half your Daily Value of protein.

Eye round roast. A lean 3-ounce serving (about the size of a deck of cards) has 143 calories, 59 milligrams of cholesterol, and just over 4 grams of fat. Protective nutrients include vitamins B_{12} and B_6, zinc, niacin, potassium, riboflavin, and magnesium.

Top loin steak. One lean 3-ounce serving with fat trimmed contains 168 calories, 65 milligrams of cholesterol, and 7 grams of fat. Protective nutrients include vitamins B_{12} and B_6, zinc, niacin, potassium, riboflavin, and magnesium.

Lamb foreshank. One lean 3-ounce serving of the meat gives you 159 calories, 88 milligrams of cholesterol, and 5 grams of fat. Protective nutrients include vitamin B_{12}, zinc, niacin, riboflavin, magnesium, and potassium.

Pork tenderloin. One lean 3-ounce serving contains 139 calories, 67 milligrams of cholesterol, and 4 grams of fat. Protective nutrients include vitamin B_{12} and B_6, riboflavin, zinc, and magnesium.

Researchers note that certain B vitamins can reduce the risk of heart disease by 10 to 25 percent. Avocados are loaded with B vitamins, including folate and vitamin B_6. Studies show that folate and vitamin B_6 may help keep down homocysteine levels, which lowers the risk of heart disease. Homocysteine tends to accumulate in the blood of people who eat meat, and it can harm artery walls.

Half an avocado gives you more than 9 percent of the Daily Value for magnesium, which also bolsters heart health. Avocados are also rich in soluble fiber, which helps control cholesterol. Plus, avocados contain potassium, which helps lower blood pressure and reduces your risk of stroke.

BANANAS

Voted America's favorite fruit, bananas are almost fat-free. They are easy to digest, except when they are green. At their peak, the skin is yellow flecked with brown spots.

■ **Fighting Cancer**—The B vitamins—one banana has 33 percent of the Daily Value of vitamin B_6—help strengthen your immune system to fight off cancer-causing interlopers. The 1.4 grams of insoluble fiber found in one banana reduces your risk of colon cancer.

Scientists think that a healthy helping of other substances in bananas—vitamin C and the powerful antioxidant glutathione—can help cut your risk of cancer of the mouth and strengthen your immune system. When glutathione was added to the white blood cells of both older and younger people, it increased their infection-fighting ability. The benefit was especially strong in the white blood cells of the older people.

■ **Fighting Heart Disease and Stroke**—In a study of 859 men and women, those who ate just one potassium-rich fruit, such as a banana, every day had a 40 percent lower risk of stroke.

Folate, a B vitamin that protects against cancer, also safeguards your heart by lowering levels of the harmful amino acid homocysteine, a risk factor in heart disease and heart attack. Vitamin C increases beneficial HDL cholesterol while it reduces harmful LDL cholesterol and triglycerides. You get 17 percent of the Daily Value of vitamin C from one banana.

BARLEY

Barley has been a staple of good health from time immemorial, even getting a "thumbs-up" in the Bible, which describes the good land as one of "wheat and barley." With that kind of endorsement, what are you waiting for?

■ **Fighting Cancer**—One serving of barley (1/2 cup cooked) gives you almost 2 grams of insoluble fiber to fight cancer.

■ **Fighting Heart Disease and Stroke**— A 1/2-cup serving of cooked barley gives you 1.2 grams of soluble fiber, which is great news for your heart.

BEANS

The butt of many jokes, beans are superheroes of disease protection. Take your pick: black, garbanzo, cranberry, navy, pink, pinto, kidney, white, or yellow. You can't beat them.

■ **Fighting Cancer**—Research shows that women who eat a diet that is rich in beans have lower rates of breast cancer, thanks to substances in beans that block estrogen. Natural chemicals in green and wax beans, and even in the juice from beans, keep cells from mutating. They also destroy enzymes that give cancer its start.

Beans boost your immune system. One-half cup of canned garbanzo beans (chickpeas), for instance, provides 10 percent of the Daily Value of copper and 8.4 percent of the Daily Value of zinc. You get protection from colon cancer with almost 4 grams of insoluble fiber in 1/2 cup of cooked beans.

■ **Fighting Heart Disease and Stroke**— A high-bean diet cuts the risk of heart disease because it lowers cholesterol levels. Even bean sprouts help your heart. In one study, people with very high cholesterol levels ate 1 1/2 cups of cooked beans daily for three weeks and made no other dietary changes. Their cholesterol levels fell by an average of 60 points.

One-half cup of cooked garbanzo beans gives you 1.3 grams of soluble fiber, the heart-protecting stuff. And 35 percent of the Daily Value of folate further cuts your risk of heart disease and stroke. Plus, you get magnesium and potassium. These nutrients help prevent blood clots and reduce high blood pressure.

BEETS

On the surface, beets don't look all that remarkable. But research reveals that beets are rich in the protective plant compounds known as phytochemicals.

■ **Fighting Cancer**—It's true: Beets have an impressive lineup of vitamins, minerals, and fiber. Just 1/2 cup of canned beets gives you a very beneficial 1.5 grams of insoluble fiber and 6.4 percent of the Daily Value for folate to protect your cells and DNA coding. But that isn't what has been impressing lab researchers. Beets contain at least 11 (and probably more) phytochemicals that fight cancer, including genistein, a substance that keeps estrogen from linking up with cancer cells to start tumor construction.

■ **Fighting Heart Disease and Stroke**— One serving (1/2 cup) gives you more than 0.5 gram of the soluble fiber that helps lower your cholesterol levels and keeps plaque in the arteries from becoming a problem. Plus, you get 6.4 percent of your daily needs of the ever-important folate, lowering your risk of heart disease.

Don't forget the green stalk and leaves that top the beet itself. One-half cup of the cooked greens (especially when they're young) will give you 2.2 milligrams of beta-carotene, 2 grams of dietary fiber plus some calcium to lower blood pressure and cholesterol levels, magnesium to ease heart arrhythmia, and vitamin C to prevent oxidation of blood cholesterol. What's more, that same serving of beet greens provides 9 percent of the Daily Value of copper—a boon to your immune system.

BLACKBERRIES AND BLUEBERRIES

Black or blue, you can't go wrong. Ever notice that when blueberries are exposed to acid (in lemon juice or yogurt, for example), they turn red? Exposed to baking soda, they turn a little green. But fear not—the change in color won't affect the protection they give you.

■ **Fighting Cancer**—Blackberries pack more fiber than any other summer fruit (3.6 grams in 1/2 cup). Blueberries and blackberries both contain important cancer fighters, including the phytochemicals catechins, flavonoids, and phenolic acids. Blackberries also contain ellagic acid, which neutralizes three different cancer-causing agents. Blackberries are high in vitamin C, which helps reduce your risk of cancers of the breast, cervix, esophagus, lung, mouth, pancreas, rectum, and stomach.

■ **Fighting Heart Disease and Stroke**— One-half cup of blackberries provides more than 25 percent of the Daily Value of vitamin C. (Blueberries contain slightly less.) The vitamin C in these berries helps keep your HDL cholesterol levels high, which lowers the risk of your arteries becoming blocked by plaque.

BREADS AND CEREALS

The name of the game is whole grain. Get out your reading glasses and check the fine print on packages. Look for the words "whole wheat" as the first ingredient on your bread wrapper— that means the bread contains whole-wheat flour. Other good ingredients to look for are things like oat bran, soy flour, seeds, nuts, or whole grain flour.

About 22 nutrients in breads and cereals are diminished because of processing. And manufacturers only put a few nutrients back in. For example, enriched flour has had niacin, iron, thiamin, and riboflavin added to it. But the best way to get the full value of breads and grains is to shop for whole-grain products.

■ **Fighting Cancer**—Consuming breads and cereals made from whole grains may help lower the risk of colon cancer. Insoluble fiber speeds up the time it takes food to travel through the intestinal tract, so potential cancer-causing substances may be moved out of the body more quickly. It could also be that insoluble fiber lowers colon cancer risk because the fermentation of the fibers in the colon lowers the pH levels. Lower pH in the colon has been associated with lower colon cancer risk. Two studies have found that something in oats keeps cells from mutating, although the compounds that provide the protection have not yet been identified.

■ **Fighting Heart Disease and Stroke**— One slice of whole-wheat bread contains about 2 grams of dietary fiber. Fiber lowers cholesterol levels partly because it slows the absorption of cholesterol. Oats, rye, and barley are good sources of soluble fiber.

While there's little calcium in breads, yeast makes it easy for your body to take full advantage of what's there, according to a study at Creighton University in Omaha, Nebraska. And some bread and cereal products are fortified with vitamins and minerals for added protection against disease. Look for cereals fortified with folic acid, the supplemental form of folate, as well.

BROCCOLI

This is the workhorse of the food world. A serving (¹/₂ cup) of chopped raw broccoli contains only 12 calories and just a tiny bit of fat. Cooking destroys a few nutrients, but broccoli is worth its weight in gold in just about any form.

■ **Fighting Cancer**—One serving (¹/₂ cup) of cooked broccoli provides you with 97 percent of the Daily Value of vitamin C, which is a very effective fighter against cancer of the breast, cervix, esophagus, lung, mouth, pancreas, rectum, and stomach.

You also get a sizable portion of folate, which helps keep your cells healthy and able to fight off cancerous agents. Researchers have found that folate plays an important role in cell division. It also helps keep the genetic coding in DNA intact. People whose diets are rich in folate have lower rates of cervical, colon, rectal, lung, and possibly esophageal cancer.

Cancer-fighting substances in broccoli also include such tongue twisters as flavonoids, isothiocyanates, sulphoraphane, indoles, carotenoids, dithiolthiones, glutathione (in uncooked broccoli), monoterpenes, plant sterols, phenolic acids, glucobrassicin. In fact, researchers have catalogued more than 30 substances in broccoli that seem to have cancer-fighting abilities—and they're not done yet.

■ **Fighting Heart Disease and Stroke**— A lot of the cancer-fighting substances also help your heart. Vitamin C can prevent the LDL particles in blood from becoming oxidized, which helps lessen the risks of heart disease. A 13-year study of men with high cholesterol levels revealed that the higher their carotenoid levels were, the lower their risk for heart disease and strokes. The carotenoids shoot down harmful LDL cholesterol, while the flavonoids lower the risk of heart disease and heart attack.

Cooked broccoli gives you 1.2 grams of heart-saving soluble fiber, which lowers LDL cholesterol levels and helps control blood sugar.

Broccoli provides a high amount of vitamin A, which may help decrease your risk of heart disease. Unlike some foods, broccoli contributes calcium that your body can use easily, which is important because calcium helps to reduce mild high blood pressure and lower harmful LDL cholesterol. The higher your LDL levels, the bigger your risk of heart disease.

BRUSSELS SPROUTS

A close relative of broccoli, brussels sprouts deliver many of the same low-fat, low-cal benefits.

■ **Fighting Cancer**—A serving (about four sprouts) gives you 3 grams of insoluble fiber for protection from colon cancer.

You also end up with an array of natural chemical protectors with long, complicated names. Indoles destroy the estrogen that helps breast cancer get started. They also help activate your body's protective forces. Isothiocyanates help eliminate or neutralize cancer-causing agents. Flavonoids inhibit the hormones that help cancer grow. Sulforaphane bolsters the body's natural defenses. Carotenoids work as antioxidants to stop damage to healthy cells.

Eat a serving of fresh, cooked brussels sprouts and get 80 percent of the Daily Value of vitamin C. More than 30 studies have shown that if you eat foods rich in vitamin C, you cut your risk of cancer. Brussels sprouts are also a good source of vitamin A and folate. And vitamin B₆ helps maintain your immune system.

■ **Fighting Heart Disease**—Heading the list of protective compounds are the 1.4 grams of soluble fiber that you get in ¹/₂ cup, helping to reduce cholesterol in your blood. You also get a good amount of folate, which lowers your levels of homocysteine, an amino acid in the blood that seems to add to the buildup of harmful cholesterol in your arteries.

Vitamin C also reduces the artery-clogging LDL cholesterol while keeping levels of the protective HDL cholesterol high. Vitamin A weighs in to protect your heart. Several studies show that even some people with heart disease may be able to cut their risks when they add foods that are good sources of vitamin A to their diets.

CABBAGE

In Lewis Carroll's Through the Looking Glass, *a talking walrus speculates about cabbages and kings. It might have sounded like nonsense to put the two together, but the walrus had a point. Cabbage is a king of disease protection.*

Any way you slice it, coleslaw it, steam it, boil it, or soup it, cabbage is a powerful disease-fighting food. And savoy cabbage, the crinkly kind, is the leader of this protective pack.

■ **Fighting Cancer**—Researchers at the Strang-Cornell Cancer Research Lab in New York City found that women who eat lots of cabbage and other cruciferous vegetables (broccoli, brussels sprouts, and cauliflower) have lower levels of a type of estrogen that stimulates breast cancer. Estrogen levels declined just five days after the women started eating more cruciferous vegetables, and the levels stayed down for the three months of the study. Those women who ate the equivalent of 1/3 of a head of cabbage daily got the most benefit. Researchers attribute the drop to a particular substance in this family of vegetables, indole-3-carbinol.

The list of heavy-duty cancer fighters in cabbage also includes flavonoids, other indoles, monoterpenes, phenolic acids, plant sterols, and sulforaphane. Each of these hard-to-pronounce natural chemicals helps to stop cancer at every

stage of development. Some keep cancerous agents from getting the slightest toehold in cells. Others keep healthy cells from mutating, block tumor development, or cut off the blood supply to tumors. Raw, cruciferous vegetables such as cabbage also contain glutathione, which helps counter cellular destruction by free radicals.

■ **Fighting Heart Disease and Stroke**—One cup of shredded raw cabbage gives you 37.6 percent of the vitamin C that you need each day, increasing your protective HDL cholesterol and lowering hazardous LDL cholesterol levels. That cup of shredded raw cabbage also provides some folate, which helps decrease your risk of heart disease.

CANTALOUPE

One of the food world's Southern belles, cantaloupe tastes sweet, but it gets tough in your system. There is a mouthful of protection from disease in every bite.

■ **Fighting Cancer**—You get a healthy 1.5 milligrams of beta-carotene from 1/2 cup of cubed cantaloupe or about 2.5 milligrams from 1/4 of the melon. Plus, that 1/2 cup gives you a little over 50 percent of the Daily Value of two nutritional heavy hitters against cancer: vitamin A and vitamin C.

Cantaloupe's folate content weighs in for the fight against cancers of the cervix, colon, rectum, lung, and possibly the esophagus. It also helps keep cells healthy and prevents DNA from getting damaged and passing on mutations to new cells. Glutathione may cut your risk of oral cancer, and it helps your immune system work as well as it did when you were a whole lot younger.

■ **Fighting Heart Disease and Stroke**—Beta-carotene may help clear your arteries of the harmful LDL cholesterol that can clog up the works and increase your risk of heart disease and stroke. In one major study, people whose diets included high levels of beta-carotene had half the number of fatal heart attacks and strokes as those subjects whose levels were low.

The potassium in cantaloupes helps lower your blood pressure. Cantaloupe provides more than 56 percent of the Daily Value of vitamin C, which increases the good cholesterol, drops the bad, and helps lower your risk of developing arterial plaque.

CARROTS

In the 1800s, an art critic predicted a revolution in painting, all because of the way artist Paul Cézanne painted some simple little carrots. The result? Modern art. Now carrots may be at the center of another revolution—the discovery of important disease fighters.

■ **Fighting Cancer**—Their orange color highlights carrots' protective compounds. Bright oranges, yellows, reds, and greens in fruits and vegetables signal the presence of carotenoids, a powerful class of cancer-fighting substances. A single raw carrot gives you more than 12 milligrams of beta-carotene, which in turn provides 405 percent of the Daily Value of vitamin A. Scientists note that beta-carotene may actually reverse cancers of the cervix and uterus. And it protects against cancer of the lung, breast, cervix, esophagus, stomach, colon, and mouth. Vitamin A is also an essential component of the mucous membranes that line the digestive, respiratory, urinary, and reproductive tracts, your body's first lines of defense against many invaders.

Researchers at Johns Hopkins University in Baltimore discovered that people who have little beta-carotene in their blood have four times the risk of developing lung cancer. The Harvard Nurses' Study found that women who eat less than one serving a day of foods that are

rich in beta-carotene have a 20 percent higher risk of breast cancer.

Carrots contain other beneficial substances, including limonene, to protect against cancer of the mouth. In studies, this substance has actually reduced the size of tumors. So far, more than 50 cancer-fighting compounds have been isolated in Bugs Bunny's favorite food.

■ **Fighting Heart Disease and Stroke**— Beta-carotene and its chemical cousin vitamin A do wonders for your heart. Studies show that people who get a lot of this nutrient suffer fewer heart attacks. One theory is that the beta-carotene may keep dangerous LDL cholesterol from attaching to artery walls. In the Physicians Health Study, men who took in high levels of beta-carotene had half as many strokes and fatal heart attacks as those who didn't. One-half cup of cooked carrots also gives you 1.1 grams of soluble fiber, which lowers blood cholesterol levels.

Carrots carry vitamin B_6 for possible heart protection and some copper to help maintain heart structure. One raw carrot gives you 11 percent of the Daily Value for vitamin C.

CAULIFLOWER

The plain Jane of the vegetable world, cauliflower looks and tastes somewhat colorless. But that plain-Jane exterior is just a front—the substances in cauliflower go a long way toward protecting you from disease.

■ **Fighting Cancer**—In the cruciform vegetable family, which claims cauliflower as a member, researchers have identified substances that are powerful cancer fighters. Some of these substances help the body counteract dangerous mutations in DNA. Others make it hard for cancer-causing agents to zero in on healthy cells. And they cut off supplies to tumors. Raw cauliflower is also a good source of glutathione, an antioxidant, which in the lab has increased the ability of protective white blood cells to divide.

You also get the usual front runners for cancer prevention: insoluble fiber, folate, and vitamin C. A cup serving of raw cauliflower has 2 grams of insoluble fiber, and $\frac{1}{2}$ cup of cooked cauliflower has almost 1 gram. There's some vitamin B_6 in a serving of raw cauliflower as well. It keeps your immune system strong.

■ **Fighting Heart Disease and Stroke—** Here's a good pair of protectors: Vitamin B_6, (which helps lower your risk of heart attack and stroke) and folate, an important B vitamin (which helps reduce your levels of homocysteine, one of the amino acids linked to plaque buildup in the arteries that leads to heart attack and stroke).

One-half cup of cooked cauliflower has nearly 0.5 gram of soluble fiber, which lowers LDL cholesterol levels and heart attack risk. It also provides about 40 percent of the Daily Value of vitamin C, which helps increase levels of the good HDL cholesterol while it shoots down the bad LDL kind.

CELERY

A dieter's delight, a serving of disease-fighting celery (three stalks or 1 cup diced) gives you only 19 calories, less than 0.1 gram of fat, and no cholesterol.

■ **Fighting Cancer—** Studies have shown that compounds in celery actually neutralize toxic substances and prevent tumors from developing. There's a group of chemicals called the phthalides that may protect you from stomach cancer. When researchers in Minneapolis looked closely at one form of the chemical, called 3-n-butyl phthalide, they found that it (along with another substance in celery, called sedanolide) interferes with the development of cancer tumors and helps activate an enzyme that detoxifies harmful substances in the body's tissues.

You get additional protection from cancer thanks to celery's insoluble fiber, folate, vitamin C, and vitamin B_6 content.

■ **Fighting Heart Disease and Stroke—** Butyl phthalide in celery may lower blood pressure by helping to relax the muscles that line the blood vessels. In the laboratory, the chemical seems to reduce stress hormones that cause blood vessels to constrict and blood pressure to rise. The vitamin C in celery also helps raise beneficial HDL cholesterol levels, lowering your risk of heart disease and stroke.

CHERRIES

"Life is just a bowl of cherries," goes the song first belted out by Ethel Merman in 1931. Eat them and you'll sing a song of disease protection.

■ **Fighting Cancer—** A 1-cup serving of sour cherries gives you almost 1 milligram of protective beta-carotene and is a source of 26 percent of the Daily Value for vitamin A, which may combat cancer-causing substances and disable them before they can invade your body's cells. Scientists discovered that a diet high in foods containing beta-carotene helps to reduce the risk of lung cancer in both smokers and nonsmokers.

One-half cup of canned red sour cherries gives you almost 1 gram of protective insoluble fiber. There is some vitamin C in canned sweet cherries. It protects you from cancer of the breast, cervix, esophagus, lung, mouth, pancreas, rectum, and stomach. There is also some cancer-fighting beta-carotene in cherries; the sour ones contain more beta-carotene than the sweet ones, and they're lower in calories, too.

■ **Fighting Heart Disease and Stroke—** Vitamin C in cherries also helps raise your beneficial HDL cholesterol levels and lower your risk of heart disease and stroke. At the same time, it cuts the amount of harmful LDL cholesterol and the triglycerides that leave you vulnerable to plaque buildup in your arteries. The potassium in cherries helps keep your blood pressure under control.

CHESTNUTS

You probably remember a song about chestnuts, open fires, and holidays. Mel Torme penned the lyrics in 1946. As a disease fighter, chestnuts can help you enjoy many holidays to come.

■ **Fighting Cancer**—Just eight chestnuts give you 9 grams of dietary fiber for protection against colon cancer and only 1.5 grams of fat. Additionally, chestnuts contain copper to protect your immune system and vitamin C to help lower your risk of cancer of the breast, cervix, esophagus, lung, mouth, pancreas, rectum, and stomach.

■ **Fighting Heart Disease and Stroke**—Heart helpers in chestnuts include potassium, magnesium, vitamin C, and the beneficial B vitamins: folate, riboflavin, and vitamin B_6. You end up with lower blood pressure, decreased risk of developing a clot that could lead to a heart attack or stroke, less harmful LDL cholesterol, and more protective HDL cholesterol.

CHICKEN BREAST

It's a deal you shouldn't pass up: The breast part of the chicken (without the skin) gives you only half the fat that you would get from a similar portion of well-trimmed, choice-grade T-bone steak, and it helps you fight disease.

■ **Fighting Cancer**—Your immune system gets a boost, thanks to zinc and vitamin B_6. Chicken breasts are also rich in niacin, which some scientists think may help prevent cancer.

■ **Fighting Heart Disease and Stroke**—Half a breast gives you a lot of vitamin B_6, which, when combined with folate, can drop your risk of heart disease by 10 to 25 percent, doctors say.

You also get smaller amounts of other B vitamins, such as riboflavin. Chicken meat provides potassium and magnesium, which help to lower high blood pressure.

CHICORIES

On your next visit to the vegetable aisle of your supermarket, keep an eye peeled for the various chicory greens—Belgian endive, curly endive, escarole, and raddichio. They're all good protectors against disease.

■ **Fighting Cancer**—You get 72 percent of the Daily Value of vitamin C in 1 cup of raw chicories, decreasing your risk of a variety of cancers. Almost half of the Daily Value of folate is found in chicories, which helps protect you against cancer of the cervix, colon, rectum, lung, and possibly the esophagus. Folate also helps keep cells healthy, making it harder for cancerous invaders to attack. Plus, the calcium in chicories seems to provide protection from colon cancer.

■ **Fighting Heart Disease and Stroke**—Chicories are a hotbed of heart protection. A rich supply of vitamin C means that your levels of good HDL cholesterol get a boost while you beat down levels of the harmful LDLs and blood fats. Chicories also give you 18 percent of the Daily Value of calcium, which may help lower blood pressure and LDL cholesterol levels. Potassium in chicories also helps lower blood pressure.

CHINESE CABBAGE AND BOK CHOY

They come from different groups within the cabbage family, but both protect you from diseases that kill.

■ **Fighting Cancer**—Researchers note that people in Asia have lower rates of some forms of cancer. They theorize that compounds such as indole-3-carbinol in Asian cabbages change the body's estrogen metabolism and stop the growth of small virus-caused tumors.

These cabbages provide fiber as well: A 1-cup serving of shredded raw bok choy contains 0.7 gram. It also gives you the important B vitamin folate, which may protect against cancer of the cervix, colon, rectum, lung, and possibly the esophagus. You also need folate to keep your cells healthy.

One-half cup of cooked bok choy is a source for more than 42 percent of the Daily Value of vitamin A, which strengthens your body's defenses against cancer. The almost 8 percent of the Daily Value of calcium in a $^{1}/_{2}$ cup of bok choy helps lower your risk of colon cancer. Your body absorbs calcium from bok choy a bit more easily than it does from milk.

■ **Fighting Heart Disease and Stroke—** You get potassium to help lower your blood pressure. The vitamin A content decreases your risk of stroke—one theory is that it keeps LDL cholesterol from getting a grip on artery walls. Plus, in $^{1}/_{2}$ cup of boiled bok choy, you get 37 percent of the Daily Value of vitamin C to further reduce LDL and harmful fat levels in the blood and increase beneficial HDL cholesterol.

CLAMS

Remember when people used to call money "clams"? Well, for disease-preventing benefits, real clams are worth a lot—especially since, when canned, they're less expensive than a lot of other seafoods. But don't go overboard: One 3-ounce serving of canned clams gives you 23 milligrams of iron or 264 percent of your requirements for iron. Men and postmenopausal women should aim for an average of 9 milligrams or less of iron a day. Your body stores more iron as you age, so you don't want to risk too big a buildup, which can be a potentially serious problem.

■ **Fighting Cancer—** One serving gives you 29 percent of your Daily Value of copper and almost 16 percent of your Daily Value of zinc to help strengthen your immune system. You'll also get more than 31 percent of your Daily Value of vitamin C, which helps reduce your risk of cancer of the breast, cervix, esophagus, lung, mouth, pancreas, rectum, and stomach. And the calcium in clams can cut your risk of colon cancer.

■ **Fighting Heart Disease—** You get bigtime heart protection from the B vitamins. One serving of clams gives you more than 1,400 percent of your Daily Value of vitamin B_{12}, plus some folate. Researchers theorize that these B vitamins can lower your risk of heart disease by 10 to 25 percent. They also help reduce levels of homocysteine, an amino acid that is linked to high risk of heart disease.

Researchers say that clams and some other seafoods are high in omega-3 fatty acids, which may protect the heart. Omega-3's seem to lower the body's production of triglycerides—fats in the blood that are harmful in excess amounts. Plus, omega-3's help get triglycerides out of the bloodstream. Scientists have linked low levels of triglycerides to high levels of HDL cholesterol. It's a one–two punch that may help protect you from heart disease.

COLLARDS

A member of the cabbage family, and closely related to kale, collards give you disease-fighting benefits along with a mild taste.

■ **Fighting Cancer—** Indoles, isothiocyanates, sulforaphane, and quercetin—that's not the name of some blue-chip law firm. It's a lineup of cancer-preventing substances that get into your system when you take a bite of collards.

You also build up your body's first line of defense with vitamin A, which helps strengthen the membranes that line your body's vital organs and helps keep cancerous invaders at bay. A serving of collards provides a decent amount of the antioxidant vitamin E, which protects red blood cells and cells of the lungs. A deficiency of vitamin E may cause the initiation of some cancers.

Several studies show that the consumption of high levels of vitamin E decreases levels of prostaglandin E_2, a substance that limits the efficiency of the immune system. Although these studies used supplements, food sources of vitamin E like collards work, too.

■ **Fighting Heart Disease**—One serving of collards ($\frac{1}{2}$ cup frozen, chopped, or cooked) provides more than 3 grams of beta-carotene, which your body can convert into 101 percent of the Daily Value of vitamin A. These important nutrients may help keep your arteries from getting clogged up with dangerous cholesterol. It also contains more than 37 percent of the Daily Value of vitamin C, which helps increase the protective HDL cholesterol while it lowers the harmful LDLs that can clog your arteries. Collards are also a source of vitamin E. A lack of vitamin E has been associated with the early stages of heart disease.

CORN

In Mitchell, South Dakota, people know how to show some appreciation for corn. Each year, the outside of the Corn Palace in Mitchell is covered in patterns, colors, and designs, all made from ears of corn. It's a big building. More than 3,000 bushels of corn are used for the project. And why not? In terms of disease protection, corn deserves a palace.

■ **Fighting Cancer**—Scientists have identified certain substances in corn that fight off cell mutations, the first step in cancer production. Corn protects in other ways, too. One ear gives you almost 9 percent of the folate that helps your cells stay healthy. High folate levels are also linked to lower rates of cancer of the cervix,

colon, rectum, lung, and possibly the esophagus. Vitamin C cuts your risk of cancer of the breast, cervix, esophagus, lung, mouth, pancreas, rectum, and stomach. Almost 2 grams of insoluble fiber protect against colon cancer.

■ **Fighting Heart Disease and Stroke**— Potassium in corn helps lower high blood pressure. You get a helping of the heart-protecting B vitamins and more than 14 percent of the Daily Value of vitamin C to help keep HDL cholesterol levels high and harmful LDLs on the low side. In addition, vitamin C works to prevent the buildup of plaque in your arteries.

CRANBERRIES

You may think of cranberries only at Thanksgiving, but—fresh or dried, in pies or breads, as sauces or juices, on salads or cereals—cranberries do more than give a tang to your taste buds. They can provide you with year-round disease protection.

■ **Fighting Cancer**—It's time for a reprise of the song about disease prevention due to ellagic acid, a polyphenol. In the lab, this substance fights cancer of the lung, skin, esophagus, and liver. It decreases the number of tumors and even keeps cancers from forming. Among fruits and nuts tested for ellagic acid content, cranberries rank high. Such polyphenols work as antioxidants to fight cancer-causing agents and may even counteract some of the effects of aging.

Cranberries also belt out 1.2 grams of insoluble fiber per $\frac{1}{2}$ cup of chopped raw berries, which protects against colon and breast cancer.

■ **Fighting Heart Disease and Stroke**— A serving contains more than 0.5 gram of soluble fiber, which helps keep blood pressure down. Plus, it has 12 percent of your Daily Value of vitamin C, which clears your arteries of the nasty fats and cholesterol that clog things up and lead to heart attacks and strokes. Also, the same polyphenols that protect you from cancer may help stave off heart disease, too.

CUCUMBERS

Cool as a cucumber, so the saying goes. But cucumbers are definitely hot stuff when it comes to disease prevention.

■ **Fighting Cancer**—Chlorogenic acid—this tongue twister may be the substance in cucumbers that makes them a powerful weapon against cell mutation. Cucumbers contain other important chemicals that protect you from cancer—coumarins, phenolic acids, monoterpenes, and triterpenes.

About a third of a cucumber (an average serving) gives you close to 9 percent of the Daily Value of vitamin C to help protect against cancer of the breast, cervix, esophagus, lung, mouth, pancreas, rectum, and stomach.

■ **Fighting Heart Disease and Stroke**—The boost from vitamin C also helps keep your levels of protective HDL cholesterol high.

CURRANTS

Run against the current of disease with currants. (We're talking about the berries here, not dried currants, which are really a type of raisin that is made from the Black Corinth grape.)

■ **Fighting Cancer**—One-half cup of raw red currants gives you more vitamin C than 1/2 cup of blackberries, or about as much as in a tangerine, to help lower your risk of cancer of the breast, cervix, esophagus, lung, mouth, pancreas, rectum, and stomach. Add to that more than 1.5 grams of insoluble fiber to guard against colon and breast cancer. Studies in Germany found that currants can prevent genetic damage to cells. There is evidence that the vitamin E in currants gives a boost to the immune system.

■ **Fighting Heart Disease and Stroke**—You get heart protection, thanks to almost 0.5 gram of soluble fiber per serving, which helps to lower your cholesterol. One cup of fresh black currants provides you with 11 percent of the Daily Value for vitamin E. There is evidence that this nutrient fights heart disease.

FIGS

The fig leaf provided Adam and Eve with coverage of one kind. And figs can also keep you covered against disease, while fitting into most diets. Two fresh, medium-size figs contain only 74 calories and less than 0.5 gram of fat.

■ **Fighting Cancer**—Two sweet medium figs give you almost 1.5 grams of insoluble fiber to protect you from colon and breast cancer. (A serving of five dried figs has almost 4 grams of insoluble fiber.) Those five dried figs supply you with 15 percent of the Daily Value for copper to help your immune system fend off invaders. The calcium in figs helps protect against colon cancer.

■ **Fighting Heart Disease and Stroke**—You get a lot of cholesterol-lowering soluble fiber from two fresh figs (1.7 grams). Plus, the potassium in figs helps lower your blood pressure.

A serving of five dried figs gives you over 3.5 grams of soluble fiber as well as more than 13 percent of the Daily Value for calcium, and 11 percent of the Daily Value of the heart-saving vitamin B_6.

FLOUNDER AND FAMILY

From a health standpoint, you just can't go wrong with flounder and its popular relatives—sole, turbot, and fluke. Beyond providing nutrients that protect you from disease, they're also low in fat. One average serving of 3 ounces weighs in with 1.3 grams of fat and 100 calories.

■ **Fighting Cancer**—These flat-bodied, bottom-feeding fish are full of disease prevention. One 3-ounce serving (the size of a deck of cards) gives you vitamin B_6 to help keep your immune system working effectively.

■ **Fighting Heart Disease and Stroke**—Flounder have a good amount of omega-3 fatty acids, which may help to decrease your risk of heart attack by lowering triglyceride levels. You get the heart-protecting B vitamins, namely vitamin B_6 and B_{12}. These nutrients reduce your risk of heart disease by up to 25 percent. Add to that magnesium, which helps to prevent the blood clots that can cause heart attacks or strokes. Magnesium also brings down blood pressure levels.

GARLIC

In World War II, Russian soldiers used garlic as an antiseptic. Not the sort of information that you'd care to share over dinner, but it should give you an inkling of how garlic powers up more than your breath.

■ **Fighting Cancer**—In lab animals, garlic reduces tumor growth by 60 percent. Researchers note that it even keeps cells from mutating. Antioxidants in garlic help keep harmful substances in the body from damaging healthy cells. The anti-tumor-promoting activity in garlic may be due to ajoene, quercetin, or other phytochemicals in the bulb. In the lab, researchers at Penn State University showed that a compound in garlic, DATS, slowed the growth of lung cancer cells. Aged garlic extract inhibited the growth of human breast cancer cells in the test tube.

■ **Fighting Heart Disease and Stroke**—Study after study has shown that people who eat $1/2$ to one clove of garlic a day see their cholesterol levels drop by an average of 9 percent. And when scientists studied the results of eight previous garlic tests, they found that in half the

tests, the people who ate garlic regularly experienced a significant reduction in their blood pressure readings.

A study at Tulane University Medical Center in New Orleans found that people who took a special garlic tablet experienced a 6 percent drop in their total cholesterol levels compared with those who did not take the tablet.

GRAPEFRUIT

It wasn't given the scientific name Citrus paradisi *for nothing. Grapefruit is certainly a fruit of paradise in terms of disease protection.*

■ **Fighting Cancer**—Lycopene, carotenoids, limonene, flavonoids, glutathione, terpenes. Sounds like the mutterings of a mad scientist, right? But these natural chemicals all show cancer-preventing promise, and you get a healthy dose of them in ruby red grapefruit. This is especially good since your lycopene levels decrease as you age.

All grapefruit contain terpenes, substances that encourage enzymes in your system to block carcinogens. Grapefruit of every color are also rich in vitamin C to protect you from cancer of the breast, cervix, esophagus, lung, mouth, pancreas, rectum, and stomach. Half of a white grapefruit gives you nearly 69 percent of the Daily Value of this important nutrient (you get about 13 percent more from red). You'll get extra fiber if you eat your grapefruit like an orange, consuming the membrane that encases each segment along with the pulp. You get 1.3 grams of insoluble fiber from half a pink grapefruit with the membrane to help fight colon and breast cancer. But if you spoon out the grapefruit without eating the membrane, you'll still get 0.5 gram of insoluble fiber.

■ **Fighting Heart Disease and Stroke**—The flavonoid naringin found in half a grapefruit may help prevent excessive clumping of red blood cells in your arteries. That same serving size of any grapefruit equips you with just over a gram of the soluble fiber to help lower your cholesterol. It also contains some potassium, which protects you from another hazard to your heart by reducing high blood pressure. Vitamin C helps lower the harmful LDL cholesterol levels to keep arteries clear of the plaque that can pave the way for heart attacks and strokes. It also helps keep levels of protective HDL cholesterol high.

GRAPES

Dionysus, the Greek god of wine, supposedly sailed in a ship outfitted with grape vines flowing from the mast. The gods of antiquity really didn't need disease protection, but you do. And the grape can provide it.

■ **Fighting Cancer**—Grapes are a good source of flavonoids, substances that scientists theorize may fight cancer. Plus, there's vitamin C to further cut your risk. Vitamin C seems to lessen your chances of developing certain cancers, including those of the cervix, breast, lung, mouth, pancreas, rectum, and stomach.

■ **Fighting Heart Disease and Stroke**—Flavonoids in grapes help protect you from heart disease. In a study of 805 men ages 65 to 84, researchers found that those whose diets were highest in flavonoids had a 32 percent lower risk of dying of heart disease than those who ate lower amounts. Researchers believe that flavonoids keep blood platelets from clumping together and forming a clot.

One-half cup of grapes (that's about 16 grapes) gives you enough vitamin C to raise the levels of good cholesterol, lower the bad, and keep your arteries clear. You also get more than 0.5 gram of heart-protecting soluble fiber, which helps lower cholesterol.

GREEN BEANS

They're just immature beans, still in the pod (or just out of it). Left in the garden, they would eventually grow up to be Great Northern, kidney, or pinto beans, depending on the variety. But while they are still immature, they're richer in beta-carotene and vitamin C than dried mature beans.

■ **Fighting Cancer**—Researchers have found that juice from beans keeps cells from mutating. They contain beta-carotene, which becomes vitamin A in our bodies and works as an antioxidant, fighting cancer-causing substances that your body produces or those that come from pollutants like car exhaust and tobacco smoke. In one study of lung cancer in nonsmokers, high intakes of the carotenes in green vegetables and fruits, which include beta-carotene, seemed to help protect against lung cancer. Vitamin A helps disable hazardous substances that can cause cancer—before those substances go to work in your body. A ½-cup serving of beans also gives you 1 gram of insoluble fiber to help prevent colon cancer.

■ **Fighting Heart Disease and Stroke**—The vitamin A in green beans does double duty. Not only does it help protect you against cancer, but it also helps lower your risk of heart attack and stroke. Beta-carotene, which gets converted into vitamin A, works as an antioxidant that may help keep the harmful LDL cholesterol from forming. This is the stuff that forms plaque buildup on artery walls and can pave the way for heart attacks and strokes.

GUAVAS

These tropical-fruit disease fighters are available in varying quantities, almost all year, especially during the late fall and early winter.

■ **Fighting Cancer**—Guavas look like big limes with smooth skin, but they contain six times more vitamin C. In one fruit, you get more than

How to Be a Crack Snacker

Remember: The terms *snack* and *junk food* are not at all the same. Here's how to satisfy your munchies and get disease prevention at the same time:

Plant the seeds for disease prevention. Seeds don't seem like healthy foods, since they're pretty high in fat. But, in moderation, they offer you a lot of protection from cancer, heart disease, and stroke.

Sunflower seeds—They're a good source of fiber and vitamin E, an important nutrient that protects against heart attacks, cancer, and stroke. Eating foods that contain vitamin E can help in the fight against heart disease. A ¼-cup serving provides almost 3 grams of fiber. But use them with caution in your diet: You also get almost 16 grams of fat from that ¼ cup.

Sesame seeds—There's that trade-off again: High calories, high fat (1 ounce gives you 13 grams). You also get iron that you probably don't need, since your body stores more iron as you get older. On the positive side, in a 1-ounce serving, you get almost 4 percent of the Daily Value of calcium, 20 percent of the Daily Value of copper, almost 5 grams of fiber, almost 25 percent of the magnesium that your heart needs daily, and 115 milligrams of the potassium that helps to control your blood pressure. Plus, you get riboflavin, niacin, and folate (the natural form of a folic acid supplement).

Ice the fruit. Make fruit ices. Put a serving of your favorite fruit in a blender and mix it until smooth. Pour it into a bowl or shallow pan, and put it in the freezer. Stir every 15 minutes or so to break up ice crystals and keep it from freezing solid too fast. It will take 1 to 1½ hours (and six to eight vigorous stirrings—try your food processor if you like).

Pop the corn. Three cups of air-popped, unbuttered popcorn—enough to get you through even the longest movie—gives you 92 calories, 1 gram of fat, and more than 3 grams of fiber.

Soirée with sorbet. If you're on the prowl for a healthful after-dinner treat, try fruit sorbet with some fresh fruit thrown in. Not only will you stoke up on the goodness of fruit, you will also take in less fat and cholesterol than you would with ice cream.

Pear it down. Grate a crispy Bosc pear and put it on hot breakfast cereal for a taste treat. Slice a Comice pear and use it in cereals and salads, or even for dessert.

Eat potato chips. Do what? Surprise—fat-free or baked potato chips are readily available these days, so you can have the snack that you crave without the high fat, sodium, and calories. Look for brands with zero fat and low sodium and calories.

---

275 percent of the Daily Value of this important nutrient to help sideline your cancer risk.

One guava also gives you more than 4 grams of insoluble fiber to help reduce your risk of colon and breast cancer.

■ **Fighting Heart Disease and Stroke**— In one doctor-supervised study, 120 people who were taking medication to lower their blood

pressures cut out the medicine and ate several guavas a day. Their blood pressures went down, and their levels of harmful cholesterol and triglycerides dropped even further on guavas than on medication.

A guava gives you nearly 1 gram of soluble fiber and is a source of 14 percent of the Daily Value of vitamin A and vitamin B_6—nutrients that cut cholesterol, drop blood pressure, and help keep your heart healthy.

HALIBUT

Get in the halibut habit, and you'll be swimming in heart protection. One 3-ounce serving of this healthy source of protein gives you less than 3 grams of fat and only 35 milligrams of cholesterol.

■ **Fighting Cancer**—A study found that lab animals developed smaller breast tumors when fed omega-3 fatty acids from fish like halibut than those that were fed a fatty acid from corn oil.

■ **Fighting Heart Disease and Stroke**— Several studies show that eating one to two servings of fish a week (one serving is the size of a deck of cards) may cut your risk of stroke in half. An Australian study showed that a fish-rich diet may actually get rid of the dangerous triglycerides that pave the way for coronary problems.

A lot of the benefit comes from a particular kind of fat in fish. Researchers have found that people who eat one to two servings of fish a week have less heart disease than people who eat none, and they think that it may be partly due to the omega-3 fatty acids in fish.

The potassium in halibut helps to lower high blood pressure. One serving of halibut gives you almost 20 percent of the Daily Values for vitamins B_6 and B_{12}. As you get older, you need more of these important B vitamins. One serving also contains 22 percent of the Daily Value for magnesium, which may help prevent blood clots and lower blood pressure. Halibut's calcium content may help lower blood pressure, too.

HONEYDEWS

Whether at a summer roadside stand or in the grocery store, people searching for honeydew do a strange dance as they pick up melon after melon to shake them and poke them, looking for those melons that are perfectly ripe. And it's worth going to all that trouble because honeydews are great at protecting you from disease.

■ **Fighting Cancer**—One-half cup of cubed honeydew provides you with 35 percent of the Daily Value of vitamin C, an antioxidant that helps protect your body from various cancers.

■ **Fighting Heart Disease and Stroke**— Just a sliver of this melon packs a punch: Its vitamin C helps keep the heart-protecting HDL cholesterol levels high while sending the harmful LDL levels into the cellar. Studies show that high levels of vitamin C keep your arteries from getting clogged and make you less vulnerable to strokes and heart attacks. Honeydew also provides potassium, which helps lower your blood pressure.

KALE

You know the plot line—if Joe Average gets a chance, he can become a hero. Sort of like kale. This powerful disease fighter doesn't usually get the opportunity to show its stuff. You will often find it relegated to nothing more than an ornamental role at restaurant salad bars. But it pays to steam it and serve it as part of a meal.

■ **Fighting Cancer**—Kale is one of the best sources of lutein, an antioxidant associated with lower rates of lung cancer. Isothiocyanates activate protective enzymes that carry carcinogens out of the system before they can damage cells. In the lab, these processes have kept tumors from forming and have neutralized cancerous agents.

Other potent disease fighters, among them indole-3-carbinol and sulforaphane, may protect against breast cancer. Kale also shores up your defenses with a good amount of dietary fiber, beta-carotene, and vitamins A and C. And kale gives you calcium in a form that your body can use easily to protect against colon cancer.

Kale is a good source of vitamin E. Some studies show that consuming high levels of vitamin E decreases levels of prostaglandin E_2, a substance that limits the efficiency of your immune system. Although these studies used supplements, dark green leafy vegetables like kale are recognized sources of vitamin E.

■ **Fighting Heart Disease and Stroke—** Kale is rich in the flavonoids linked to lower rates of fatal heart attacks. One-half cup of frozen kale, cooked, provides 27 percent of the Daily Value for vitamin C and 2.5 milligrams of beta-carotene.

With ½ cup of cooked kale, you get almost 9 percent of the Daily Value of calcium, which helps lower blood pressure. Studies show that people with high levels of vitamin E, abundant in kale, are less likely to suffer heart attacks.

KIWIFRUIT

What taste would you get if you crossed a banana with a strawberry and added a touch of tartness? The kiwifruit—a brown, fuzzy-skinned fruit with emerald green pulp that hails from California and New Zealand.

■ **Fighting Cancer—** Kiwifruit are packed with vitamin C—in an ounce-for-ounce contest, the kiwi even beats out oranges. One large fruit gives you almost 150 percent of the Daily Value of that cancer-fighting nutrient. Studies show that high intakes of vitamin C lower the risk of breast cancer. You also get a gram of insoluble fiber to guard against colon and breast cancer. Research has found that substances in the kiwifruit also keep cells from mutating.

■ **Fighting Heart Disease and Stroke—** Vitamin C, so abundant in kiwi, may be the food world's workaholic. Not content with protecting against cancer, it also helps your heart by lowering the levels of harmful fats and triglycerides in your blood. This means less buildup of debris that

would narrow arteries and increase your risk of a heart attack or stroke.

From kiwis, you get more than 0.5 gram of soluble fiber plus two other nutrients that keep your heart healthier: 6.8 percent of the Daily Value of magnesium, plus some potassium to help lower blood pressure.

KOHLRABI

Kol-rab-ee. If you think that pronouncing kohlrabi is a hoot, just wait until you get a load of the science-speak that sums up how the substances in this wonder food can protect you.

■ **Fighting Cancer—** On the cancer front, let's sample this strange use of the English language: Antimutagenic, desmutagenic, and inducers of glutathione-S-transferease. Translation: All are methods by which your body fights off tumor initiation, and kohlrabi contributes to them all.

You also get the usual lineup of protection that comes with any cruciferous vegetable. One-half cup cooked kohlrabi contains 74 percent of the Daily Value of vitamin C to help protect you from cancer of the breast, cervix, esophagus, lung, mouth, pancreas, rectum, and stomach. Your immune system gets pumped up with copper and vitamin B_6. If you like to nibble kohlrabi raw, a 1-cup serving provides some folate, which may protect against cancer of the cervix, rectum, colon, lung, and possibly the esophagus.

■ **Fighting Heart Disease and Stroke—** Beyond weighing in with the vitamin C that helps block the formation of the LDL cholesterol that can build up in your arteries, kohlrabi helps lower your blood pressure with potassium.

LEEKS

Okay, these relatives of onions and garlic are a nuisance to prepare. You have to clean them really well, or you end up eating dirt, literally.

But it's worth it—their taste is sweeter and milder than onions, yet their protective qualities are just about as strong.

■ **Fighting Cancer**—A close relative of garlic, leeks give off a mildly pungent scent. But they'll give you a lot of protection against cancer. Two studies identified compounds in leeks that may help to slow or halt tumor growth. Among them are the important sulfur compounds that stop carcinogens before they can do damage. When researchers in Belgium studied the eating habits of 3,669 people, they found that those who ate leeks were 66 percent less likely to develop colon cancer than those who didn't eat leeks.

Other substances take the fight out of dangerous free radicals that damage healthy cells. Plus, you get more than 0.5 gram of insoluble fiber to help protect against colon and breast cancer.

■ **Fighting Heart Disease and Stroke**—The same sulfur compounds that cancel carcinogens also help cut down blood pressure. Substances in leeks called flavonoids neutralize LDL cholesterol to help keep your arteries from clogging up. They also seem to help keep levels of the beneficial HDL cholesterol high. You get more heart protection from the 1.3 grams of soluble fiber per serving that leeks contain.

LEMONS

"I would like a medium vodka dry martini— with a slice of lemon peel. Shaken and not stirred, please." Leave it to James Bond, master of high-tech weaponry, to figure out the protective qualities of the piquant lemon and its peel.

■ **Fighting Cancer**—The spray of oil from a twist of lemon releases limonoids, powerful substances that, in animal studies, prevent oral cancer. But the twist isn't the only way to get protection. You can grate the zest (the colored part of the peel) and use it as a flavor enhancer.

Lemons put the squeeze on cancer: Flavonoids inhibit the hormones that promote cancer. Monoterpenes work as antioxidants to neutralize harmful substances. Phenolic acids keep dangerous nitrosamines from forming. Terpenes help enzymes block carcinogens.

Vitamin C gets into the act, too—when you eat a wedge, one-quarter of a lemon, you get close to 13 percent of the Daily Value, lowering your risk of oral cancer. And you pick up just under 0.5 gram of dietary fiber to guard against colon cancer.

■ **Fighting Heart Disease and Stroke**— Lemons fight heart disease with a payload of vitamin C, which helps prevent cholesterol from accumulating and blocking your arteries.

LENTILS

Whether you choose red, brown, or green lentils, this bean is such a star that it deserves to shine on its own, rather than get lumped with the rest of the beans. Lentils are often sold as an Indian dish called "dahl," but this isn't the best buy for protection, since the fiber-rich outer skins have been removed.

■ **Fighting Cancer**—One-half cup of cooked lentils serves up over 4.6 grams of insoluble fiber to help protect against colon cancer. You also get almost 45 percent of the Daily Value of folate, which may protect you against cancer of the cervix, colon, rectum, lung, and possibly the esophagus. Folate also helps your cells stay healthy, making it harder for cancers to attack, and keeps the important DNA intact. Plus, you get 12.5 percent of the Daily Value of copper and 8.4 percent of the Daily Value of zinc to help strengthen your immune system.

■ **Fighting Heart Disease and Stroke**— This little bean is a beacon of heart protection. In one study, people with high cholesterol who added 1½ cups of lentils or other legumes to their diets each day for three weeks experienced an average 60-point drop in cholesterol. Add to that some soluble fiber to help lower your LDL cholesterol and 9 percent of the Daily Value of vitamin B_6, which may help keep homocysteine levels low. The magnesium and potassium in lentils work together to lower high blood pressure and keep blood from clotting, which could prevent a heart attack or stroke.

LETTUCE AND OTHER SALAD GREENS

Lettuce is a mixed bag in terms of benefits. You don't get many nutrients from the pale green stuff that most of us put on our sandwiches, although even that contains some protective substances. Rule of the green thumb: The darker the leaf's green color, the more protection you'll get from it.

■ **Fighting Cancer**—Scientists have found that even the juice of lettuces contain substances that fight cell mutation and interfere with the development of tumors.

Romaine lettuce, with its broad, dark leaves, is a noble cancer fighter. One-half cup, shredded, gives you more than 9 percent of the Daily Value of folate. This valuable B vitamin may protect you against cancer of the cervix, colon, rectum, lung, and possibly the esophagus. It also helps cells stay healthy and strong to fight off cancerous agents.

Romaine gives you 11 percent of the Daily Value of vitamin C, reducing your risk of cancer of the breast, cervix, esophagus, lung, mouth, pancreas, rectum, and stomach. More good news: Endive does just as well.

■ **Fighting Heart Disease and Stroke**— One cup of romaine weighs in with lots of potassium. Arugula is a heavyweight in beta-carotene, a substance that may block harmful LDL

cholesterol. It also reduces your risk of stroke, packing 2 milligrams into a 1-cup serving.

LIMES

In the 1700s, British naval ships packed limes to protect the sailors from scurvy. Thus, British seamen earned the nickname "limeys." Scurvy's not a disease that we worry about anymore, but limes protect against diseases that we do fret over.

■ **Fighting Cancer**—Limes are rich in a lot of substances that keep cancer from getting a foothold: flavonoids that inhibit the hormones that help cancers get started, limonoids that trigger enzymes to protect you, monoterpenes that work as antioxidants, phenolic acids that keep dangerous nitrosamines from forming, and terpenes that block carcinogens. Limes also give you vitamin C, which helps decrease the risk of breast cancer.

■ **Fighting Heart Disease and Stroke**— Like other citrus fruits, limes are particularly rich in vitamin C, which lowers the risk of stroke, especially in people age 65 and over.

LOBSTER

Who says that healthy eating can't be fun? Steamed or boiled, lobster contains 0.5 gram of fat and just 83 calories per serving.

■ **Fighting Cancer**—Eat lobster and you do a favor for your immune system as well as your taste buds. Three ounces of lobster (about the size of a deck of playing cards) gives you 83 percent of your Daily Value for copper and more than 16 percent of your Daily Value for zinc, both of which keep your immune system at its best. Calcium in lobster helps fight against colon cancer.

■ **Fighting Heart Disease and Stroke**— Lobster is the catch of the day in terms of heart protection. A rich helping of omega-3 fatty acids may work to lower your risk of heart attack by bringing down your triglyceride levels. Plus, you get a lot of nutrients that may help to combat high blood pressure: 5 percent of the Daily Value of calcium, more than 7 percent of the Daily Value of magnesium, and some potassium.

High levels of homocysteine in the blood are linked to a high risk of heart attack. Some B vitamins, such as B_{12}, plentiful in lobsters, reduce homocysteine levels. You get 44 percent of the Daily Value of vitamin B_{12} in a serving.

MACKEREL

You know the routine: On one hand, the benefits; on the other, the problems. Mackerel is that kind of fish, swimming in both directions. On the plus side, mackerel is rich in disease preventers. It is also rich in calories, fat, and cholesterol. One 3-ounce serving loads you up with 15 grams of fat. Fortunately, more than a third of that is mono-unsaturated fat, the kind that helps, not hurts. You also pull in 64 milligrams of cholesterol and 223 calories. Even so, from a disease-prevention standpoint, mackerel has a lot going for it.

■ **Fighting Cancer**—The zinc found in mackerel builds up your body's defenses by strengthening the immune system and disabling substances that could cause cancer.

■ **Fighting Heart Disease and Stroke**— Several studies have revealed that people who eat one serving of fish each week may cut their risk of stroke in half. Part of the reason may be that high levels of protective omega-3 fatty acids are tied to lower rates of heart disease. Researchers note that the higher a fish's fat content, the more omega-3 fatty acids it provides, which makes mackerel a winner.

One serving of mackerel gives you 269 percent of the Daily Value of vitamin B_{12}. That's important because, as you age, you don't absorb this important nutrient as efficiently as you used to. You also get vitamin B_6 to help keep your heart healthy, plus 21 percent of the Daily Value of magnesium and some potassium to help keep your blood pressure low.

MANGOES

A taste sensation, mangoes remind some people of a fruit assortment of apricots and melons. Others characterize it as a cross between peaches and pineapple. But however you slice it, you get the taste of a healthful fruit cocktail in just one fruit.

■ **Fighting Cancer**—Just half a mango is an excellent source of vitamin A, providing you with almost 78 percent of its Daily Value and almost 6 percent of the Daily Value for vitamin E. Vitamins A and E are heavyweight cancer fighters, protecting your body from cancer-causing substances such as nitrosamines.

A serving of $1/2$ a mango gives you 5 percent of the Daily Value for copper, which boosts your immune system, and more than 2.3 milligrams of beta-carotene. Researchers have found that a diet high in beta-carotene–rich foods protects both smokers and nonsmokers from lung cancer.

■ **Fighting Heart Disease and Stroke**— Half a mango gives you 1.5 grams of the soluble fiber that keeps high blood pressure down. The same nutrients that lower your cancer risk also help your heart: Vitamin E helps disarm fats before they can latch onto artery walls and clog up the works. Vitamin A and beta-carotene also work to protect your arteries from the plaque buildup that leaves you at risk for heart attacks and strokes. In addition, you get 46 percent of the Daily Value for vitamin C, which helps decrease your risk of stroke.

MILK

It has a well-deserved rep for building bone, but that's not all it does. Milk deserves a place high on your list of protectors against cancer, heart disease, and stroke—especially skim milk.

Okay—you've tried skim milk, and it tastes watery and looks worse. You can fix that. Have a decaf café latte. It's pretty much hot milk with a little espresso mixed in. Less than 80 calories and 0.5 gram of fat are in it, plus it protects your heart (and your bones) with 264 milligrams of calcium.

Or give the milk a richer taste and creamier look by stirring 2 to 4 tablespoons of instant nonfat milk powder into each cup of skim milk. You get extra calcium that way, too.

■ **Fighting Cancer**—The skim in skim milk isn't something to take lightly. One study links high rates of breast cancer in mice to a high-fat diet.

Beyond cutting down on fat for cancer protection, drinking skim milk provides calcium, which may reduce your risk of breast and colon cancer; and zinc, which helps your immune system stay strong. Skim milk is a source of vitamin A and beta-carotene, which may help disarm cancerous agents that invade your cells. One study suggests that beta-carotene, when derived from foods, reduces the risk of lung cancer in nonsmokers.

■ **Fighting Heart Disease and Stroke**—One cup of skim milk that is fortified with vitamin A gives you almost 10 percent of the Daily Value for this important vitamin, plus some beta-carotene, which may help keep cholesterol from attaching to your artery walls and increasing your risk of heart attack and stroke.

Note: Buy milk in cardboard cartons that block light—fluorescent lights in supermarket refrigerator cases can destroy up to 90 percent of vitamin A in milk after 24 hours.

Skim milk makes a three-pronged attack on high blood pressure: You get more than 30 percent of the Daily Value of calcium (which many researchers believe to be a countermeasure to mild high blood pressure), close to 7 percent of the Daily Value of magnesium, and more than 405

milligrams of potassium. Calcium may also help lower levels of the harmful LDL cholesterol.

In milk, you also get a sampling of three B vitamins: riboflavin, B_{12}, and B_6, which are all important for reducing your risk of heart disease, heart attack, and stroke.

MUSHROOMS

The mushroom may be a lowly fungus, but it has been a favorite food of royalty since ancient Egypt. And it defends your body nobly with antibacterial and medicinal substances.

■ **Fighting Cancer**—Mushrooms contain antibacterial properties that help keep tumors from growing.

Shiitake mushrooms are especially rich in nutrients. Four cooked mushrooms (72 grams) give you almost 33 percent of the Daily Value of copper to make your immune system's defenses, well, mushroom. You also get almost 2 grams of dietary fiber to help protect you from colon cancer and heart disease, and you receive more than 6 percent of the Daily Value of zinc to help protect your immune system.

Button mushrooms also give you immunity-building protection: 1/2 cup gives you 8.5 percent of the Daily Value of copper.

■ **Fighting Heart Disease and Stroke**—Just four cooked shiitake mushrooms equip you with more than 84 milligrams of potassium, lowering your blood pressure. The vitamin C mushrooms contain does double duty against both cancer and heart disease, as it raises your blood levels of beneficial HDL cholesterol and drops the levels of the harmful LDL cholesterol and triglycerides (fats, in the blood). You end up with a lower risk of plaque buildup in the arteries that can lead to a heart attack or stroke. You also get small amounts of heart-helping folate and vitamin B_6, which have both been shown to lower the production of homocysteine—the substance that promotes the formation of dangerous blood clots.

Regular raw mushrooms aren't nearly as powerful defensively as cooked shiitakes, but with a quarter cup of them, you still end up with a very respectable 42 milligrams of potassium to fight heart disease.

MUSSELS

Mussels muscle up your body's protective systems. These delicate shellfish are very sensitive to pollution in the water along the coastlines where they naturally grow, so the best of them are now cultivated in clean-water farms.

■ **Fighting Cancer**—One serving of $3\frac{1}{2}$ ounces of cooked mussels provides vitamin A, which may help strengthen your body's defenses and protect against lung cancer. Its vitamin C helps ward off cancer of the breast, cervix, esophagus, lung, mouth, pancreas, rectum, and stomach. Almost 18 percent of the Daily Value of zinc and a bit of copper assist your immune system. You get almost 19 percent of the Daily Value of folate, which may lower your risk of cancer of the cervix, colon, rectum, lung, and possibly the esophagus. Folate also helps cells stay healthy.

■ **Fighting Heart Disease and Stroke**— Mussels are rich in omega-3 fatty acids, which may help keep your cholesterol levels low and fight heart disease. Some studies have found that vitamin A and beta-carotene block the harmful LDL cholesterol and lower your risk of stroke. Vitamin C from mussels keeps the beneficial HDL cholesterol levels high and also helps knock down the nasty LDLs and triglycerides in your blood. Potassium weighs in at almost 266 milligrams, keeping your blood pressure low.

The innards of these deep blue shells are rich in B vitamins. High levels of B_{12}, B_6, and folate in the blood have been shown to lower the production of homocysteine—a substance that activates clotting, making blood more prone to adhere to arterial walls. So getting the proper daily dose of these vitamins helps lower your heart disease risk. Mussels contain almost 19 percent of the Daily Value of folate, 397 percent of the Daily Value of the important vitamin B_{12}, and 5 percent of vitamin B_6. These tasty mollusks also contain more than 24 percent of the Daily Value of riboflavin, which has been shown to control cholesterol levels.

MUSTARD GREENS

Hey, the seeds that are ground up to make mustard for sandwiches and salad dressings have to come from somewhere. As you might expect, the mother plant of mustard—this leafy green vegetable—has a fragrant, tangy taste.

■ **Fighting Cancer**—Researchers working with the National Cancer Institute have been busy isolating substances in mustard greens that, at least in the lab, put a lid on cancer. Here's what some of these substances do: They interfere with cancer's start-up process, propelling your protective enzymes into action. They even get in the way of estrogen, helping to reduce the likelihood of breast cancer.

A good source of fiber when eaten raw, mustard greens lower the risk of colon cancer. A $\frac{1}{2}$-cup serving, cooked and chopped, is a source of almost 42 percent of the Daily Value of vitamin A and a respectable amount of beta-carotene, which may strengthen the mucous membranes that keep cancer-forming agents from damaging healthy cells. Also, there is nearly 30 percent of the Daily Value for vitamin C, lowering your risk of cancer of the breast, cervix, esophagus, lung, mouth, pancreas, rectum, and stomach.

You get almost 13 percent of the Daily Value of folate, which may protect you from cancer of the cervix, colon, rectum, lung, and possibly the esophagus. This vitamin also protects DNA's genetic codes. At the most basic level, your cells rely on folate to help them divide and replicate properly. Doctors note that damaged cells are easy prey for carcinogens.

■ **Fighting Heart Disease and Stroke**— Mustard greens are a source of vitamin E, an important antioxidant that several studies say helps reduce your risk of heart attack and stroke. Researchers at Harvard Medical School looked at 1,795 women who'd had a heart attack or angina. Over a 10-year period, the women who ate the most foods containing vitamin E, beta-carotene, vitamin C, and riboflavin had a 71 percent lower risk of a stroke and a 33 percent lower risk of a second heart attack. You get all these nutrients in mustard greens.

The benefits continue with mustard greens, providing more than 141 milligrams of potassium to lower your blood pressure, and a healthy dose of magnesium to help keep blood pressure down and prevent the blood clots that could lead to a heart attack or stroke. Calcium may help by lowering mild high blood pressure and the harmful LDL cholesterol levels. Mustard greens also contain B_6 and folate, which help to reduce your risk of heart disease by lowering blood pressure and homocysteine levels.

NECTARINES

The name probably comes from the Greek word for "drink of the gods." The ambrosial nectarine should be celebrated for its disease-fighting capabilities as well as its taste.

■ **Fighting Cancer**—Researchers working with the National Cancer Institute found that substances in nectarines help prevent cancers from getting started and growing.

Your immune system will like the taste of nectarines—the fruit is a source of copper,

vitamin B_6, and vitamin A, which all help to keep cancerous agents away. More than 12 percent of the Daily Value of vitamin C is in a nectarine, which helps protect you against cancer of the breast, cervix, esophagus, lung, mouth, pancreas, rectum, and stomach. And it has close to 2 grams of insoluble fiber to cut your risk of colon and breast cancer.

■ **Fighting Heart Disease and Stroke**— Eat a nectarine and give high blood pressure a downward push, thanks to more than 288 milligrams of potassium. Nearly a gram of soluble fiber helps send cholesterol down, too. Vitamin C helps lower the level of LDL cholesterol that tends to promote the buildup of plaque in your arteries.

OLIVE OIL AND CANOLA OIL

Wait a minute—how can oils be on a healthy foods list? Easy. Eaten in small quantities, their health benefits outweigh their caloric challenge.

■ **Fighting Cancer**—Next time you measure out a tablespoon of olive oil, look at it this way: You're getting almost 8.5 percent of the Daily Value of vitamin E, which helps your infection-fighting T cells do their job. You're also keeping the rest of your immune system up to par. Plus, vitamin E seems to reduce the risk of oral cancer.

■ **Fighting Heart Disease and Stroke**— When researchers at the University of Milan examined the relationship between the Mediterranean diet and low rates of heart disease, they decided to investigate oleuropein, a component of olive oil. They found that it blocks some of the conditions that contribute to chronic heart disease.

Canola oil is rich in omega-3 fatty acids (the same stuff that makes fish the dish of protective choice) that may combat cholesterol and protect you from heart disease.

Both olive and canola oil are good sources of vitamin E. Several large studies have shown that vitamin E reduces the risk of heart disease by preventing the oxidation of cholesterol and the formation of blood clots. Although these studies used vitamin E supplements, foods that contain vitamin E can always help.

Not surprisingly, both of these oils are high in monounsaturated fat, the kind that doesn't clog up your arteries. In fact, this type of fat has been linked to lower levels of both cholesterol and blood pressure.

ONIONS

In Shakespeare's A Midsummer Night's Dream, *one character advises, "Eat no onions nor garlic, for we are to utter sweet breath." That may be good advice for a romantic evening, but not for a disease-free life.*

■ **Fighting Cancer**—Onions come in all shapes, sizes, and colors. You'll get more cancer protection from red onions because they contain the most flavonoids, substances that studies show help fight cancer. But any onion contains a wealth of cancer protection. Compounds in onions block or suppress carcinogens, help keep cells from mutating, and interfere with tumor growth. Onions have even been reported to protect against radiation damage.

■ **Fighting Heart Disease and Stroke**— Substances in onions called flavonoids may lower blood pressure. They also help neutralize the LDL cholesterol that leads to clogged arteries and increases your risk of heart attack or stroke.

ORANGES

Christopher Columbus carried orange seedlings with him across the Atlantic. What would Florida and California look like today if he had forgotten that part of his cargo? Your personal health would certainly lack an important protector.

■ **Fighting Cancer**—Orange juice is loaded with limonoid glucosides, natural chemicals that reduce the growth of cancer in animals. You also get glutathione, which may lower the risk of oral and throat cancer and help your immune system work more efficiently. Eat an orange and get almost 2 grams of insoluble fiber to help prevent colon and breast cancer. You'll also get more than 116 percent of the Daily Value of vitamin C to protect against cancer of the breast, cervix, esophagus, lung, mouth, pancreas, rectum, and stomach. Look for calcium-fortified orange juice, which may combat colon cancer.

■ **Fighting Heart Disease and Stroke**— Calcium-fortified orange juice gives you about 33 percent of the Daily Value of calcium. In some studies, calcium has been shown to also help lower your blood pressure. Plus, that healthy dose of vitamin C lowers bad LDL cholesterol levels and raises good HDL levels. Another excellent reason to reach for orange juice is for the fiber it contains. A ¾-cup serving gives you almost 0.5 gram of soluble fiber to protect your heart.

Oranges give you 237 milligrams of potassium to help keep your blood pressure in check. Eat the white part just under the outer peel as well as the center core of the orange, and you'll get an extra dose of heart-protecting flavonoids.

OYSTERS

Crack open that stubborn little shell, and you will discover an elegant seafood that contains an abundance of disease protection.

■ **Fighting Cancer**—Oysters help make your immune system a hard shell for cancer to crack. Six medium steamed oysters provide you with 159 percent of the Daily Value of copper and 509 percent of the Daily Value of zinc. Talk about defenses. Plus there's vitamin C, which contributes to the protective elements. Oysters are also a good source of vitamin A, which may cut your risk of cancer as well.

Spice It Up for a Dash of Protection

How nice—what's good for your taste buds is also great for your body. The spices that transform bland foods into sublime culinary treats also protect you from cancer, heart disease, and stroke.

Chilies. Hot peppers, the source of dried chilies and cayenne, contain capsaicin, a chemical that not only gives your taste buds a buzz but also fights bacteria and mutes your system's pain receptors. Chilies are rich in vitamin C—1/2 ounce of the red variety gives you more than 57 percent of the Daily Value. It never hurts to keep your taste buds happy by using chilies or cayenne when you eat low-salt and low-fat foods.

Curry. Turmeric, derived from a plant root, gives a characteristic flavor to many Indian curry dishes. It contains curcumin, which in the lab prevents cancerous lesions of the skin, breast, and colon. It also helps keep blood platelets from sticking together and causing clots, and helps stop fats in the blood from oxidizing and turning into harmful low-density lipoprotein cholesterol.

Horseradish. This condiment will not only wake up your taste buds, but may also provide disease prevention. A cruciferous vegetable (meaning it's a cousin to broccoli and cauliflower), fresh horseradish contains beta-carotene and vitamin C, along with the phytochemical isothiocyanate that gets your body's protective enzymes working to root out cancerous agents. Remember, fresh is best—prepared horseradish that you buy in the store is not very nutritious.

Parsley. Two sprigs offer more than 4 percent of the Daily Value of vitamin C, 2 percent of the Daily Value of vitamin A, and a little fiber. They're also a good source of protective flavonoids and beta-carotene. You benefit most from dried parsley, with its concentrated nutrients like copper and magnesium. But don't go wild: 1 tablespoon gives you 7 percent of the Daily Value for iron, and you probably don't need extra.

■ **Fighting Heart Disease and Stroke—** Oysters defend your heart, too. Just six oysters give you a lot of the important B vitamins that reduce risk of heart disease: 245 percent of the Daily Value of vitamin B_{12}, plus some riboflavin. Vitamin B_{12} is harder for your body to absorb as you age, so it's especially important that your diet contain an abundance of it.

Magnesium in oysters helps prevent the blood clots that can lead to a stroke. Oysters also provide potassium, which can help lower blood pressure levels.

PAPAYAS

Sweet and refreshing, these large fruits contain little black, peppery-tasting seeds (and, yes, they're fine to eat—some people actually use them as a substitute for capers).

■ **Fighting Cancer—**One serving, about 1 cup of cubed papaya, gives you 144 percent of your Daily Value of vitamin C—important to help cut your risk of cancer of the breast, cervix, esophagus, lung, mouth, pancreas, rectum, and stomach. It's also a source of beta-carotene as well as vitamin A, which may help strengthen your body's defenses. You also get more than 13 percent of the Daily Value of folate to help ward off cancer of the cervix, colon, rectum, lung, and possibly the esophagus. Folate helps keep cells healthy so they're less easily invaded by carcinogens.

■ **Fighting Heart Disease and Stroke—** The abundance of vitamin C in papayas raises levels of HDL cholesterol, protecting you from heart disease and heart attacks. It also lowers the harmful blood fats that attach to artery walls and increase your risk of heart attack and stroke.

Vitamin A gets into the act and has been found in some studies to block LDL cholesterol before it can become a permanent (and unwelcome) fixture in your arteries. Vitamin B$_6$ also helps lower levels of harmful LDL cholesterol, decreasing your risk of heart problems.

You get a little magnesium from papayas to reduce the blood's tendency to clot where it shouldn't. Calcium in papayas may help lower mild high blood pressure and LDL cholesterol levels. And a serving of papaya gives you 359 milligrams of potassium, which helps keep your blood pressure down, too.

PARSNIPS

Food fashions do change. Most people today probably couldn't tell you what a parsnip looks like. In the 1700s, they were one of the most commonly consumed vegetables in America. These now-exotic vegetables resemble pale, over-sized carrots. They have a celery-like scent and a vaguely nutty taste.

■ **Fighting Cancer—**Eat parsnips and you get an array of protective phytochemicals, such as coumarins, phenolic acids, monoterpenes, and phthalides. What's more, 1/2 cup of boiled parsnips contains 1 gram of insoluble fiber to guard against colon and breast cancer. Plus, it provides copper, which helps strengthen your immune system.

■ **Fighting Heart Disease and Stroke—** Parsnips aren't parsimonious when it comes to heart protection: The same phytochemicals that help prevent cancer also lower your risk of heart

disease. They prevent harmful LDL cholesterol from sticking to artery walls.

You get a healthy, heart-saving helping of the B vitamins, including folate, riboflavin, and vitamin B$_6$. You also get almost 2 grams of soluble fiber to lower LDL cholesterol levels, 286 grams of potassium to help keep blood pressure down, and more than 16 percent of the Daily Value for vitamin C to raise your levels of HDL cholesterol and lower LDL levels even more. That's hearty protection.

PEACHES

When settlers from Spain came to the New World, they brought peaches with them. "Just peachy," you might say, especially when you consider what peaches do to protect you.

■ **Fighting Cancer—**In the lab, substances in peaches make it hard for cancerous tumors to get started. Peaches contain glutathione, which may reduce the risk of oral and throat cancer. One peach gives you nearly a gram of insoluble fiber, which reduces your risk of colon and breast cancer. Vitamin C protects important organs, and the vitamin A in peaches may help keep cancerous agents from getting into your system.

■ **Fighting Heart Disease and Stroke—** One peach gives your heart all-purpose protection. It's a source of more than 9 percent of your Daily Value of vitamin A, which may help keep the harmful LDL cholesterol from adhering to artery walls.

Peaches provide you with more than just one LDL-fighting weapon—think of it as gang warfare on your behalf. Along with vitamin A, vitamin C clobbers the LDL cholesterol that leads to clots. It also increases the levels of HDL cholesterol and keeps the bad stuff from getting a grip. The potassium in peaches also protects against high blood pressure.

PEARS

If your body is shaped like a pear, you're in luck: Your risk for disease is lower than that of your apple-shaped friends. For those of you who don't sport a pear shape, and for those "pears" who want to remain healthy, eating pears—the fruit—has considerable disease-fighting effects.

■ **Fighting Cancer**—In the laboratory, substances in pears prevent cell mutations and may trip up cancer's first footholds within your body. In one medium pear, you get more than 3 grams of insoluble fiber to protect against colon cancer and a helping of copper to assist in keeping your immune system up to par.

■ **Fighting Heart Disease and Stroke**— A pear gives you almost 2 grams of soluble fiber to protect your heart. Add to that more than 350 milligrams of potassium to help drop your blood pressure, and about 11 percent of the Daily Value of vitamin C to cut harmful LDL cholesterol and raise the beneficial HDL cholesterol levels. (You'll get less benefit from canned pears because they have been peeled. The canning process also saps away some of the vitamin C.)

PEAS

Remember the story that you read to your children about the princess and the pea? If her highness had been thinking about disease prevention, she would have banished the servant who put the pea under the mattress instead of on the dinner table.

■ **Fighting Cancer**—While the princess of the story did discover the pea, many researchers remain puzzled. Peas do seem to prevent cells from mutating, although no one yet has a clue as to why that happens.

But we do know that peas are a good source of vitamins A and C. One-half cup of snow peas gives you about 64 percent of the Daily Value of vitamin C, protecting you from cancer of the breast, cervix, esophagus, lung, mouth, pancreas, rectum, and stomach.

■ **Fighting Heart Disease and Stroke**— Peas give you princely protection—one serving, about $1/2$ cup of green peas, provides almost 17 percent of the Daily Value of vitamin C to help slash the LDL cholesterol that leads to clots. This nutrient also helps raise levels of the HDL cholesterol that keeps the LDLs in check. Peas are also a good source of vitamin A, which may help keep LDL cholesterol from attaching to arterial walls. There's some vitamin B_6 and folate, which work to lower the blood levels of homocysteine, a substance that activates dangerous clotting. The magnesium in peas helps lower mild high blood pressure, and the soluble fiber keeps cholesterol down.

PECANS

Okay—they're really high in calories. Of the nuts that you are likely to see in the grocery store, only macademia nuts pack more calories per nut. Pecans are high in fat, too, although 55 percent is monounsaturated, the kind of fat that doesn't contribute to clogs in the arteries. But pecans also wield some mighty weapons against cancer, heart disease, and stroke.

■ **Fighting Cancer**—In a study using laboratory mice, the ellagic acid in pecans has been shown to be a powerful adversary that fights cancer of the lung, skin, esophagus, and liver. It detoxifies carcinogens and scavenges substances that carcinogens need to do their nasty work. It might even keep cancerous substances from damaging DNA.

One ounce of pecans—that's about a handful—also gives you almost 18 percent of the Daily Value of copper, an essential nutrient for your immune system. It provides almost 11 percent of the Daily Value for zinc, another key mineral for immunity.

■ **Fighting Heart Disease and Stroke**— That single ounce of pecans does a lot for your heart. You get 105 milligrams of potassium and more than 9 percent of the Daily Value of magnesium to lower high blood pressure. Magnesium also helps keep your blood from clotting. The monounsaturated fat in pecans helps lower cholesterol and blood pressure levels.

PEPPERS

You know John Wayne didn't talk much in films—he just mowed down villains and saved the town. Bell peppers are a lot like that. They don't get the attention, but boy do they come to the rescue. (For information about their showier cousins, the chili pepper clan, see the box on page 84.)

■ **Fighting Cancer**—Red peppers are really just green ones that got to spend more time growing on the vine—and in the process, they stocked up on extra nutrients that protect you.

You get more vitamin C in one red pepper than you do in two oranges. Low vitamin C levels have been linked to a higher risk of developing breast, cervical, esophageal, lung, oral, pancreatic, rectal, and stomach cancer. Plus, you get 2.5 milligrams of beta-carotene (more than in a cup of apricots and nine times more than in a green bell pepper). Researchers have found that beta-carotene may help cut your risk of oral cancer. You also get other carotenoids and flavonoids for added anti-cancer protection.

■ **Fighting Heart Disease and Stroke**— The flavonoids that protect against cancer also help you steer clear of heart disease and stroke. In a five-year Dutch study, older men with diets that were high in flavonoids had a lower risk of heart attack and stroke.

Peppers are loaded with other nutrients for your heart: 1/2 cup sweet green peppers gives you 74 percent of your Daily Value of vitamin C to help keep your arteries clear of debris. Eating peppers also gives you some vitamin B_6 and folate, which a study involving older adults found may reduce the risk of heart disease.

PERSIMMONS

Persimmons are the Jekyll and Hyde of the food world: Bite into an unripe persimmon, and you'll get a taste more bitter than three-day-old coffee. When ripe, persimmons turn sweet and spicy— and healthy.

■ **Fighting Cancer**—One medium-size Japanese persimmon weighs in with a lot of disease protection. It contains more than 2 milligrams of beta-carotene, and it is a source of almost 73 percent of the Daily Value of vitamin A. Several studies have shown that these nutrients may protect against cancer. You get 9.5 percent of the Daily Value of copper to help your immune system, and more than 6 grams of dietary fiber to lower your risk of colon cancer.

■ **Fighting Heart Disease and Stroke**— The vitamin C in persimmons helps keep the levels of HDL cholesterol high while it decreases harmful LDL cholesterol. Your arteries get the benefit: Less plaque buildup means less stuff that can lead to a stroke or heart attack. Persimmons also have some potassium to help lower blood pressure.

PINEAPPLES

Pop quiz: Where do pineapples come from, really? South America. By the time Columbus arrived, they had spread to the Caribbean. Other explorers soon carried them to China and the Philippines. Finally, they landed happily in Hawaii, where most of these healthful fruits are now grown.

■ **Fighting Cancer**—This globe-trotting fruit packs a lot of disease-preventing power. Researchers working with the National Cancer Institute have discovered that substances in pineapple fight cell mutations.

One-half cup of diced raw pineapple gives you almost a gram of dietary fiber to help protect against colon and breast cancer. There's also a little folate to help keep your cells healthy and less vulnerable to a cancerous attack. Folate may also help reduce your risk of cancer of the cervix, colorectum, lung, and possibly the esophagus. You also get some copper to help strengthen your immune system.

■ **Fighting Heart Disease and Stroke**— One helping gives you almost 20 percent of the Daily Value of vitamin C. It helps raise levels of beneficial HDL cholesterol, the stuff that keeps harmful LDL cholesterol from doing damage. Having a low level of HDL cholesterol may be the most accurate indicator that you're at risk for a heart attack or stroke.

PLUMS

When you think "plum," you think "purple," right? Not so—colors range from almost green to red to so-purple-they-look-black. And plums have great names, such as President, Empress, Tragedy, Freedom, and Elephant Heart, which are mainly used in gardening catalogs. Take your pick—they're all plum protection.

■ **Fighting Cancer**—One medium plum gives you almost 1 gram of insoluble fiber to help fight colon and breast cancer. The vitamin C in plums protects against cancer of the breast, cervix, esophagus, lung, mouth, pancreas, rectum, and stomach. A little vitamin B_6 helps round out the anti-cancer forces by boosting your immune system.

■ **Fighting Heart Disease and Stroke**— Plums give you some of the cholesterol-lowering soluble fiber that protects your heart. They also contain a cornucopia of heart protection from riboflavin, vitamin B_6, and vitamin C. The result? Higher amounts of protective HDL cholesterol, lower levels of the harmful LDL cholesterol that clogs your arteries, and less risk of blood clots that trigger heart attacks and strokes.

POLLOCK

This lean fish is eaten more often in the U.S. than any of its cousins. Pollock sometimes masquerades as fish sticks or imitation crabmeat (often labeled "surimi"). One 3-ounce serving gives you just over 1 gram of fat and 77 milligrams of cholesterol, and plenty of disease protection. (But watch the fat content on those breaded, fried fish sticks.)

■ **Fighting Cancer**—Pollock provides a healthy helping of vitamin B_6, weighing in at 14 percent of your Daily Value, which strengthens your immune system. Folate, another B vitamin in pollock, may help lower your risk of cancer of the cervix, colon, rectum, lung, and possibly the esophagus. You need folate to protect DNA's genetic codes and to help cells divide and multiply properly, since damaged cells are attractive targets for cancerous invaders.

■ **Fighting Heart Disease and Stroke**— People who eat one serving of fish a week can lower their risk of stroke by about half. A $3\frac{1}{2}$-ounce serving of Atlantic pollock, for example, gives you 421 milligrams of omega-3 fatty acids, along with just over 1 gram of fat. In several studies, omega-3 has been shown to fight heart disease. A healthy 77 milligrams of calcium in one serving of pollock contributes close to 7 percent of your Daily Value and may help to lower your levels of hazardous LDL cholesterol while it keeps your blood pressure under control.

One 3-ounce serving deals out disease protection in the form of 19 percent of the Daily Value of magnesium, which is another weapon in the fight against high blood pressure. It also helps keep blood from clumping and forming clots that increase your risk of a heart attack or stroke.

POTATOES

Pop quiz: What food makes up the leading source of vitamin C in the American diet?

Yup—potatoes.

■ **Fighting Cancer**—Eat one medium baked potato with its skin, and you will take in more than 43 percent of the Daily Value of vitamin C, which helps stave off cancer of the breast, cervix, esophagus, lung, mouth, pancreas, rectum, and stomach. There are also substances in potatoes that help prevent cell mutation.

■ **Fighting Heart Disease and Stroke**—That baked potato also gives you 844 milligrams of potassium to help bring down high blood pressure. (To get the full benefit, eat the skin.) And its vitamin B_6 helps lower your risk of heart disease.

PRUNES

Why all the fuss? Prunes are just dried-up plums, right? When water gets removed during processing, nutrients become more concentrated. If foods received Academy Awards for disease protection, prunes would be working on an acceptance speech for their leading role.

■ **Fighting Cancer**—One-half cup of these dried delectables contains more than 2 grams of insoluble fiber to help prune your risk of colon and breast cancer. They are a source of vitamin A and beta-carotene, which may help keep cancers from invading healthy cells. Some studies also suggest that these nutrients may offer protection against lung cancer. You get 10 percent of the Daily Value of copper as well, which helps strengthen your immune system.

■ **Fighting Heart Disease and Stroke**—In an ounce-per-ounce comparison, prunes contain more fiber than most dried beans, fruits, and vegetables. A lot of it is soluble, which will protect your heart. You get 354 milligrams of potassium, plus an assortment of powerful defenders against heart disease: calcium, folate, magnesium, riboflavin, vitamin A, vitamin B_6, and vitamin C.

PUMPKINS

The kind of pumpkin that you and your grandchildren carve out at Halloween isn't the kind that usually goes into a pie, bread, or soup. Smaller, sweeter (and less stringy) sugar pumpkins are the kind that get used instead.

■ **Fighting Cancer**—A mug full of pumpkin soup can give you about 1.4 grams of nutritious fiber. One-half cup of mashed pumpkin is a source of more than 26 percent of the Daily Value of vitamin A and some beta-carotene, which may reduce your risk of cancer of the esophagus, stomach, colon, breast, cervix, uterus, and lung. You get cancer-fighting, immune-strengthening copper, too. Researchers working with the National Cancer Institute also note that substances in pumpkins keep cells from mutating.

■ **Fighting Heart Disease and Stroke**—A 10-year study of 1,795 female heart-attack or angina survivors found that those who ate the highest amounts of beta-carotene, vitamin C, vitamin E, and riboflavin had 71 percent less risk of stroke and a 33 percent reduced risk of a second heart attack. Fortunately, pumpkins contain all these nutrients.

Pumpkins are one of the few foods that give you even a moderate amount of vitamin E. Several large studies show that consuming vitamin E may reduce the risk of heart disease. It helps prevent the oxidation of cholesterol and the clumping of platelets in blood vessels. These studies used vitamin E supplements, but foods that contain vitamin E will help, too. And one-half cup of canned pumpkin contains more than 251 milligrams of potassium, along with magnesium, to help keep your blood pressure from going through the roof.

RADISHES

What movie features the leading actress brandishing a radish? Here's a clue: "As God is my witness, I'll never be hungry again." Sure, you remember: Vivien Leigh as Scarlett O'Hara in Gone with the Wind, *and the vegetable that many of us use to garnish salads. Radishes kept Scarlett going, and the substances in them will help your body fight off disease.*

■ **Fighting Cancer**—Researchers working with the National Cancer Institute have found that eating more than one radish a day may keep tumors from developing and cells from mutating. Radishes are a rich source of vitamin C for protection against cancer.

■ **Fighting Heart Disease and Stroke**—Just 1/2 cup of sliced radishes gives you 22 percent of your Daily Value of vitamin C to raise the levels of the important HDL cholesterol that helps keep your arteries clean. HDL levels are often used as an indicator of whether you're likely to suffer a heart attack—the lower the levels, the greater your risk. Vitamin C also helps lower the dangerous LDL cholesterol that clings to artery walls—which, over time, leaves them narrow and easily clogged, increasing the risk of heart attack and stroke.

RAISINS

People have been drying grapes in the sun to make health-protective raisins for more than 3,000 years. Talk about wisdom of the ages!

■ **Fighting Cancer**—A 1/2-cup serving gives you almost a gram of insoluble fiber to help

prevent colon cancer. You also get 11 percent of the Daily Value of copper and more than 9 percent of vitamin B_6 to boost your immune system.

■ **Fighting Heart Disease and Stroke**—Imagine a David and Goliath setup: Little raisins battle big diseases. The winner? The little guys, of course. A 1/2-cup serving of raisins contains more than 544 milligrams of potassium to help keep your blood pressure low. You get additional heart protection from magnesium. Riboflavin and vitamin B_6 gang up on LDL cholesterol and other heart-damaging substances to keep your body healthy.

RASPBERRIES

These delicate berries won't keep for long in the refrigerator, so what are you waiting for? Pop them in your mouth for disease protection.

■ **Fighting Cancer**—Like other berries, raspberries give you a healthy dose of ellagic acid. In the lab, this substance fights cancer of the lung, skin, esophagus, and liver. It may even keep cancerous substances from damaging DNA, the first step in cancer's growth.

One-half cup of raspberries provides more than 1 gram of insoluble fiber to help protect against colon and breast cancer, and more than a quarter of the Daily Value of vitamin C to defend you from cancer of the breast, cervix, esophagus, lung, mouth, pancreas, rectum, and stomach.

■ **Fighting Heart Disease and Stroke**—A healthy dose of vitamin C helps protect your heart by raising your HDL cholesterol levels, thus preventing buildup of plaque in your arteries. It also helps reduce levels of LDL cholesterol and other blood fats that lodge in your arteries. You will also get almost 0.5 gram of soluble fiber to help fight bad cholesterol.

RHUBARB

Talk about a confusing plant. Those stalks that look like pink celery protect you from disease—

but the leaves are poisonous. Most people don't eat the roots, but they were prized for medicinal use in ancient China.

■ **Fighting Cancer**—One-half cup of raw rhubarb has more than 1 gram of dietary fiber to help protect you from colon cancer. You also get some vitamin C that helps lower your risk of cancer of the breast, cervix, esophagus, lung, mouth, pancreas, rectum, and stomach.

■ **Fighting Heart Disease and Stroke**—One-half cup of cooked rhubarb gives you more than 17 percent of your Daily Value of calcium, which may help lower blood pressure and reduce levels of the harmful LDL cholesterol that sticks to your artery walls.

The vitamin C in rhubarb takes care of more than one matter of the heart, as it raises your HDL cholesterol and lowers LDL cholesterol and other blood fat.

RICE

The big question: Is there really a difference between white rice and brown rice? The big answer: Yes.

■ **Fighting Cancer**—Let's do a little math. Copper protects you from cancer because it helps build up your immune system. Eat $1/2$ cup of cooked long-grain brown rice, and you will get 5 percent of the Daily Value. If, instead, you choose white rice, you get 3.5 percent. Brown rice gives you almost 2 grams of total dietary fiber, which protects you from colon cancer. The long-grain white stuff gives you 0.4 gram.

Researchers working with the National Cancer Institute have also found that brown rice neutralizes dangerous substances that play havoc with your system and allow cancer to make inroads.

■ **Fighting Heart Disease and Stroke**—Eat $1/2$ cup of cooked brown rice and get double

protection from vitamin B_6 and magnesium. Both lessen the risk of developing a blood clot, while magnesium also helps to lower blood pressure.

RUTABAGA

If the name of this hearty, healthy vegetable sounds a little foreign to your ear, there's a reason: It comes from a Swedish word that means "round root."

■ **Fighting Cancer**—This round root harbors a lot of protective substances: indoles, isothiocyanates, sulforaphane, and some genistein—cancer fighters all. There are compounds in rutabaga that keep cells from mutating and block the formation of tumors. More than 26 percent of the Daily Value of vitamin C, found in $1/2$ cup of cooked rutabaga, protects you from oral cancer. As a source of vitamin A, rutabaga may help prevent cancerous agents from taking hold in your system.

■ **Fighting Heart Disease and Stroke**—Eat a $1/2$-cup serving of cooked rutabaga and take in more than 26 percent of the Daily Value of vitamin C, which helps lower levels of LDL cholesterol while raising the HDL. More than 277 milligrams of potassium helps keep your blood pressure low. As a source of almost 10 percent of the Daily Value of vitamin A, rutabaga may help keep LDL cholesterol from getting a grip on artery walls.

SALMON

As one of the much-touted sources of omega-3 fatty acids, salmon swims against the current of disease.

■ **Fighting Cancer**—Half of a filet of fresh cooked coho salmon has high levels of vitamin B_6 along with some copper and zinc, which have been shown to heighten cancer-resisting immunity. Salmon has more than 7 percent of the Daily Value for calcium, which helps fight colon cancer.

■ **Fighting Heart Disease and Stroke**— Eating fish once a week will cut your risk of stroke in half, researchers say. Make it salmon, and you get plenty of omega-3 fatty acids, which some studies have associated with the reduced risk of heart attack and stroke.

One 3-ounce serving of fresh cooked coho salmon dishes up almost 387 milligrams of potassium, helping to lower your blood pressure. It provides almost 63 percent of the Daily Value of vitamin B_{12}, one of the important B vitamins that can help to reduce your risk of heart disease by lowering the amount of homocysteine, a substance that activates the clotting system in your blood. Other B vitamins in salmon include riboflavin (more than 8 percent of the Daily Value) and vitamin B_6 (almost 24 percent of the Daily Value). Your body doesn't absorb vitamin B_{12} very well now that you're older, so it's important to make sure that you get a good supply through your diet.

Salmon also gives you magnesium (almost 8 percent of the Daily Value) and a little folate, which, combined with B_{12} and B_6, may lower the homocysteine levels in your blood, to help prevent clogged arteries. Eat salmon and you're going to get calcium, which in some studies has been shown to lower slightly high blood pressure. Get extra calcium by eating canned sockeye salmon, which contains edible chunks of bone.

SARDINES

When you peel back the lid on a can of sardines, you let out a crowd of disease fighters as dense as a school of these small fish.

■ **Fighting Cancer**—That canned cluster of tightly packed fish provides a healthy dose of zinc and copper to help your immune system function at its peak and to neutralize dangerous invaders. From one can of sardines, you get more than 5 percent of the Daily Value of calcium, which may lower your risk of developing colon cancer.

■ **Fighting Heart Disease and Stroke**— The calcium in sardines may help keep your blood pressure and levels of harmful LDL cholesterol down. One can, or about 3 ounces, gives you a heart-helping assortment of the B vitamins that cut down your risk of a heart attack or stroke. It adds up to 137 percent of the Daily Value of vitamin B_{12} and almost 8 percent of the Daily Value of vitamin B_6 to help control clots in the blood vessels.

SEA BASS

Sea bass, or grouper, swim in just about any ocean and include a lot of species, most of which have firm, white, lean meat. One 3-ounce serving contains just over 2 grams of fat.

■ **Fighting Cancer**—The zinc in a serving of sea bass helps protect you against cancer by keeping your immune system strong.

■ **Fighting Heart Disease and Stroke**— One 3-ounce serving of sea bass gives you 650 milligrams of omega-3 fatty acids, which some studies have found to fight cholesterol. You get almost 279 milligrams of potassium to help lower blood pressure. A generous helping of magnesium also works to keep clots from forming and lower blood pressure. As a source of vitamin A, sea bass may elevate the levels of the beneficial HDL cholesterol. It also contains an assortment of the valuable B vitamins, which help reduce your overall risk of heart disease, heart attack, and stroke.

SHALLOTS

Shallots look like a cross between garlic and an onion. So you won't be surprised to find out that they offer just about as much protection as their close relatives.

■ **Fighting Cancer**—In the lab, substances in shallots block and suppress cancer-causing carcinogens. Shallots also contain beta-carotene and are a source of vitamin A, which may keep cancerous agents from invading healthy cells. In one study, beta-carotene is linked to lower rates of lung cancer in nonsmokers. Some scientists believe that they also protect other important organs from cancer invasion.

■ **Fighting Heart Disease and Stroke**— The same vitamin A and beta-carotene that may protect you from cancer could also help your heart. One study found that beta-carotene keeps the harmful LDL cholesterol from oxidizing— the first step in latching onto the walls of your arteries, where it can turn into dangerous plaque that increases your risk of heart attack and stroke.

SOYBEANS

Yes, we're talking about tofu and sprouts. But before you roll your eyes toward the ceiling, consider all of the good things that these foods do.

■ **Fighting Cancer**—Soy products contain genistein, a chemical that attacks cancer the way that a comic-book superhero goes after bad guys. It blocks the formation of blood vessels around new tumors, stops cancer cells from multiplying, and prevents the absorption of tumor-promoting estrogen. In the lab, it keeps breast cancer cells and precancerous prostate cells from growing.

You get protection from other foreign-sounding substances: isoflavones, phytosterols, protease inhibitors, saponins, and phytic acid. The bottom line? Soy helps to keep cancer-causing substances from taking hold in your body, stop cancerous cells from reproducing, and slow down tumor growth. One-half cup of boiled soybeans provides a healthy amount of calcium, 13 percent of the Daily Value, which may protect you from colon cancer.

■ **Fighting Heart Disease and Stroke**— Soybean products give you the same high level of protection from heart disease as they do from cancer. Calcium may help lower your blood pressure and reduce the nasty LDL cholesterol that leads to clogged arteries, heart attacks, and strokes. In 1/2 cup of boiled soybeans, you get almost 14 percent of your Daily Value of magnesium to help keep blood from clotting and gumming up your arteries. Magnesium also helps lower blood pressure. The beans weigh in with 485 milligrams of potassium to help with your blood pressure, too.

Vitamin C in soybeans (more than 25 percent of your Daily Value) helps raise your HDL cholesterol, which keeps fatty deposits from blocking your arteries.

SPINACH

Popeye was no fool. Spinach is low in calories and high on disease prevention.

■ **Fighting Cancer**—Researchers working with the National Cancer Institute note that some of the stuff in spinach keeps cells from mutating. Antioxidants also neutralize the substances that help cancer get started.

One cup of raw spinach (green and tender, not brown and wilted) has more than 27 percent of the Daily Value of folate, which protects you against cancer of the cervix, colon, rectum, lung, and possibly the esophagus. Folate also helps keep cells strong and healthy, so they are better able to fend off a cancerous attack.

Some studies show that the consumption of high levels of vitamin E decreases the levels of prostaglandin E_2, a substance that limits the efficiency of the immune system. Although these studies used supplements, dark green leafy vegetables are a known source of vitamin E.

■ **Fighting Heart Disease and Stroke**— When Popeye fought Bluto, he may have looked as though his blood pressure was about to go through the roof, but the potassium in the spinach he loved probably helped keep his pressure down. Other heart-helping nutrients include vitamin C, magnesium, folate, and vitamin E. Several large studies note that vitamin E can actually slow the development of heart disease by preventing the oxidation of cholesterol and the formation of blood clots. Although these studies used vitamin E supplements, foods that contain vitamin E can always help.

SQUASH

If you just think of winter squash as a decoration for your Thanksgiving table, you're in for a low-calorie, disease-fighting treat. For that matter, summer squash gives you similar protection — just in smaller doses.

■ **Fighting Cancer**—Winter squash—of any shape and color—is rich in beta-carotene, an important antioxidant that may help stop cancer before it gets started. One study found that it provides protection against lung cancer. One serving (about 1/2 cup, cubed) of butternut squash gives you more than 3 milligrams of beta-carotene. The same amount of Hubbard squash dishes out almost 2 milligrams of beta-carotene.

As if that weren't enough, researchers have found that something in squash keeps tumors from developing, but they haven't yet identified the substance with this disease-squashing ability.

■ **Fighting Heart Disease and Stroke**— Acorn squash dishes up heart protection, too. A 1/2-cup serving, baked and cubed, gives you about 18 percent of the Daily Value of vitamin C to maintain high levels of beneficial HDL cholesterol. It also reduces levels of the harmful LDL cholesterol that lodges in your arteries and can lay the groundwork for a heart attack or stroke.

Other nutrients, such as folate, magnesium, and potassium, team up to lower levels of LDL cholesterol, raise levels of protective HDL cholesterol, drop high blood pressure, and keep blood from forming those nasty clots that can lead to heart attacks and strokes.

STRAWBERRIES

"Strawberry fields forever," sang the Beatles when you were young. Strawberries will get your immune system humming, too.

■ **Fighting Cancer**—In one study involving lab animals, researchers discovered that ellagic acid, found in strawberries, fights cancer of the lung, skin, esophagus, and liver. It also decreases the number of tumors in animals. When applied to the skin of animals, it prevents cancer. Ellagic acid seems to keep carcinogens from damaging the DNA of healthy cells. It's even possible that it eats up substances that carcinogens need to go into action inside your body.

Glutathione may help boost your cells' ability to divide, thereby launching a strong counter-attack against cancer. And the best news is that glutathione works best in older folks. You also get 1 gram of insoluble fiber to help protect you from colon and breast cancer.

■ **Fighting Heart Disease and Stroke**— One cup of strawberries gives you 247 milligrams of potassium, keeping your blood pressure down, and 140 percent of the Daily Value of vitamin C, helping to lower your cholesterol. You also get soluble fiber to keep cholesterol low and folate to help reduce homocysteine levels, preventing blood clots. Magnesium in strawberries also helps prevent blood clots and lower blood pressure. Studies show that the pantothenic acid in strawberries may lower cholesterol and triglycerides. And there is riboflavin, which lowers cholesterol.

SWEET POTATOES

Let's get the confusion cleared up: Sweet potatoes and yams are different critters that belong to different families. And, chances are, you have never seen an actual yam. These giants of the vegetable world hail from Africa and Asia, and they can weigh up to 100 pounds. Now, sweet potatoes—that's a whole different story. These vegetables have their roots in the United States and undoubtedly kept more than one family of frontier homesteaders alive. Anytime you go to the grocery store, you're going to come home with sweet potatoes, not yams.

■ **Fighting Cancer**—One 4-ounce baked sweet potato is a source of 249 percent of the Daily Value of vitamin A, which may help protect you against cancer of the mouth. And the bright orange color tells you that beta-carotene is on board. So is almost half the Daily Value of vitamin C, which strengthens your defenses against cancer of the breast, cervix, esophagus, lung, mouth, pancreas, rectum, and stomach. A healthy amount of fiber protects against colon cancer. Researchers working with the National Cancer Institute have also discovered that substances in sweet potatoes actually keep cells from mutating, at least in the laboratory.

■ **Fighting Heart Disease and Stroke**—A common misconception about soluble fiber is that some of the best sources are tasteless and often involve oats. It doesn't have to be that way, since sweet potatoes are an excellent source of cholesterol-fighting soluble fiber. There's also plenty of beta-carotene, which may help shut out the harmful LDL cholesterol that leads to plaque buildup and clotting in the arteries. Vitamin C in sweet potatoes raises HDL levels, which protects you from heart disease. It disarms the harmful LDL and gets rid of triglycerides. Your blood pressure may decline, thanks to a lot of potassium—397 milligrams in a 4-ounce baked sweet potato.

TANGERINES

They're a lot like oranges, but easier to eat. You don't get as much vitamin C in a tangerine as in an orange—although, at 43 percent of the Daily Value, the amount you do get is nothing to sneeze at.

■ **Fighting Cancer**—Substances in tangerines can keep cells from mutating. Other components may keep nitrites in the stomach from being converted into dangerous carcinogens, or strengthen the production of enzymes that make the carcinogens more water-soluble so that the body gets rid of them quickly.

In one tangerine, you also get more than 43 percent of your Daily Value of vitamin C to help prevent cancer of the breast, cervix, esophagus, lung, mouth, pancreas, rectum, and stomach. Its vitamin B_6 beefs up your immune system, and its fiber lowers your risk of colon cancer.

■ **Fighting Heart Disease and Stroke**—Tangerines are a source of vitamin C and vitamin A, which may knock down the levels of the dangerous LDL cholesterol and raise the levels of the valuable HDL. Vitamin C and potassium in tangerines also help lower your blood pressure.

TEA

The American colonists started a war by dumping a load of tea into Boston Harbor. If they had known about its disease-preventing properties, they might have selected something else to throw overboard. Whether you drink green, black, or decaf, tea protects.

■ **Fighting Cancer**—Substances in tea help enzymes neutralize cancer-causing agents and may repair damaged DNA. One study showed that tea drinkers have a lower risk of breast and stomach cancer. In other studies, substances in tea block skin cancer.

■ **Fighting Heart Disease and Stroke—** Drink tea and cut your risk of heart disease: Many varieties of black and green tea (though not herbal teas) are rich in flavonoids, substances that protect your heart and lower your risk of heart disease. In a Dutch study, researchers found that the antioxidant quercetin, found in tea, lowers the risk of stroke by one-third. The effects of tea were reportedly most beneficial to older folks. You get the biggest benefit from bagged tea because the leaves are more thoroughly crushed.

TOMATOES

Until the 1800s, people believed that tomatoes were poisonous. After all, they are related to the nightshade family of plants known for poisonous leaves, berries, flowers, and fruit. But now that we're eating them with gusto, researchers have found that tomatoes protect, whether on a pizza, in a sandwich, or fresh off the vine.

■ **Fighting Cancer—** Substances in tomatoes fight cell mutation. And uncooked tomatoes arm your defenses with glutathione, which may reduce the risk of oral and throat cancer and make your immune system work better. You also get the powerful cancer fighter lycopene in tomatoes. Other substances battle nitrosamines, compounds in our bodies that can lead to cancer.

■ **Fighting Heart Disease and Stroke—** One ripe tomato offers a generous 399 milligrams of potassium to lower blood pressure, and 57 percent of the Daily Value of vitamin C, which helps control bad LDL cholesterol. You also get vitamin B_6, which may help reduce the incidence of blood clots.

TROUT

As game fish, trout have been highly prized for their fighting spirit. As food, they're equally fierce at helping your body fight disease.

■ **Fighting Cancer—** Your immune system gets a boost from trout with 17 percent of the Daily Value of vitamin B_6. A serving of trout also gives you more than 5 percent of the Daily Value of folate, which is known to reduce the risk of developing cancer of the cervix, colon, rectum, lung, and possibly the esophagus.

■ **Fighting Heart Disease and Stroke—** Some researchers have zeroed in on fish as an easy way to help your heart. One study reported that people who eat $2/3$ ounce of any type of fish a day can cut their risk of stroke in half. In a 3-ounce serving of baked trout, you'll also get heart protection from calcium, folate, magnesium, riboflavin, thiamin, vitamin B_{12}, and vitamin B_6. An impressive 375 milligrams of potassium will help to lower mildly high blood pressure.

TUNA

Pop quiz: Name the most popular fish in the U.S. Yes, it's tuna. But not all tuna is equal. Look for fresh bluefin or canned albacore.

■ **Fighting Cancer—** A 3-ounce serving of baked, fresh bluefin tuna is a source of almost 43 percent of the Daily Value of vitamin A, which in some studies has been shown to reduce the risk of cancer. (Compare that figure to just over 1 percent of the Daily Value of vitamin A from the same amount of canned tuna.) You also get more than 22 percent of the Daily Value of vitamin B_6 to build up your immunity—that's 4 milligrams more than the canned tuna. Canned tuna contains about 8 milligrams of copper, however, compared with fresh bluefin's 4.

■ **Fighting Heart Disease and Stroke—** Bluefin tuna provides a rich source of the omega-3 fatty acids that may help lower your cholesterol and protect you from heart disease. Albacore, or white tuna, also gives you a good helping of protection from omega-3's.

A heart-healthy portion of magnesium lowers your blood's tendency to clot and reduces your risk of a heart attack or stroke. Magnesium also lowers blood pressure. The assortment of B vitamins in tuna makes it a champion for heart protection. Three ounces of fresh baked bluefin tuna provide more than 15 percent of the Daily Value of riboflavin, a B vitamin that helps other heart-saving nutrients work harder and more efficiently. Even better, you get more than 154 percent of the Daily Value for vitamin B_{12}, another important heart protector, and 274 milligrams of potassium to help lower your blood pressure.

TURKEY

Ben Franklin had such high regard for the turkey that he wanted to make it the official bird of the United States. We ended up with the eagle on our coins and the turkey on our table, which is good for you, since eating turkey cuts your risk of heart disease, cancer, and stroke.

■ **Fighting Cancer**—A 3-ounce serving of turkey is low in fat (2 grams) and cholesterol (30 milligrams); it's the leanest of all meats. And that's important to reduce your risk of cancer. Plus, turkey gives you more than 8 percent of your Daily Value for zinc, a mineral that's important to your immune system. You also boost your immune system with 9 percent of the Daily Value of vitamin B_6.

■ **Fighting Heart Disease and Stroke**—Turkey provides an assortment of heart-protecting B vitamins: pantothenic acid, riboflavin, vitamin B_{12}, and vitamin B_6. Working together, they lower your risk of heart disease. They increase the HDL cholesterol that protects your arteries from plaque buildup and lower the levels of homocysteine. You'll also benefit from potassium, which protects you from deadly high blood pressure.

TURNIPS

Ever want to step back in history? Eat what the ancients ate? Well, you can do that with turnips, the food of choice in ancient Rome and medieval Europe. And it probably protected as well then as it does today. Don't ignore the leaves—turnip greens protect you, too.

■ **Fighting Cancer**—In the laboratory, substances in turnip greens keep tumors from developing and cells from mutating, meaning that cancers can't get started easily. Chemicals such as indoles, isothiocyanates, and sulforaphane combat carcinogens. Researchers believe that sulforaphane activates an enzyme that removes cancerous agents from your body's cells.

One-half cup of mashed turnips gives you almost 5 grams of insoluble fiber, an important protector against colon cancer.

■ **Fighting Heart Disease and Stroke**—More than 2.5 grams of soluble fiber makes turnips a top pick for heart protection. You also get 22 percent of your Daily Value of vitamin C to help lower levels of harmful LDL cholesterol and raise levels of protective HDL cholesterol.

WALNUTS

You could call them the royal nuts. In ancient Rome, for instance, walnuts were consumed by the nobility and dedicated to the god Jupiter. They're good for us commoners, too.

■ **Fighting Cancer**—Walnuts are rich in ellagic acid. In lab animals, this substance fights cancer of the lung, skin, esophagus, and liver. The same tests determined that it decreases the number of tumors. When ellagic acid was applied to the skin of mice, it kept cancers from forming.

Researchers at Ohio State University believe that ellagic acid keeps cancerous substances from starting the process of DNA damage. It may also neutralize cancer-causing substances before they do damage. These researchers also believe that ellagic acid may actually beat cancerous substances to the punch by sopping up substances they need to grow.

■ **Fighting Heart Disease and Stroke—** Don't like fish but want to get the potential benefits of the omega-3 fatty acids found in fish? Eat English or black walnuts and you may be taking steps to help lower your cholesterol levels and protect your heart. While ⅓ cup of walnuts will load you up with almost 25 grams of fat, the nuts contain no cholesterol. Walnuts also give you folate and vitamin B₆—two vitamins that lower your risk of heart disease. One-third cup of walnuts provides 201 milligrams of potassium to help lower blood pressure.

WATERCRESS

Upon finding this green leafy vegetable in her salad, a character in the 1939 film The Women *exclaimed, "Watercress! I'd just as soon eat my way across a front lawn." Well, obviously she had never tried it or she would have learned to relish the tangy taste. If she had been able to predict the science of the last few years, she would also treasure watercress for its disease-preventing possibilities.*

■ **Fighting Cancer—**Watercress contains one particularly powerful, naturally occurring chemical substance, PEITC (phenethyl-isothiocyanate) that blocks lung cancer in animals exposed to tobacco carcinogens. One-half cup of chopped watercress provides some beta-carotene, which may help protect you from cancer. You also get insoluble fiber, which has been shown to prevent colon cancer.

■ **Fighting Heart Disease and Stroke—** One-half cup of chopped watercress has almost 16 percent of the Daily Value for vitamin A, which may block the harmful LDL cholesterol

that can put you at risk for a heart attack or stroke. Vitamin C in watercress lowers LDL and triglyceride levels, as well as the risk of plaque buildup in your arteries. There's some calcium, too, which may lower blood pressure, and soluble fiber, which fights bad LDL cholesterol.

WATERMELON

Isn't it nice—the watermelon that's such a treat on a hot summer day is also great for disease protection? Beyond nutrients, watermelon gives you a lot of—what else?—water, which is also vital to your health.

■ **Fighting Cancer—**You get a good amount of glutathione from watermelon. Researchers at Emory University in Atlanta found that this substance may function as an anticarcinogen to reduce your risk of oral and throat cancer by up to 50 percent. A lab study at Tufts University in Boston found that glutathione helps white blood cells (in a test tube) fight off invaders. When you consider that people over age 60 have blood levels of glutathione that are about 17 percent lower than people under 40, it's possible that eating more glutathione could make your immune system work as well as that of a much younger person.

■ **Fighting Heart Disease—**One-half cup of watermelon contains more than 12 percent of your Daily Value of vitamin C, helping to lower your levels of harmful LDL cholesterol. You also get vitamin B₆, which helps deactivate your blood's clotting system. Watermelon is also a source of beta-carotene and vitamin A, which some studies show help fight heart disease.

WHEAT GERM

Wheat germ is the part of the wheatberry that is cast off when flour is refined from whole wheat to white. What a waste of such powerful protection from disease.

■ **Fighting Cancer**—Wheat germ gives you vitamin E, which helps to strengthen the T cells that protect you from disease. It also reduces prostaglandin E_2, a substance that interferes with your immune system as you age. People who get a lot of vitamin E also have a lower risk of stomach cancer.

■ **Fighting Heart Disease and Stroke**— Several studies have shown that supplemental vitamin E slows down the progress of heart disease. It helps prevent the oxidation of cholesterol and helps prevent clumping of platelets in blood vessels. These studies used vitamin E supplements, but foods that contain the vitamin are a good bet, too. In people who've had a heart attack, vitamin E helps reduce the risk of another attack.

When you eat $1/4$ cup of toasted wheat germ, you take in 25 percent of the Daily Value of folate. Researchers believe that this nutrient can help prevent heart attacks and strokes because it reduces levels of the amino acid homocysteine, which injures the walls of your arteries. In a study of 536 men, researchers found that those subjects who had the highest levels of homocysteine in their systems had a slightly elevated risk for stroke.

YOGURT

It's really just curdled milk mixed with bacteria. That may not sound so appetizing—until you think about how much good yogurt can do for you.

■ **Fighting Cancer**—A 1-cup serving of plain, low-fat yogurt gives you almost 42 percent of the Daily Value of calcium, which helps guard against colon cancer. You get folate, which protects your DNA's genetic codes so that they're able to divide and replicate properly, keeping cancer at bay. Folate may also protect against cancer of the cervix, colon, rectum, lung, and possibly the esophagus. Yogurt provides more than 13 percent of the Daily Value of zinc, which helps keep your immune system strong.

■ **Fighting Heart Disease and Stroke**— The B vitamins—folate, riboflavin, vitamin B_{12}, and vitamin B_6—protect your heart. People who get a lot of folate and vitamins B_6 and B_{12} in their diets may lower their risk of heart disease by 25 percent. One 8-ounce serving of low-fat yogurt gives you almost 29 percent of the Daily Value of riboflavin, more than 21 percent of vitamin B_{12}, and more than 6 percent of the Daily Value for folate. In addition, its 264 milligrams of potassium helps lower blood pressure.

Your Prescription for Eating the Top 100 Foods

When you get right down to it, your best recipe for the prevention of heart disease, cancer, and stroke—next to quitting smoking, of course—is right in your own kitchen, in foods you can buy cheaply and prepare easily.

Here is what you can do to lower your risk:

DO:

▶ **Eat foods from plants.** Fruits, vegetables, grains, nuts, and seeds have no cholesterol and are high in natural substances that fight disease.

▶ **Eat a variety of healthy foods.** You'll get a wide assortment of protective substances from a diversified diet.

▶ **Emphasize fresh, not processed, foods.** You'll get more nutrients that way.

DON'T:

▶ **Overcook your vegetables.** While some protective compounds are impervious to heat, others are not.

▶ **Overindulge in nuts and other foods that are high in protective substances.** Many are high in calories as well.

5

50 Recipes for Healthy, Quick, Terrific-Tasting Meals

by Linda Gassenheimer

Recipes are usually popular because they're delicious. If they can be ready in a flash, that only adds to their appeal. But there's another important criterion to consider when preparing food—is it healthy? Do the recipes use very little fat and plenty of fruits and vegetables? If so, they can help your body fight the aging process by developing strong defenses against cancer, heart disease, and stroke. Healthy eating keeps your weight down, fights off high blood pressure and diabetes, increases your good HDL cholesterol, and decreases your bad LDL cholesterol. You also get vitamins and other nutrients in the most efficient way your body can absorb them—from a variety of good, fresh food rather than supplements.

Here are more than 50 recipes that are not just good, they are good for you (and a friend—each recipe serves two people). These recipes can be part of a winning strategy in any antiaging campaign, because they're low in fat, high in fiber, and full of nutritious fruits and vegetables. And there's nothing difficult about making these healthy recipes—they were developed by Linda Gassenheimer, an expert food editor who writes a syndicated newspaper column for *The Miami Herald* called "Dinner in Minutes" and gives advice about quick meal preparation on a weekly radio food program. She's also developed eight cookbooks: *Low-Carb Meals in Minutes, More Low-Carb Meals in Minutes, Dinner in Minutes, Mix 'n Match Meals in Minutes for People with Diabetes, Vegetarian Dinner in Minutes, Simply Sauces, Keys Cuisine: Flavors of the Florida Keys,* and *Cooking to Dine: French Cuisine.*

Changing the Way You Cook

Gassenheimer created these recipes to show you how to use foods to open the door to a more healthful lifestyle. But with her kind of low-fat cooking, there's no reason to forego the two other major criteria for better eating: quick preparation and delicious flavor. These recipes are so delectable, any excess fat just won't be missed. And, they cut the time you'll spend in the kitchen. Best of all, they'll show you how to modify your own favorite recipes to fit into a low-fat eating plan that will last a lifetime. It's an easier way to develop the habit of cooking food that's good in more ways than one.

Appetizers

ROASTED RED PEPPER PESTO SPREAD

2 cups canned/jarred roasted red peppers, drained

2 garlic cloves, peeled

1/4 cup sliced almonds

2 tablespoons tomato paste

2 tablespoons olive oil

Salt and freshly ground black pepper

Make sure peppers are well drained. Blot them with a paper towel. With the food processor motor running, add garlic and almonds through the feed tube.

Remove cover, and add peppers, tomato paste, and olive oil. Process until smooth. Add salt and pepper to taste.

Spread the mixture on toasted bread triangles, or serve as a dip with fresh vegetables.

SWEET PEA GUACAMOLE

1 cup frozen peas, defrosted and drained

1 teaspoon ground cumin

1 tablespoon onion, chopped

1 tablespoon lemon juice

1 tablespoon olive oil

Several drops hot pepper sauce

Salt and freshly ground black pepper

Add peas, cumin, and onion to a food processor bowl. Process until smooth. Combine lemon juice and olive oil, and add to the processor. Process until blended, about one minute. Add hot pepper sauce and salt and pepper to taste. Process for a few seconds.

Serve with baked tortilla chips, crackers, or fresh vegetables.

CARAMELIZED ONION CROSTINI

1 tablespoon olive oil

3 cups sweet onion (Vidalia, red, or other), thinly sliced

1/2 cup water

1 large French baguette

Heat oil in a large, nonstick skillet on medium-high. Add onions, and sauté for two minutes. Add water and cover with lid. Cook for 15 minutes or until water evaporates and onions are golden and sweet. Add more water if onions become dry before they are golden. Slice baguette on the diagonal into about eight 1/2-inch slices, and toast. Spread caramelized onions on slices and serve.

STUFFED ENDIVE

1 bunch fresh dill, washed

8 ounces prepared hummus

2 large heads Belgian endive, washed

Mince fresh dill with scissors to make 1/4 cup snipped dill. Keep remainder for garnish. Mix dill with hummus. Carefully remove leaves from endive. Fill wide ends of leaves with one-half to one tablespoon hummus/dill mixture. Arrange stuffed leaves on serving platter, and place small sprig of dill on top of each.

HONEY MUSTARD YOGURT DIP OR DRESSING

1 cup plain, low-fat yogurt, drained* (dip only)

2 tablespoons honey mustard

2 tablespoons sherry wine vinegar

For dip: Mix together all ingredients.

For dressing: Do not drain yogurt. Simply mix all ingredients together.

*To drain yogurt, place it in a sieve lined with three layers of paper towel. Place over a bowl, and let drain several hours or overnight in the refrigerator to thicken.

QUICK SALSA

1 tablespoon red onion, chopped

1 medium tomato, coarsely chopped (1 cup)

¼ cup fresh cilantro, chopped

1 small jalapeño pepper, seeded and
  chopped (1 tablespoon)

½ teaspoon ground cumin

½ teaspoon sugar

1 tablespoon fresh lime juice

Salt and freshly ground black pepper

Mix ingredients together in a food processor. Add salt and pepper to taste.

Use on turkey, meat, or cheese sandwiches—or mix with low-fat mayonnaise or yogurt for salad dressing. You can spoon on small pieces of toast or baguettes and serve as an hors d'oeuvre.

Soups and Casseroles

FAST WINTER CASSEROLE SOUP

3 cups fat-free, low-salt chicken broth

2½ cups canned diced tomatoes, including
  juice

½ pound red potatoes, washed and sliced

1 cup red onion, sliced

1 cup carrots, sliced

1 cup celery stalks, sliced

1 cup white cabbage, sliced

1 cup uncooked fusilli pasta

1 tablespoon ground horseradish

1 tablespoon balsamic vinegar

2 cups fresh, washed spinach

½ cup shredded Swiss cheese (optional)

Salt and freshly ground black pepper

Bring broth, tomatoes, and potatoes to a boil in a large pot on medium-high heat.

Add onion, carrots, and celery. Cover the pot and lower heat to medium. Cook at a slow boil for 15 minutes.

Add cabbage and fusilli. Boil, uncovered, for 10 minutes.

Mix horseradish and vinegar together, and add with spinach to soup. Boil for two minutes, at which point potatoes and pasta will be cooked and spinach will just be wilted.

Add cheese if you wish, and salt and pepper to taste. If desired, serve with warm, crusty bread.

LOW-FAT WINTER STEW

¾ pound low-fat, mild turkey sausage

2 small sweet potatoes (¾ pound)

½ medium onion, sliced (1 cup)

1 medium green pepper, sliced (1 cup)

1 Granny Smith apple, peeled and sliced
  (1½ cups)

2 large tomatoes, sliced (3 cups)

12 ounces beer or ginger ale

1 teaspoon dried thyme

Salt and freshly ground black pepper

2 slices multigrain bread or 2 rolls

Cut sausages into two-inch pieces. Peel sweet potatoes and cut into one-inch cubes.

Sauté sausage, sweet potatoes, onion, and green pepper in a large, nonstick saucepan on medium high for five minutes. Add the apple, tomatoes, beer or ginger ale, and thyme.

Bring to a simmer, cover with a lid and simmer gently for 15 minutes. Add salt and pepper to taste.

While stew simmers, place bread in oven to warm.

ITALIAN PASTA AND BEAN SOUP

$\frac{1}{4}$ cup small pasta (any small size, such as orzo or acini pepi)

12-ounce can reduced-salt tomato soup (not condensed)

1 cup canned small cannellini or navy beans, rinsed and drained

1 medium garlic clove, crushed

Several drops hot pepper sauce

1 tablespoon olive oil

Salt and freshly ground black pepper

2 tablespoons grated fresh Parmesan cheese

Fresh basil leaves, torn into small pieces

Bring a medium-sized saucepan of water to a boil. Add the pasta, and cook eight minutes or according to package instructions.

Meanwhile, place tomato soup, beans, and garlic in another medium-sized saucepan. Bring to a simmer, and cook five minutes.

Drain pasta. Add the cooked pasta, hot pepper sauce, and olive oil to the tomato soup mixture. Add salt and pepper to taste. Ladle into two soup bowls. Sprinkle with Parmesan cheese and basil leaves.

NO-CREAM CREAMY WILD MUSHROOM SOUP

$\frac{1}{2}$ cup water

$\frac{1}{4}$ cup dried cepe or porcini mushrooms

1 tablespoon olive oil

$1\frac{1}{2}$ cups yellow onion, sliced

$2\frac{1}{2}$ cups portobello mushrooms, sliced

$1\frac{1}{2}$ teaspoon flour

14-ounce can fat-free, low-salt chicken broth

$\frac{1}{8}$ teaspoon ground nutmeg

Salt and freshly ground black pepper

Heat water in a microwave or small saucepan. Add the dried mushrooms to the hot water and let stand five minutes. Drain and slice.

Heat the olive oil in a large saucepan over medium-high heat. Add onion, and sauté five minutes. Stir constantly. Do not brown onion.

Add portobello mushrooms and sauté two minutes, stirring one or two times. Sprinkle flour on top and stir until absorbed, one minute. Add chicken broth and reconstituted mushrooms and bring to a boil. Simmer, covered, 10 minutes. Add nutmeg and salt and pepper to taste.

Remove a $\frac{1}{2}$ cup of the soup to a blender or food processor and purée. Return to the soup.

COLD GAZPACHO SOUP

1 cup low-salt tomato juice

1 cup ripe tomatoes, diced, or 1 cup canned tomatoes, drained

$\frac{1}{4}$ cup Vidalia or red onion, diced

$\frac{1}{4}$ cup plus 2 tablespoons peeled cucumber, diced

1 teaspoon curry powder (optional)

Several drops hot pepper sauce

2 teaspoons extra-virgin olive oil

2 teaspoons balsamic vinegar

Place all ingredients—except the two tablespoons of diced cucumber—in the bowl of a food processor or blender. Process until smooth.

Serve with reserved diced cucumber sprinkled on top. The soup can be served immediately—or prepare it up to one day in advance and let the flavors blend together.

WATERCRESS AND ZUCCHINI SOUP

1 teaspoon extra-virgin olive oil

$1\frac{1}{2}$ cups red onion, sliced

$1\frac{1}{2}$ cups zucchini, sliced

2 cups fat-free, low-salt chicken broth

Salt and freshly ground black pepper

1 cup watercress leaves, washed

2 tablespoons chives, snipped

Heat olive oil in a nonstick medium-sized saucepan. Add onion and sauté for three minutes on medium high. Add zucchini and sauté for three additional minutes.

Pour in broth and simmer for 10 minutes. Season with salt and pepper to taste.

Remove from heat, add watercress and purée in a blender until smooth. Cool slightly, store in the refrigerator and serve at room temperature. Sprinkle chives on top before serving.

Salads

ROASTED SALAD GREENS

1 tablespoon olive oil

1 pound radicchio or endive

Roast, grill or pan-sear radicchio or endive in a light coating of oil.

Turn leaves once and cook until lightly browned.

Cooked radicchio goes well with beef. Endive, which soaks up flavor if cooked in liquid, goes well with pork and poultry.

BLACKBERRY AND CHICKEN TOSSED SALAD

$\frac{1}{2}$ cup blackberries

$\frac{1}{2}$ pound salad greens

$\frac{1}{8}$ cup oil-and-vinegar dressing

1 chicken breast, cooked and sliced

Add blackberries to salad greens and toss them with an oil-and-vinegar dressing. Top the salad with cooked chicken slices.

YOGURT CUCUMBER DRESSING

$\frac{1}{2}$ cucumber

1 cup plain, low-fat yogurt

2 medium cloves garlic, crushed

2 tablespoons red onion, chopped

Salt and freshly ground black pepper

Seed and chop cucumber. Drain. Mix all ingredients together.

Serve with grilled meat, chicken, or fish, It can also be served as a sandwich spread, mixed into tuna or chicken salad, or as a dip with crackers or cut vegetables.

STRAWBERRIES WITH GREENS

2 tablespoons fresh basil

1 tablespoon grated Parmesan cheese

$\frac{1}{4}$ cup oil-and-vinegar dressing

$\frac{1}{2}$ pound field greens

1 cup strawberries, quartered

Add basil and Parmesan cheese to the dressing. Purée in a blender or food processor. Toss with field greens and strawberries.

BLACKBERRY RELISH

$\frac{1}{4}$ cup Vidalia onion, diced

2 cups blackberries

3 tablespoons balsamic vinegar

2 tablespoons sugar

Salt and ground black pepper to taste

If using a food processor, coarsely chop the onion to measure $\frac{1}{4}$ cup. Return measured quantity to the processor, and add remaining ingredients.

Or dice onion and berries by hand, and mix with remaining ingredients. Let sit at room temperature for 20 minutes.

Serve over grilled chicken, beef, or pork— or use as a condiment on sandwiches.

CHUNKY STRAWBERRY SALSA

2 cups strawberries, hulled and cut into $\frac{1}{4}$-inch pieces

1½ teaspoon sugar

¼ cup red onion, chopped

1 small jalapeño pepper, seeded and
   chopped (about 1 tablespoon—use
   more jalapeño if you like it spicy)

1 small green pepper, cut into ½-inch
   chunks (about 1 cup)

½ teaspoon ground cumin

2 Tbsp fresh lime juice

¼ cup fresh cilantro, chopped

Salt

Place strawberries in a medium bowl and sprinkle with sugar. Add onion, jalapeño pepper, and green pepper.

Mix cumin and lime juice together, and drizzle over ingredients. Add salt to taste. Toss well and sprinkle with cilantro.

Serve over grilled chicken, beef, or pork, or use as a condiment on sandwiches, or as a dip with baked tortilla chips.

GARDEN-FRESH PASTA SALAD

½ pound uncooked tricolor fusilli or other
   short-cut pasta (about 3 cups)

1 cup pecan pieces

4 scallions, sliced

1 medium cucumber, peeled and cut into
   ½-inch cubes (about 2 cups)

2 cups grape tomatoes

2 cups dried cranberries

4 tablespoons low-fat vinaigrette dressing

Salt and freshly ground black pepper to
   taste

½ cup snipped parsley leaves

Cook pasta according to package instructions.

While pasta boils, toast pecan pieces in a toaster oven or under a broiler for two minutes or until golden. Drain pasta, run cold water over it until cool, and place in a bowl.

Add pecans, scallions, cucumber, tomatoes, cranberries, and dressing to pasta.

Toss well. Add salt and pepper to taste. Sprinkle parsley on top.

BROCCOLI SLAW

2 tablespoons reduced-fat mayonnaise

¼ cup distilled white vinegar

2 teaspoons sugar

Salt and freshly ground black pepper

4 cups ready-to-eat sliced broccoli slaw mix
   (one-half of a 10-ounce bag)

2 cups frozen corn kernels

½ cup mild salsa

Mix mayonnaise, vinegar, and sugar in a medium-size bowl. Add salt and pepper to taste. Add broccoli slaw mix, corn, and salsa.

Toss well. Add more salt and pepper if needed.

ROASTED CHICKEN POTATO SALAD

¾ pound red potatoes (do not peel)

¾ pound roasted chicken breast, boned
   and skinned

½ cup low-fat vinaigrette dressing

½ cup red onion, diced

1 celery stalk, diced

Salt and freshly ground black pepper

½ cup fresh parsley, chopped

½ small head romaine lettuce, washed and
   torn into bite-sized pieces

1 medium tomato, cut into wedges

½ French baguette

Wash potatoes and cut into one-inch chunks. Place in a medium saucepan and cover with cold water. Cover with a lid and boil for about 15 minutes, until potatoes are cooked.

Meanwhile, cut the roasted chicken breast into 1-inch pieces. Place dressing in a large bowl and add chicken, onion, and celery.

When potatoes are cooked, drain and add them, still warm, to the bowl. Toss. Add parsley. Add salt and pepper, if needed.

Place a layer of lettuce on a serving platter. Spoon salad onto lettuce. Place tomatoes around edge. Sprinkle tomatoes with salt and pepper. Serve with baguette.

MEDITERRANEAN COUSCOUS SALAD

2 tablespoons olive oil

½ yellow onion, sliced

¼ medium zucchini, cut into 1-inch cubes (½ cup)

2 medium cloves garlic, crushed

1 cup water

¾ cup uncooked couscous

2 tablespoons low-fat vinaigrette dressing

2 tablespoons orange juice

⅛ teaspoon cayenne pepper

¼ teaspoon ground cinnamon

1 cup fresh strawberries, sliced

¾ cup canned chickpeas, drained

Salt and freshly ground black pepper

¼ cup fresh mint, coarsely chopped

2 tomatoes, cut into quarters

2 pita breads

Heat olive oil in a saucepan on medium-high heat. Add onion, zucchini, and garlic. Sauté five minutes. Add water and bring to a boil. Remove from heat and add couscous. Stir and cover. Let sit five minutes.

Mix vinaigrette dressing, orange juice, cayenne, and cinnamon together in a medium bowl. Add strawberries and chickpeas and toss well. Add couscous mixture and toss well. Add salt and pepper to taste.

Place on plates. Sprinkle mint on top. Arrange tomato quarters on the side. Serve with warm pita bread.

TUSCAN TUNA SALAD

1⅓ cups small, white canned beans (cannellini, navy, or Great Northern), rinsed and drained

3 6½-ounce cans water-packed, solid white tuna, drained (about 3 cups)

2 medium red bell peppers, seeded and diced

1½ cups fresh basil leaves, torn into bite-sized pieces

8 tablespoons olive oil

3 tablespoons balsamic vinegar

Salt and freshly ground black pepper to taste

Place beans, tuna, red pepper, and basil in a salad bowl. Toss with olive oil, vinegar, and salt and pepper.

TOMATO TAPENADE SALAD

2 medium garlic cloves, crushed

2 tablespoons capers, drained

8 green olives, pitted

2 teaspoons balsamic vinegar

2 teaspoons olive oil

2 medium-sized ripe tomatoes

2 tablespoons pecans, chopped

¼ cup Vidalia onion, diced

Place garlic, capers, olives, balsamic vinegar, and olive oil in a food processor until they are finely chopped. Slice tomatoes and place on a serving platter.

Place pecans on a tray in a toaster oven for about one minute…or toast in a dry skillet over medium heat for one or two minutes, until golden brown.

Spoon tapenade on top of tomatoes. Sprinkle Vidalia onion and pecans over tapenade. Add salt and pepper to taste. Serve at room temperature.

Chicken and Turkey

BARBECUED CHICKEN AND PORTOBELLO SANDWICH

4 medium garlic cloves, crushed

½ cup balsamic vinegar

¾ pound boneless, skinless chicken breast

¼ pound whole Portobello mushrooms

2 slices Vidalia onion

4 slices brioche bread (or any egg-based bread)

Olive oil spray

Salt and freshly ground black pepper

Mix garlic and balsamic vinegar in a self-sealing plastic bag. Add chicken and mushrooms. Marinate 15 minutes in the refrigerator, flipping the bag once during that time.

Heat stove-top grill or preheat gas grill. (If using a stove-top grill, spray with olive oil spray.) Remove chicken and mushrooms from marinade. Place on hot grill with onion slices and cook five minutes. Turn chicken, mushrooms, and onion slices, and cook five more minutes.

While the chicken, mushrooms, and onions cook, spray bread with olive oil spray and place on grill for one minute. Turn and grill one minute or until bread is golden. Slice chicken and mushrooms into thin strips, reserving the juices. Arrange on two slices of bread and place onions on top. Pour chicken juices over the top. Add salt and pepper to taste. Cover with the remaining bread slices and cut sandwiches in half.

25-MINUTE CHICKEN POT PIE

2 teaspoons canola oil

1½ cups frozen diced onion

1½ cups frozen diced green pepper

¼ pound baby bella mushrooms, sliced (1¾ cups)

2 tablespoons flour

½ cup fat-free, low-sodium chicken broth

1 tablespoon dried tarragon

1 cup frozen peas

½ cup canned, sliced sweet pimentos

Salt and freshly ground black pepper

¾ pound skinless, boneless chicken or turkey, cooked

1 small package ready-to-cook biscuit dough (6 ounces)

Preheat oven to 400°F. Heat canola oil in a large nonstick skillet on medium-high. Add onion, green pepper, and mushrooms. Sauté for five minutes.

Add flour. Mix it with onion, pepper, and mushrooms. Add chicken broth. Simmer about one minute to thicken.

Mix tarragon, peas, and pimentos into sauce. Add salt and pepper to taste.

Cut chicken into bite-sized pieces and place in a two- to three-inch-deep oven-proof pie dish or a soufflé dish about 8 inches in diameter. Pour sauce over chicken and mix well.

Open the cylinder of biscuit dough and slice each biscuit in half so they will be half as thick. Place them as close together as possible over the top of the pie. Bake for 15 minutes until biscuits have risen and are golden brown.

CHICKEN WITH SPRING HERBS

1 whole chicken breast, boned and skinned

¼ cup freshly chopped mixture of tarragon, chives, scallions, and mushrooms

Salt and freshly ground black pepper

1 pound asparagus, steamed

Make a slit in the chicken breast. Fill it with tarragon, chive, scallion, and mushroom mixture. Brown the chicken breast for two minutes per side. Lower heat, cover, and cook for three minutes—

or until chicken is cooked through. Add salt and pepper to taste. Serve with steamed asparagus.

CHICKEN WITH GARLIC GREENS

1 whole chicken breast, boned and skinned
1 teaspoon balsamic vinegar
1 pound firm lettuce (such as radicchio or romaine)
1 clove garlic, crushed
1 tablespoon olive oil
2 cups rice, cooked
1 pound asparagus, steamed

Sauté chicken breasts six minutes with balsamic vinegar. Set aside. Then sauté garlic and lettuces in the olive oil for a minute. Serve lettuce over chicken with rice and asparagus.

FAST TURKEY MEAT LOAF

Olive oil spray
½ cup onion, thinly sliced
½ cup carrots, thinly sliced
½ cup mushrooms, thinly sliced
¼ cup plain bread crumbs
¾ pound ground white meat turkey
1 egg white
Salt and freshly ground black pepper

Preheat oven to 400°F. Line a baking sheet with aluminum foil and spray with olive oil spray.

Heat a nonstick skillet, and coat with olive oil spray. Add onion, carrots, and mushrooms. Sauté for five minutes.

Mix vegetables with bread crumbs, ground turkey, and egg white. Add salt and pepper to taste.

Divide the ground turkey mixture into two portions, place on baking tray and shape into two loaves about six inches by three inches. Bake for 15 minutes.

CHINESE FIVE-SPICE CHICKEN

6 ounces boneless, skinless chicken thighs, fat removed
1 tablespoon flour
2 tablespoons no-fat, low-salt chicken broth
2 tablespoons Chinese rice vinegar
½ teaspoon Chinese five spice, which can be found in most supermarkets
2 large garlic cloves, peeled
1 tablespoon low-salt soy sauce
2 tablespoons water
1 teaspoon canola oil
¼ cup cucumber, peeled and sliced
¼ cup quick-cooking rice

Dredge chicken thighs in flour. Shake off excess. Mix chicken broth, vinegar, Chinese five spice, garlic cloves, soy sauce, and water together. Heat oil in a wok or skillet until smoking. Brown chicken on all sides, about two minutes. Add sauce and lower heat to medium.

Simmer 12 minutes, turning chicken a few times during this period. Liquid should be just at the bubbling stage. The sauce will boil down to a glaze as the chicken cooks.

Add cucumbers and continue to simmer three minutes. Meanwhile make rice according to package instructions. Serve chicken over rice.

NANTUCKET TURKEY HASH

1 teaspoon olive oil
¾ pound red potatoes (unpeeled), diced
½ medium red onion, diced (1 cup)
1 medium red bell pepper, diced (1 cup)
3½ ounces shiitake mushrooms, diced (1½ cups)
¾ pound cooked turkey (skin removed), diced (2½ cups)
2 tablespoons pine nuts
2 tablespoons white flour
½ cup skim milk or broth

2 tablespoons whipping cream (optional, if using milk)

Salt and freshly ground black pepper

Heat olive oil on medium high in a nonstick skillet. Add potatoes. Sauté 10 minutes, turning potatoes after five minutes. Add onion, red bell pepper, mushrooms, turkey, and pine nuts and sauté 20 minutes, turning them every five minutes. Push ingredients to the sides of the skillet, leaving a hole in the center. Add the flour and then milk or broth. Stir until sauce thickens, and combine with the ingredients to lightly bind the hash together. Add cream and stir again. Add salt and black pepper to taste.

GINGER-CRUSTED CHICKEN

Olive oil cooking spray

¾ pound boneless, skinless chicken breast

¼ cup plain bread crumbs

Salt and freshly ground black pepper

1 egg white

2 teaspoons ground ginger

Preheat oven to 450°F and line a baking sheet with foil. Spray foil with olive oil spray. Remove fat from chicken. Wrap loosely in plastic wrap, and pound with the palm of your hand or the bottom of a skillet until ½-inch thick. Mix bread crumbs with salt and pepper to taste. Break up egg white with a fork and dip chicken into egg white. Sprinkle ginger on both sides of chicken breasts. Roll chicken in bread crumbs, making sure chicken is completely coated. Place chicken on baking sheet and bake 10 minutes.

Serve the chicken with rice and asparagus tips.

SAUTEED CHICKEN AND SWEET POTATOES

½ pound sweet potatoes, peeled and cut into 1-inch cubes

½ cup fat-free, low-salt chicken stock

6 ounces boneless, skinless chicken breast, cut into 1-inch cubes

½ teaspoon curry powder

1 tablespoon Major Grey's mango chutney

1 tablespoon parsley, chopped

Heat a nonstick skillet on medium high and sauté potatoes for one minute. Add half the chicken stock, cover, and sauté for five to eight minutes. Add chicken and sauté for two minutes. Add the remaining chicken stock and curry powder and sauté for three minutes. Add chutney and toss well. Serve with parsley sprinkled on top.

BALSAMIC TURKEY WITH MUSHROOMS AND PINE NUTS

2 teaspoons extra virgin olive oil

1 cup red onion, chopped

2 garlic cloves, crushed

12 ounces turkey breast slices (¼-inch thick)

½ cup balsamic vinegar

¼ cup water

¼ pound button mushrooms, sliced (about 1½ cups)

¼ cup pine nuts (or pecans or walnuts)

2 teaspoons sugar

Salt and freshly ground black pepper

2 cups rice, cooked

Heat olive oil in a nonstick 12-inch skillet on medium heat. Add onion and garlic. Sauté for two minutes. Raise heat to high and add turkey slices. Sauté for one minute. Turn and sauté for another minute.

While each side cooks, add salt and pepper to the other side. Remove turkey and set aside. Add balsamic vinegar and water to the skillet. Reduce liquid for one minute. Add mushrooms, pine nuts, and sugar. Cook for two minutes. Add salt and pepper to taste. Spoon sauce over turkey and serve with rice.

Vegetables and Other Side Dishes

SWEET-AND-SOUR MUSHROOMS

3 ounces (1½ cups) portobello
    mushrooms, cut into chunks

2 tablespoons cornstarch, sifted

1 egg white

1 small green pepper (½ cup sliced)

½ cup canned pineapple chunks, drained

1 small tomato, quartered

1 tablespoon canola oil

½ cup low-salt sweet-and-sour sauce

¼ cup quick-cooking rice

1 scallion, sliced (2 tablespoons)

Toss mushrooms in cornstarch. Separate egg and discard yolk. Break up the egg white with a fork. Add the mushrooms and lightly toss in egg white and in cornstarch again.

Heat canola oil in a wok or skillet until smoking. Stir-fry mushrooms in hot oil for three minutes. Add green peppers and stir-fry two minutes. Add pineapple, tomato, and sweet-and-sour sauce, then toss all vegetables together for one minute. Cook rice according to package instructions. Drain rice and place on individual plates. Then sprinkle scallion over rice. Serve vegetables over rice.

BULGUR WHEAT WITH RAISINS AND PINE NUTS

2 cups fat-free, low-salt chicken broth

1 cup coarse bulgur wheat (cracked wheat)

1 tablespoon olive oil

¼ cup raisins

¼ cup pine nuts

Bring broth to a boil in a medium saucepan. Add bulgur. Lower heat, stir, and cover with a lid. Gently simmer 10 minutes until liquid is absorbed. Remove from heat and let stand, covered, 10 minutes.

Heat olive oil in a nonstick skillet and add raisins and pine nuts. Sauté about one minute, until pine nuts are golden. Toss with cooked bulgur.

ORANGE BARLEY

2 cups fat-free, low-salt chicken broth

1 cup quick-cooking pearl barley

1 tablespoon olive oil

1 cup onion, sliced

½ teaspoon dried thyme

½ teaspoon dried sage

2 tablespoons orange juice

Bring broth to a boil in a medium saucepan and add barley. Boil 10 minutes, uncovered.

Heat olive oil in a nonstick skillet and sauté onion for five minutes. Drain the barley and toss with onion. Add thyme, sage, and orange juice.

PAN-ROASTED ASPARAGUS AND BABY TURNIPS

½ pound fresh asparagus

4 teaspoons olive oil

½ pound baby turnips, peeled and cut into
    1-inch cubes (about 2 cups)

1 medium-sized garlic clove, crushed

Cut or snap off the fibrous stem on the end of each asparagus spear and discard. Slice asparagus into 2-inch pieces (about 2½ cups total).

Heat olive oil in a medium-sized nonstick skillet on medium-high. Add turnips and sauté five minutes, turning to brown all sides. Add asparagus and garlic. Continue to sauté five minutes for thin asparagus, 10 minutes for thicker stalks.

GINGER-SPICED APPLESAUCE

2 Granny Smith apples, cored and cut into eighths

½ cup water

2 tablespoons freshly squeezed lemon juice

2 envelopes sugar substitute

1 or 2 tablespoons fresh ginger, grated

½ teaspoon ground cinnamon

Place the apples and water in a medium saucepan. Cover with a lid and bring to a boil. Cook for 10 minutes. (To prepare in a microwave: Place the apples and water in a microwave-safe bowl. Cover and cook on high for five minutes. Let stand three minutes.)

Place the cooked apples and water in the bowl of a food processor. Add lemon juice and sugar substitute. Grate the ginger over the bowl, making sure to catch any ginger juice. Process until thoroughly mixed. Spoon into two dessert bowls and sprinkle with cinnamon.

Pasta and Pizza

SWEET ONION PASTA

Olive oil spray

1 medium Vidalia onion, sliced (2 cups)

½ pound sugar snap peas, trimmed (about 2½ cups)

2 medium cloves garlic, crushed

2 tablespoons pine nuts

¼ pound uncooked rotelle or fusilli pasta (about 1½ cups)

2 teaspoons olive oil

1 tablespoon tomato paste

Salt and freshly ground black pepper

Bring three to four quarts of water to a boil in a large pot.

While the water comes to a boil, heat a large nonstick skillet on medium-high and spray with olive oil spray. Sauté onions for five minutes—do not brown. Add sugar snap peas, garlic, and pine nuts. Sauté another five minutes. Remove from heat and spoon into a large bowl.

Meanwhile, cook pasta for about 10 minutes. Remove ¼ cup pasta water, and mix with olive oil and tomato paste. Set aside. Drain pasta and add to bowl with onion mixture. Pour tomato mixture over pasta and toss well. Add salt and pepper to taste.

MACARONI PIE

⅔ cup small elbow macaroni

Olive oil spray

¼ medium yellow onion, grated (½ cup)

½ medium green bell pepper, grated (½ cup)

½ cup fat-free ricotta cheese

2 ounces shredded sharp cheddar cheese (½ cup), divided

Several drops hot pepper sauce

Salt and freshly ground black pepper

Heat a large pot containing two to three quarts of water. When water boils, add macaroni and boil for 10 minutes.

Meanwhile, spray a nonstick skillet and sauté onion and green pepper for five minutes. Remove from heat.

Combine ricotta and 1 ounce of the cheddar cheese in a bowl. Add hot pepper sauce and mix in onion and green pepper. Drain macaroni and add to cheese mixture. Add salt and pepper to taste.

Return to skillet and sprinkle remaining cheddar evenly over the top. Cover with a lid, and heat on medium for 10 additional minutes.

PEPPER, MUSHROOM, & ONION PIZZA

1 medium-sized onion (1 cup sliced)

1 small green pepper (1 cup sliced)

1 small red pepper (1 cup sliced)

1½ cups water

10 medium-sized mushrooms (2 cups sliced)

2 tablespoons olive oil and olive oil spray

2 large or 4 small pizza bases (ready-to-bake prepared dough)

8 ounces pizza sauce

1 cup grated Parmesan cheese

Preheat oven to 400°F. Add the onion, peppers, and 1½ cups water to a hot nonstick skillet. Simmer for about 10 minutes—or until onions are golden, not black. Add mushrooms and sauté three minutes. Toss cooked vegetables with olive oil.

Line baking tray with foil and spray with olive oil spray. Place pizza bases on the tray, and spoon sauce over each pizza base. Sprinkle onions, peppers, and mushrooms evenly on top. Sprinkle Parmesan over the top. Spray the pizza with olive oil spray. Place pizza in hot oven for five minutes.

PENNE PUTTANESCA

1 cup bottled marinara sauce

½ pound chicken breast, cut in 1-inch cubes

1 medium garlic clove, chopped

1 tablespoon capers, drained

¼ cup pitted olives, sliced

2 cups penne pasta, cooked

½ cup grated Parmesan cheese

Heat marinara sauce in a nonstick skillet. Add chicken cubes, garlic, capers, and olives. Simmer until chicken cubes are cooked through—about four to five minutes. Toss with penne pasta and sprinkle with Parmesan cheese.

FAST HOMEMADE PIZZA TOPPINGS

Olive oil spray

2 to 4 pizza bases (ready-to-bake prepared dough), or slices of Italian bread, or English muffins

Pizza toppings (as shown below)

Heat the oven to 400°F. Spray pizza base, Italian bread, or English muffin with olive oil spray. Add one of the topping combinations below and place in oven for five minutes.

California pizza. Goat cheese, sun-dried tomatoes, and smoked turkey on top of a bed of sliced yellow tomatoes.

Mixed pepper pizza. Yellow, red, and green peppers sautéed with diced chopped tomatoes. Sprinkle with shaved Parmesan curls.

Sicilian pizza. Tomato, oregano, black olives, anchovies, garlic, mozzarella, and ham.

Southwestern pizza. Cooked corn, black beans, Monterey jack cheese, jalapeño peppers, and ground sirloin flavored with chili powder. (Broil five minutes or until meat is cooked.)

Spanish roasted pepper pizza. Turkey sausage, roasted peppers, green olives, Manchego cheese, and tomato sauce. (Broil five minutes or until sausage is cooked.)

Spring pizza. Vidalia onion, mushrooms, diced tomatoes, and shredded mozzarella.

Tuscan pizza. Grilled chicken, pine nuts, wild mushrooms, basil, tomato sauce, and olive oil.

PASTA PRIMAVERA

Any combination of vegetables can be used. The list of ingredients is per person.

1 teaspoon olive oil

4 peeled baby carrots, sliced

4 broccoli florets, cut in half

½ cup zucchini, sliced

2 tablespoons fresh or frozen diced onion

1 medium clove garlic

1 cup bottled pasta sauce (low fat/low salt)

1 tablespoon light cream (optional)

Salt and freshly ground pepper

1 sourdough roll or 2 slices Italian bread

¼ pound fresh linguine

1 tablespoon grated Parmesan cheese

1 tablespoon fresh basil

Heat a large pot of water to boil. Preheat the oven to 350°F. Heat olive oil in a small nonstick skillet. Add baby carrots, broccoli florets, zucchini, onion, and garlic to pan. Sauté for five minutes. Add sauce.

Bring to a simmer, cover, and cook for five minutes. Add cream and salt and pepper to taste. Place bread or roll in oven to heat.

Add linguine to boiling water. Boil according to package directions. Drain and place in bowl. Add sauce and toss well. Remove bread from oven.

Sprinkle Parmesan on linguine. Tear basil into pieces and sprinkle on top.

Fish and Seafood

GINGER-SOY STEAMED FISH WITH CHINESE NOODLES

2 tablespoons low-salt soy sauce

1 scallion, sliced (2 tablespoons)

½ tablespoon fresh ginger, chopped

1½ teaspoons canola oil

6 ounces fish fillet (any light non-oily fish such as snapper, cod, grouper, flounder, or sole)

Small head bok choy or romaine lettuce, leaves washed

¼ pound steamed or fresh Chinese noodles, which can be found in the supermarket produce section

Mix soy sauce, scallion, ginger, and oil together. Pour half over fish and marinate five minutes. Reserve remaining sauce.

Meanwhile, place water in steamer bottom or saucepan large enough to hold steaming basket, and bring to a boil. Spread noodles over base of basket and place bok choy leaves on noodles.

Put marinated fish on leaves. Place basket over boiling water and cover. Steam for about eight minutes.

To serve, place fish on plate with the noodles and bok choy beside it. Pour remaining sauce over noodles and bok choy.

BAHAMIAN DELIGHT SPICY SHRIMP

(Ingredients listed are per person.)

6 ounces large shrimp

2 teaspoons butter or olive oil

½ cup yellow onion, sliced

¼ cup tomato paste

½ cup water

1 tablespoon fresh thyme

¼ or ⅛ teaspoon crushed red pepper

½ teaspoon sugar

¼ cup quick-cooking rice

Salt and freshly ground pepper

½ cup canned pigeon peas or frozen green peas

1 teaspoon butter or olive oil

Shell and devein shrimp. Cut into half-inch pieces. Heat one teaspoon butter or olive oil in a small nonstick skillet. Sauté onion, without browning, for about five minutes.

Mix tomato paste with ½ cup water and add to the skillet with shrimp, thyme, and red pepper. Simmer for five minutes. Sprinkle sugar over mixture. Salt and pepper to taste.

Make rice according to package instructions. Add peas to the rice one minute before the end of the rice's cooking period. Toss with butter or olive oil, salt and pepper to taste.

Serve shrimp over rice and peas.

SALSA SNAPPER WITH LINGUINE

Vegetable oil spray
6 ounces of snapper or other light fish fillet
1 cup any type of salsa
½ pound linguine
½ teaspoon olive oil
Salt and freshly ground black pepper

Heat oven to 400°F. Place a large pot of water on to boil. Line baking tray with foil and spray with vegetable oil. Place the fish on the tray and spoon ½ cup of salsa over each fillet. Bake for 10 minutes.

Meanwhile, boil linguine for seven minutes. Drain, leaving a little water on pasta. Return pasta to the cooking pot. Toss with olive oil and salt and pepper to taste. Serve the fish over the pasta.

BALSAMIC SWORDFISH WITH DILLED RED POTATOES

2 tablespoons balsamic vinegar
¼ cup fresh cilantro, chopped
2 cloves garlic, crushed
10 ounces swordfish steak
1 pound baby red potatoes (do not peel)
1 tablespoon butter or margarine
1 teaspoon fresh or dried dill
Salt and freshly ground black pepper
¼ pound asparagus or broccoli

Mix balsamic vinegar, cilantro, and garlic in a self-sealing bag. Add the swordfish steaks and seal. Marinate in the refrigerator for 15 minutes.

Discard the marinade. Broil or grill the swordfish 10 minutes per inch of thickness.

Wash and boil the red potatoes about 20 minutes or until soft. Mix with butter or margarine, dill, and salt and pepper.

Microwave asparagus or broccoli in ¼ cup water for two to three minutes on high, or boil five minutes or until tender.

Serve vegetables alongside the fish.

GRILLED SALMON WITH GREEK CUCUMBER SAUCE

¼ cucumber, peeled and seeded
½ cup plain nonfat yogurt
1 clove garlic, crushed
2 teaspoons fresh dill—or ½ teaspoon dried
1 tablespoon red onion, chopped
½ teaspoon fresh lemon juice
Salt and freshly ground black pepper
10 ounces salmon steak

Chop the cucumber and drain. Mix with yogurt, garlic, dill, onion, and lemon juice. Add salt and pepper to taste.

Grill the fish in the broiler or over hot coals. Serve with a dollop of the cucumber sauce.

BOILED SHRIMP WITH SPICY HORSERADISH SAUCE

¼ cup nonfat or low-fat mayonnaise
½ tablespoon horseradish
1 teaspoon fresh lemon juice
½ teaspoon sugar
½ tablespoon Dijon mustard
2 teaspoons seeded, chopped jalapeño pepper
10 ounces jumbo shrimp, shelled and deveined

Mix ingredients in a medium-sized bowl. Taste for seasoning, and add more lemon juice or pepper to taste.

Boil shrimp in 4 cups water. Drain and cool. Serve with sauce on the side.

Breakfast

OATMEAL—3 VERSIONS

Oatmeal Base

⅓ cup oats (quick or old-fashioned)

½ cup skim milk

Place in a microwave-safe bowl and microwave on high for three minutes.

Add any one of the following combinations:

Banana-Maple

1 small ripe banana, sliced

½ tablespoon maple syrup

2 tablespoons walnut pieces (toasted in a toaster oven for one minute)

Pear-Ginger

1 small ripe pear, cored and cut into cubes

2 tablespoons crystallized ginger, cut into small pieces

Fig-Apricot

⅓ cup dried figs, cut into small pieces

1 tablespoon apricot jam

Cook oats and skim milk in a microwave oven on high for two minutes. Add figs and cook for one additional minute. Remove from microwave and stir in apricot jam.

TOASTED WALNUT OATMEAL

1 cup oatmeal

2 cups water

¼ cup walnuts

1 cup skim milk

2 envelopes sugar substitute (optional)

Combine oatmeal and water in a microwave-safe bowl. Microwave on high for four minutes. (To prepare on the stovetop: Combine oatmeal and water in a small saucepan over medium-high heat and bring to a boil. Reduce heat to medium. Cook about five more minutes, stirring occasionally.)

Place walnuts on a foil-lined tray and toast in toaster oven for one minute. Stir milk, sugar substitute, and walnuts into oatmeal. Divide between two bowls and serve warm.

BANANA STRAWBERRY SHAKE

1 peeled frozen banana, cut into 2-inch pieces

1 cup frozen strawberries (not packed in sugar syrup)

1 cup skim milk

2 teaspoons honey

4 tablespoons whey protein powder, plain or vanilla flavor (in health food stores)

Place ingredients in a blender, and mix until smooth, about 45 seconds. If too thick, add more milk to taste.

(Keep different types of frozen and/or fresh fruit on hand, and mix and match as you please. Ripe fruit brings out the most flavor.)

PEACH SMOOTHIE

2 medium-size ripe peaches, pitted and cut into large cubes (about 2 cups)

1 cup light peach yogurt

1 teaspoon almond extract

2 teaspoons sugar

4 cups ice cubes

Place peaches, yogurt, almond extract, and sugar in a blender. Blend until smooth. Add the ice cubes and blend until thick.

6

How Supplements Help You Stay Youthful

Stroll down the vitamin and supplement aisle at your local supermarket, drugstore, or health food store. You'll find neat rows of vitamins, minerals, and herbs, their contents measured in RDAs, DVs, IUs, milligrams, and micrograms. But sorting through all this stuff can be daunting. The names and numbers are all there, but how do you concoct a regimen that can reduce your risk of heart disease, cancer, and stroke?

Is Taking Supplements Really Worthwhile?

Some studies suggest that specific vitamin and mineral supplements can help reduce your risk of heart disease by 30 to 40 percent and even slow the disease's progress," says Jeffrey Blumberg, M.D., associate director and chief of the Antioxidants Research Laboratory at the U.S. Department of Agriculture Human Nutrition Research Center on Aging in Boston. Such a protective regimen involves nothing fancier than over-the-counter supplements. They're relatively inexpensive, and some of them may go a long way toward cutting high blood pressure and stopping the blood clots that lead to strokes.

Vitamins can also boost the immune system, which is important in battling cancer cells. "Older people who take vitamin and mineral supplements have stronger immune systems," says John Bogden, Ph.D., professor of preventive medicine and community health at the New Jersey Medical School in Newark. "Generally, the immune system starts to decline around age 50 and may already be compromised by age 60." If your immune system can't protect you, the door is wide open for cancer and other diseases to come in.

But it doesn't have to be this way. When researchers in Italy looked at healthy 100-year-olds, they made a surprising discovery—immune systems so strong that they could easily have belonged to people 80 years younger. "That's probably why these people got to be 100-plus. Their immune systems never deteriorated," says Dr. Bogden.

Supplements will help strengthen your immune system, but they don't work miracles. "While supplements are cheap, easy to take, and—in many cases—beneficial, they're not magic bullets," says Dr. Blumberg. "They're supplements, not substitutes for healthy eating." That means you can't do

Don't Damage Your Nutrition

Besides the specific foods you eat, the kind of life you lead will determine your nutritional needs. Here's how your lifestyle may cause damage that can require more than the average amount of some vitamins and minerals:

Sun damage. If you're retired and spend your days at the pool, in the garden, or on the tennis court, you probably need a supplement. Sunlight gives you beneficial vitamin D, but it also promotes cell damage. Your body's supply of protective antioxidants gets used up fast, notes Richard Cutler, Ph.D., president, chief executive officer, and scientific research director at Genox in Baltimore. One study showed that ultraviolet light lowered antioxidant levels. When test subjects spent 15 minutes a day under solar lamps for a two-week period, their infection-fighting T cells became less active, a sign that their immune systems weren't working as well.

Smoke damage. Cigarette smoking exposes you to millions of harmful free radicals, lead, mercury, and radioactive materials. As your body battles these invaders, you may end up with lower levels of key protective vitamins. One study showed that a smoker needs 250 milligrams of vitamin C to have a blood level comparable with that of a nonsmoker getting the Daily Value of 60 milligrams. Although you may reduce the risk by taking a multivitamin and additional supplements of vitamin C, vitamin E, and beta-carotene, the best thing to do is to quit smoking altogether, says Jeffrey Blumberg, M.D., associate director and chief of the Antioxidants Research Laboratory at the U.S. Department of Agriculture Human Nutrition Research Center on Aging in Boston.

Stress damage. You'll probably need extra vitamins and minerals if you drink even moderately, or if you exercise intensely, says Dr. Blumberg. Medical problems also cause increased stress, especially: irritable bowel syndrome, chronic diarrhea, constipation, yeast infection, surgery, radiation, chronic stress, and overuse of prescription drugs.

the bacon-and-eggs, burgers-and-fries routine, pop a pill, and think that everything will be fine. Still, researchers estimate that up to one-third of older adults may not be getting enough important vitamins and minerals through diet alone.

How Supplements Prevent Disease

You'll benefit from a vitamin supplement if you are over 55, although your system may not really register the improvement for six months to a year. That's not an excuse to procrastinate. As you get older, getting the nutrients that you need—through a combination of diet and supplements—becomes an increasingly important way to shore up your body's defenses, says Dr. Bogden.

Here's how a supplement can help:

■ **Lowering the risk of low-cal eating.** It's a catch-22: Take in too many calories and you gain weight, increasing your risk of cancer, heart disease, and stroke. But if you cut calories to lose weight or maintain your current weight, you may end up low on vitamins and minerals. So you are still at high risk, especially if you make poor food choices. But Dr. Bogden says you can replace key vitamins and minerals lost in dieting through carefully chosen supplements.

Dietitians at Utah State University tried to create balanced diets of less than 2,200 calories—probably close to the number of calories you take in. They found it nearly impossible to

What About an Antioxidant Supplement?

I recommend that older people take an antioxidant formula, in addition to a multiple vitamin," says James Goodwin, M.D., director of the Center on Aging at the University of Texas Medical Branch in Galveston. "Pick one with around 200 international units of vitamin E, 250 milligrams of vitamin C, and 30 milligrams or so of beta-carotene, plus 70 to 100 micrograms of selenium. That should give most people all the protection they need," he says. Since most multivitamins contain only 200 milligrams of calcium, you'll need an additional supplement for calcium.

do that and meet the recommended daily amount of important vitamins and minerals.

■ **Compensating as systems slow down.** As you get older, a lot of your body's systems work less efficiently. The right supplements help you compensate for the slowdown. For instance, you don't have as much of the stomach acid that helps you get nutrients from your food. That means that up to 40 percent of the nutrients you take in may go unused. You're likely to be low in such protective components as vitamins D, B_6, and B_{12} as well as riboflavin, folate (the natural form of the supplement folic acid), and calcium.

Your body's system for storing the nutrients that you take in isn't what it used to be either. That's because your percentage of body fat increases with age, notes Sharon Miller, Ph.D., associate dean of the College of Health and Human Sciences at Northern Illinois University in DeKalb.

■ **Flushing out by-products that promote aging.** "The body's metabolism keeps you alive and healthy, but it also produces harmful by-products. It's very much like the fire that gives you warmth—along with the unpleasant smoke," says Richard Cutler, Ph.D., president, chief executive officer, and scientific research director at Genox in Baltimore, where he specializes in antioxidant research. The

body's "smoke" includes free radicals and other compounds that damage the cells' DNA and lead to many of the effects of old age.

Your body makes antioxidants to fight off these harmful substances. As you get older, the production levels of antioxidants drop, probably because your metabolism slows down. It becomes harder and harder to get enough antioxidant protection from food alone. Supplements can make big contributions to the cause.

Warning: Although you can get most of the nutrients you need from a multivitamin, Dr. Blumberg suggests you might want to take extra supplements of certain vitamins and minerals to promote optimum health. However, he cautions that you should always keep your doses within the recommended range—some vitamins and minerals are toxic when taken in large doses. It's a good idea to consult your physician about any supplements you're considering—he/she can determine the specific nutrients you need and in what amount, and can ensure that supplementation will not interfere with any other medication or treatment he has prescribed.

As a general rule, do not exceed published Daily Values (DV), which are the U.S. government's general guidelines for basic daily nutritional needs. Some recommendations for protection offered by the experts who were interviewed for this chapter may exceed the DVs, so be sure to check with your doctor.

Monitor Your Medications

If you take medication, especially any of those listed below, ask your doctor whether you ought to take supplements. Some vitamins and minerals can interfere with your body's ability to use certain medicines, says Jeffrey Blumberg, M.D., associate director and chief of the Antioxidants Research Laboratory at U.S. Department of Agriculture Human Nutrition Research Center on Aging in Boston. The clash can work in reverse, too. Some drugs, such as alcohol, as well as other medications, may make vitamins pass through your system more quickly than they should—or make them stick around too long.

Drug	Interferes with
Alcohol	Folic acid, Niacin, Thiamin, Vitamin B_6, Zinc
Aluminum hydroxide (antacids)	Vitamin A, Calcium, Phosphate
Amphetamines	Vitamin C
Anticonvulsants	Folic acid, Vitamin D, Calcium
Antidepressants	Vitamin C
Antihypertensives (treat high blood pressure)	All nutrients
Calcitonin (treats Paget's disease)	Calcium
Chelating agents (treat metal poisoning)	Vitamin B_6
Cholestyramine (reduces cholesterol)	Folic acid, Vitamin A, Vitamin B_{12}, Vitamin D, Vitamin E, Vitamin K, Calcium
Colchicine (treats gout)	Vitamin B_{12}
Corticosteroids (steroids such as cortisone)	Calcium
Cycloserine (fights tuberculosis)	Vitamin B_6, Estrogen, Folic acid, Calcium
Hydralazine (fights high blood pressure)	Vitamin B_6
Isoniazid (prevents and treats tuberculosis)	Vitamin B_6
Laxatives containing phosphate	Calcium
Levodopa or L-DOPA (treats Parkinson's disease)	Vitamin B_6
Methotrexate (treats psoriasis, rheumatoid arthritis)	Folic acid, Vitamin B_{12}
Mineral oil (a component of many drugs)	Vitamin A, Vitamin D, Vitamin E, Calcium, Phosphorus
Neomycin (treats infections)	Vitamin B_6, Vitamin B_{12}, Iron
Phenobarbital (relieves anxiety and tension)	Folic acid, Vitamin B_6, Vitamin B_{12}, Vitamin D
Phenytoin (prevents seizures)	Folic acid, Vitamin B_6, Vitamin D
Sulfasalazine (treats inflammatory bowel disease)	Folic acid
Sulfonamides (antibiotics)	Vitamin C
Tetracycline	Calcium
Theophylline (treats bronchial asthma, emphysema)	Vitamin B_6
Triamterene (diuretic)	Folic acid, Potassium
Warfarin (anticoagulant)	Vitamin A, Vitamin E, Vitamin K

The Must-Have Micronutrients

Some researchers think that deficiencies in the diet pave the way for heart disease, stroke, and cancer. Many experts believe that an extra dose of key vitamins and minerals—often difficult to get through diet alone—provides maximum protection from this trio of killers.

Here are the major vitamins and minerals that can help protect you:

VITAMIN A/BETA-CAROTENE

Daily Values:
> Vitamin A—5,000 international units
> Beta-carotene—no Daily Value

Experts recommend:
> Vitamin A—5,000 international units
> Beta-carotene—6–20 milligrams

Is a multivitamin likely to contain enough?
> Vitamin A, yes.
> Beta-carotene, no.

Multivitamins may contain vitamin A, beta-carotene, or a combination of the two. To the body, beta-carotene and vitamin A are one and the same. But experts note that it's safer to take beta-carotene. That's because the body stores this substance and converts it into vitamin A whenever it needs it. If you take vitamin A, it stays in the system, where an excess can cause damage to your liver. With beta-carotene, you will know if you take too much—it will turn your skin orange.

You can get the recommended levels by adjusting your diet instead of taking a supplement. "You can get the equivalent of the Daily Value of vitamin A just by eating a carrot a day," says James Goodwin, M.D., director of the Center on Aging at the University of Texas Medical Branch in Galveston.

Here's how vitamin A and beta-carotene protect you:

■ **Fighting Heart Disease**—Beta-carotene keeps the harmful low-density lipoprotein (LDL) cholesterol from getting a grip on artery walls. In the Harvard Physicians' Health Study, doctors with heart disease took 50 milligrams of beta-carotene on alternate days for six years—and had half as many fatal heart attacks and angioplasties as doctors who didn't supplement their diets.

■ **Fighting Stroke**—The Harvard study also showed that the doctors who took beta-carotene had half as many strokes over the six-year period.

■ **Fighting Cancer**—Vitamin A contributes to the body's first line of defense against bacteria and viruses by maintaining the protective mucous membranes that line the digestive, respiratory, urinary, and reproductive tracts. It also produces the bacteria-fighting chemicals in tears, saliva, and sweat.

In one study, smokers with precancerous oral lesions took 30 milligrams of beta-carotene for eight weeks. Seventy percent of their lesions stopped growing or actually got smaller.

In a study conducted in Linxian, China, the diets of 30,000 people aged 40 to 69 were supplemented with either a placebo or different combinations of vitamins and minerals in doses that were one to two times higher than the U.S. Recommended Dietary Allowances. After five years of daily supplementation, those taking a combination of beta-carotene, vitamin E, and selenium had cancer death rates 13 percent lower than other study subjects.

Warning: Take a vitamin A/beta-carotene supplement with a meal or snack. Because it's a fat-soluble nutrient, it needs a little fat to get into your system.

THE B VITAMINS

Daily Values:

Vitamin B_6—2 milligrams

Vitamin B_{12}—6 micrograms

Folic acid—400 micrograms

Niacin—20 milligrams

Riboflavin—1.7 milligrams

Pantothenic acid—10 milligrams

Experts recommend:

Vitamin B_6—2–10 milligrams

Vitamin B_{12}—2–10 micrograms

Folic acid—400–800 micrograms

> (*Note:* Some experts maintain that 400 or more micrograms of folic acid can interfere with your body's ability to use zinc.)

Niacin—20 milligrams

Riboflavin—1.7 milligrams

Pantothenic acid—10 milligrams

Is a multivitamin likely to contain enough?

Yes.

Getting older usually means ending up with lower levels of the protective B vitamins. It just becomes harder for the body to get them in and use them. If you're a vegetarian, you're probably particularly low on vitamin B_{12}, since it's found primarily in animal products.

Here's how B vitamins work for you:

■ **Fighting Heart Disease**—"We see evidence that folic acid and vitamins B_6 and B_{12} reduce heart disease by 10 to 25 percent, and since heart disease is a major disease of aging, it's important that older people get enough," says Dr. Blumberg.

Low levels of the B vitamins could saddle you with high blood levels of homocysteine, increasing your risk for heart disease and heart attack. "The relationship of high homocysteine levels to low levels of the B vitamins, particularly folic acid, is quite clear," says Dr. Blumberg. Homocysteine is also poisonous to your cells.

Riboflavin powers up folic acid and vitamin B_6. Niacin probably protects against heart disease, but experts caution against taking more than the Daily Value. In experiments, very high amounts of niacin raise the levels of beneficial high-density lipoprotein (HDL) cholesterol, but they can also cause liver damage and worsen stomach ulcers, diabetes, and arthritis.

■ **Fighting Cancer**—Studies of older adults show that low levels of vitamin B_6 depress the immune system. Fortunately, the system gets back in gear when it gets more B_6.

The high levels of folic acid can protect you against cervical and colon cancer, possibly by normalizing both tissue growth and the production of DNA (your cells' genetic material).

Warning: Don't exceed recommended levels. Megadoses of vitamin B_6 can cause nerve damage.

VITAMIN C

Daily Value:

60 milligrams

Experts recommend:

250–1,000 milligrams

Is a multivitamin likely to contain enough?

No.

Some researchers believe that the added boost from vitamin C supplements can give men six more years of life and women an additional two years. You can get protective levels of vitamin C from either foods or supplements. One 8-ounce glass of orange juice, for example, contains 100 milligrams.

Studies show that as you get older you absorb vitamin C less easily. To counteract this, Dr. Blumberg says that it is advisable to take vitamin

Supplement the Smart Way

The better the immune system works, the longer you live. "Older people who take a quality over-the-counter multivitamin show improved immune systems," says John Bogden, Ph.D., professor of preventive medicine and community health at the New Jersey Medical School in Newark. "Diet plus a supplement seems the best protection."

When you shop for a multivitamin, choose one with close to the Daily Value of copper, because it's a key nutrient for the immune system. Pick one with an equal percentage of zinc to make sure that you get the benefit of the copper, advises Dr. Bogden.

"Stick with the major brands," says Richard Cutler, Ph.D., president, chief executive officer, and scientific research director at Genox in Baltimore, who works extensively with antioxidants. Once you choose a multivitamin, here's how to get the most out of it:

Time it yourself. Avoid multivitamins with time-release formulas. They may release nutrients far down the intestinal tract, where absorption is poor. A better approach is to divide the dose so that you take in nutrients several times a day, says Dr. Bogden.

Store it safely. Some experts suggest storing multivitamins with your herbs and spices. Keep the bottle away from hot or humid places, suggests Dr. Bogden. That means not in the bathroom, not on a sunny windowsill, and definitely not near the sink or stove.

Take it with a meal. Some nutrients are only released with fat. Jeffrey Blumberg, M.D., associate director and chief of the Antioxidants Research Laboratory at the U.S. Department of Agriculture Human Nutrition Research Center on Aging in Boston, says that you need to take in some dietary fat with your multivitamin to get the benefits of key protectors. But there is no need to make a special effort to consume fat, explains Dr. Blumberg. You would get a sufficient amount of fat from a low-fat meal.

Check the expiration date. Buying a bucket-size container of vitamins may not be the bargain it first seemed. Make sure that you have time to use the entire bottle before the product's expiration date. Otherwise, those vitamins may lose their punch, notes Dr. Bogden.

C at doses higher than the Daily Value. Men probably need at least 125 milligrams a day and women around 75 to 80 milligrams a day.

Here's how vitamin C protects you from health problems:

■ **Fighting Heart Disease**—High levels of vitamin C in your system tend to accompany high levels of beneficial HDL cholesterol as well as low amounts of harmful LDL cholesterol and triglycerides. In a 10-year study, men who consumed 300 milligrams of vitamin C per day (partly from supplements) had almost half the death rate from heart disease as those who took less than 50 milligrams a day.

■ **Fighting Stroke**—Vitamin C helps keep arteries clear of the LDL that clogs and narrows them, leaving you less vulnerable to strokes.

■ **Fighting Cancer**—Vitamin C seems to mop up free radicals and prevent cancer-causing agents from mutating cells.

Warning: Chewable vitamin C may damage your tooth enamel. Don't over-supplement—you may end up with diarrhea. In addition, taking too much vitamin C could lead to kidney problems, and very large doses may keep your body from absorbing copper, an important immune-system protector.

Learn Your Es and Cs

A recent study indicates that supplemental vitamins E and C lower cardiovascular risk. One group of men took 200 mg. a day of vitamin E and 500 mg. a day of slow-release vitamin C. Another group took placebos. After three years, men in the supplement group had significantly less narrowing of the carotid arteries in the neck, says Jukka T. Salonen, M.D., Ph.D., professor of epidemiology at the University of Kuopio in Finland. Narrowed carotids are linked to heart attack and strokes. The observed benefit was strongest among male smokers.

Bottom Line Health

Also, if you smoke or inhale secondhand smoke, you may lose the benefits of vitamin C altogether.

VITAMIN D

Daily Value:

400 international units (10 micrograms)

Experts recommend:

400 international units (10 micrograms)

Is a multivitamin likely to contain enough?

Yes.

Vitamin D helps regulate calcium levels in the blood, and many people are deficient in this important nutrient. To get sufficient vitamin D, you need to go outdoors and get into the light—both window glass and sunscreen block the signals that start the production of vitamin D in your system.

As you get older, your skin synthesizes less vitamin D from sunlight, and it's harder for your body to convert vitamin D into its active form. Some studies suggest that up to three-fourths of all older people get less vitamin D than what they need, especially if they stay indoors most of the time during the winter months.

Warning: Don't overdo it. High levels of vitamin D can be toxic, and anything more than 400 international units should be taken only with a doctor's supervision. Check to see how much you may already be getting if you drink milk fortified with vitamin D.

Also, limit the time you spend outdoors without sunscreen to 15 or 20 minutes, and avoid going outdoors between the hours of 10 AM and 2 PM. This is when the sun's rays are the strongest—and most harmful.

VITAMIN E

Daily Value:

30 international units

Experts recommend:

100–400 international units

Is a multivitamin likely to contain enough?

No.

Vitamin E is emerging as the most important of the protective nutrients, yet few Americans get more than 6 to 12 international units in their diets, well below the Daily Value. "It's incredibly difficult to get enough vitamin E. The biggest source in the American diet is mayonnaise, followed by potato chips—foods that you want to stay away from," says Dr. Goodwin. Vitamin E is also plentiful in eggs and oils, which can be troublesome if you're following a low-fat diet.

Here's how vitamin E can protect you:

■ **Fighting Heart Disease**—In study after study, vitamin E has been shown to protect against

Future Science: Antioxidant Self-Test

You can test your blood pressure and cholesterol levels with home kits, so why can't you test your levels of protective antioxidants?

Emerging products may allow you to do just that. Researchers are busy perfecting inexpensive take-home tests that you can buy at the grocery store to get a reading of your body's levels of important antioxidants. If you're low, a change in diet may bring up your protective levels.

If necessary, a made-to-order supplemental package might be concocted to meet your specific needs. "We're working on that now," says Richard Cutler, Ph.D., president, chief executive officer, and scientific research director at Genox in Baltimore. "You'll get the most protection that way because you're taking in exactly what you need. If you repeat the test periodically, you can also tell that the supplements you take are actually benefiting your body by raising the levels of important protective substances."

heart disease, partly because it seems to travel alongside the harmful LDL cholesterol in the bloodstream and ambush it before it can clog arteries. In one study, researchers conducted an eight-year study of the eating habits of more than 87,000 nurses between the ages of 34 and 59. They found that those who took at least 100 international units of vitamin E a day for two years had 36 percent fewer heart attacks than those who did not supplement their diets. Scientists have also found that vitamin E actually helps slow the development of heart disease in cardiac patients by reducing the size of lesions.

■ **Fighting Stroke**—Vitamin E can help keep your blood from clotting and sticking to artery walls. In an East Carolina University Medical School study, 52 people who had experienced small strokes, or transient ischemic attacks, took aspirin (the standard treatment) plus 400 international units of vitamin E. After two years, it turned out that the vitamin E group had 25 percent fewer strokes than people in a control group who just took aspirin.

■ **Fighting Cancer**—Some researchers theorize that, as you get older, your body produces prostaglandin E2 (PGE2), which may interfere with the infection-fighting T cells. Vitamin E reduces PGE2 levels and jump-starts the immune system. At the U.S. Department of Agriculture Human Nutrition Research Center on Aging at Tufts University in Boston, people ages 62 to 70 took 800 international units of vitamin E for 30 days—and ended up with improved immune responsiveness.

In addition, vitamin E probably protects cells, particularly their membranes, making it harder for cancer-causing substances to get a toehold. In a study of 35,215 women, researchers found that those who took in more than 66 international units of vitamin E had a 68 percent lower risk of developing colon cancer. In another study, the likelihood of a common skin cancer dropped by 70 percent in people who took 100 international units of vitamin E daily.

Warning: "The fact that vitamin E is safe and potentially effective against a variety of chronic diseases is good enough reason to consider taking it as a supplement," says Dr. Blumberg. But don't give yourself megadoses—one report suggests that very high levels of vitamin E ingested over a long period of time may activate latent immune and autoimmune diseases.

You Can't Get Kidney Stones from Calcium

It's true, most kidney stones contain calcium oxalate, a sediment that forms in the urine. Based on that fact, many urologists have suggested a low-calcium diet for their patients. But according to Barbara Levine, Ph.D., R.D., co-director of the Human Nutrition Program at The Rockefeller University in New York City, new studies now show that normal levels of calcium in the diet (1,000 mg. daily) actually decrease the level of oxalate in the urine, reducing the risk for kidney stones.

Bottom Line Health

Because vitamin E is fat-soluble, taking it with a meal will give you the most benefit, advises Dr. Blumberg. Even most low-fat meals will contain the amount of fat you need.

CALCIUM

Daily Value:

1,000 milligrams

Experts recommend:

1,500 milligrams for women over age 50 and men over age 65

1,000 milligrams for men under age 65

Is a multivitamin likely to contain enough?

No.

Calcium does a lot more than ward off osteoporosis, and few people consume enough to get the protection they need. "Everybody has bought the cholesterol phobia and avoids dairy products —which are high in calcium—like the plague," says Dr. Goodwin. "In one study, we found that healthy women past menopause get only about 350 milligrams of calcium from their diets."

Besides strengthening your bones, here's what calcium can do for you:

■ **Fighting Heart Disease**—Calcium may help cut high blood pressure as well as LDL levels. In one study, men who took 1,800 milligrams of a calcium supplement had an 11 percent

drop in LDL—and a 20 percent lower risk of having a heart attack. Calcium also keeps the levels of harmful triglycerides in the body low, unlike some cholesterol-lowering medications.

Warning: Each 8-ounce serving of milk, yogurt, or calcium-fortified orange juice or 1 1/2-ounce serving of cheese contains about 300 milligrams of calcium. Figure out how much extra you need by deducting the amount that you get in your diet from your goal of 1,500 milligrams a day. Take no more than 500 milligrams of a calcium supplement at a time. That's probably as much as your body can absorb, says Dr. Goodwin.

Since calcium interferes with your body's ability to use other substances (zinc, for example), don't take your calcium and multivitamin supplement together, says Ananda S. Prasad, M.D., Ph.D., professor of medicine at Wayne State University School of Medicine in Detroit.

Calcium also blocks your body's ability to use tetracycline. More important, remember that the reverse is also true, cautions Dr. Blumberg. Tetracycline inhibits calcium function in the body.

Fiber keeps your body from absorbing calcium, so don't take your calcium supplement with high-fiber foods, suggests Dr. Goodwin. If, for example, you take your supplement along with a high-fiber wheat-bran cereal (containing 10 grams or more of fiber), your body will get 25 percent less calcium than it would otherwise.

Take More Calcium to Lose Weight

If you don't consume enough calcium, your body overproduces calcitriol. Scientists at the University of Tennessee recently discovered that this hormone promotes fat storage in the body. To verify these findings, researchers analyzed the calcium intake and weight levels of more than 10,000 Americans. People with an average intake of 255 mg. a day were 75% more likely to be overweight than those averaging 1,350 mg. a day.

But calcium supplements aren't as beneficial for weight loss as dietary calcium. People who get calcium from dairy products lose more weight than those who get calcium from supplements. Based on these findings, dieters should consume four daily servings of nonfat or low-fat dairy products, which supply about 1,300 mg. of calcium.

Bottom Line Personal

Some experts prefer calcium citrate because it's easily absorbed by the body, can be taken on an empty stomach, and seldom causes gas or constipation. Take the other form of calcium—calcium carbonate—with meals for better absorption. You might also try chewable calcium products, citrus-flavored drinkable supplements, and calcium-fortified orange juice.

Warning: Calcium supplements made from bonemeal, dolomite, or oyster shells may contain high amounts of arsenic and lead.

CHROMIUM

Daily Value:
50 micrograms

Daily Value:
120 micrograms

Experts recommend:
50–200 micrograms

Is a multivitamin likely to contain enough?
No.

Most people don't get enough chromium, although you find it in a wide range of foods, including meats, whole grains, broccoli, black pepper, brewer's yeast, and barbecue sauce.

Here's how chromium can protect you:

■ **Fighting Heart Disease**—Low levels of chromium are linked to glucose intolerance, a risk factor for heart disease. Chromium may also

help increase the beneficial HDL cholesterol levels. In one study, 76 heart disease patients took 250 micrograms of chromium a day for seven to 16 months. Their HDL levels increased to potentially give them a 30 percent reduction in their risk of heart disease.

COPPER

Daily Value:
2 milligrams

Experts recommend:
2 milligrams

Is a multivitamin likely to contain enough?
Yes.

You get copper in foods such as nuts, cocoa, shellfish, mushrooms, and gelatin. But most people don't come close to meeting the Daily Value through diet alone, say experts.

Here are some of the benefits you get from copper:

■ **Fighting Heart Disease**—Copper is part of the protective antioxidant enzyme system. It helps kill destructive free radicals.

■ **Fighting Cancer**—Scientists believe that copper may play an important part in keeping the immune system healthy.

A Little Powerhouse of Vitamins

Sesame seeds are a good source of calcium, iron, zinc, and vitamin E, as well as other nutrients. Like other seeds, sesame seeds are high in fat, but moderate consumption is fine. According to *Environmental Nutrition,* a New York City–based newsletter, you should eat several servings a week of up to an ounce a day. That adds up to $1/4$-cup of ground or hulled kernels. Sprinkle the seeds on salads, cereals, and pasta or add them to trail mix or yogurt.

Warning: It's important to match your copper and zinc intakes. If you take a supplement that contains 75 percent of the Daily Value of zinc, be sure you get 75 percent of the Daily Value of copper, too, says David B. Milne, Ph.D., research chemist at the U.S. Department of Agriculture Grand Forks Human Nutrition Research Center in Grand Forks, North Dakota. Otherwise, you won't get the full benefits from these nutrients.

IRON

Daily Value:

18 milligrams

Experts recommend:

10 milligrams or less

Is a multivitamin likely to contain enough?

Yes—perhaps even too much.

Warning: Take care when you consider iron supplements, or even multivitamins containing iron. As you age, your body stores more iron. Some studies show that high levels of iron increase heart attack risk, but the evidence is not conclusive. There's some evidence that extra iron means added risk of cancer, too.

Choose a multivitamin that either doesn't contain iron or contains no more than half the Daily Value, recommends Dr. Bogden. Regardless of your gender, avoid "women's supplements"

because of their high iron content—they are meant for younger women who lose iron during menstruation.

MAGNESIUM

Daily Value:

400 milligrams

Experts recommend:

400 milligrams

Is a multivitamin likely to contain enough?

Yes.

You get magnesium from a variety of sources, including foods and hard drinking water.

Within recommended amounts, here's what magnesium can do for you:

■ **Fighting Heart Disease**—Magnesium helps lower blood pressure and may improve insulin sensitivity. Researchers note that people who drink hard water—which is rich in magnesium—have lower rates of sudden, fatal heart attacks.

■ **Fighting Stroke**—Researchers believe that magnesium helps prevent the clotting which can lead to strokes.

Warning: People with kidney disease or who have kidney problems and who consume a lot of products that contain magnesium, such as combined antacid/anti-gas drugs (like Maalox Antacid Plus Anti-Gas or Mylanta), some laxatives (like Correctol), and some pain relievers (like Arthritis-Strength Bufferin), can actually develop magnesium poisoning. Products that slow the digestive system, including some antidepressants, can also provide you with too much magnesium.

POTASSIUM

Daily Value:
    3,500 milligrams

Experts recommend:
    3,500 milligrams

Is a multivitamin likely to contain enough?
    Perhaps.

You get this mineral in a variety of fruits, vegetables, and meats, and, according to Dr. Blumberg, supplementing potassium is unnecessary. But some drugs lower potassium levels, including diuretics, digitalis, and steroids.

Here's how potassium works for you:

■ **Fighting Heart Disease**—Potassium helps lower blood pressure, so it's not surprising that people with high blood pressure often have low levels of potassium (as well as calcium and magnesium).

Warning: If you're taking medications, such as diuretics, check with your doctor before taking more than the Daily Value of potassium.

SELENIUM

Daily Value:
    70 micrograms

Experts recommend:
    70–100 micrograms

Is a multivitamin likely to contain enough?
    Yes.

"Some antioxidant supplements contain a little extra selenium for protection. That's fine," says Dr. Bogden. But the mineral is toxic at levels higher than 1 milligram per day.

Selenium protects you in several ways:

■ **Fighting Heart Disease**—Selenium may play a role in lowering heart disease risk. In Italy, deaths from heart disease rose dramatically among residents of a village whose public water supply was changed from wells high in selenium to wells with a lower selenium content.

■ **Fighting Cancer**—Evidence indicates that getting enough selenium may cut your risk of most cancers, including lung, skin, breast, and prostate cancer. A study in the Netherlands found that people with high levels of selenium had half the rate of lung cancer compared with those with low selenium levels.

ZINC

Daily Value:
    15 milligrams

Experts recommend:
    15 milligrams

Is a multivitamin likely to contain enough?
    Yes.

"A significant number of older people have zinc deficiency," says Dr. Prasad. If you're low in this mineral, you may have a loss of taste or smell. Sometimes zinc deficiency also results in loss of appetite.

Zinc can be helpful in building immunity:

■ **Fighting Cancer**—Some studies show that zinc supplements improve signs of immune function. But other studies suggest that too much zinc can also weaken your immune system.

Prescription for Smart Supplementation

While supplements aren't a substitute for healthy eating, they can help reduce your risk of heart disease by 30 to 40 percent. They also strengthen your immune system, which is particularly important as it becomes less efficient with age.

DO:

▶ **Choose a high-quality multivitamin.**

▶ **Check the expiration date** to make sure that you'll use up the vitamins before that date arrives.

▶ **Add an antioxidant supplement** containing 100 to 400 international units of vitamin E, 250 to 1,000 milligrams of vitamin C, 6 to 20 milligrams of beta-carotene, plus 70 to 100 micrograms of selenium.

▶ **Add a calcium supplement** or be sure to get enough calcium through your diet. For women over age 50 and men over 65, take a total of 1,500 milligrams per day (1,000 milligrams a day for men aged 60 to 65). Be sure to take calcium in divided doses so that it is fully absorbed.

▶ **Buy a product that contains equal percentages of the Daily Value for copper and zinc.**

▶ **Choose a multivitamin that contains little or no iron.**

▶ **Take your multivitamin and antioxidant supplement with meals** or low-fat snacks to get the full benefit of fat-soluble and water-soluble vitamins.

▶ **Buy dairy products fortified with vitamin D.**

DON'T:

▶ **Take doses larger than those recommended** by experts of any vitamin or mineral without approval from your doctor. Some can be dangerous at high levels or interfere with other medication.

▶ **Take calcium and your multivitamin supplement together.**

▶ **Take calcium without checking with your doctor if you're on tetracycline.**

▶ **Overconsume magnesium products, such as certain laxatives,** antacid/anti-gas combination drugs, and pain relievers if you have kidney problems.

▶ **Increase your current consumption of supplements** without checking with your doctor first, especially if you're on other medications.

7

Thin Down to Trim Your Disease Risk

When Orson Welles wasn't acting or directing classic films like *Citizen Kane,* he ate. Reportedly, it wasn't uncommon for him to eat four to five large portions of caviar a day, and three huge steaks and mounds of rich desserts for dinner. His lifetime of gluttony weakened his heart and dangerously elevated his blood pressure. Welles died at age 70 of a massive heart attack.

"To my mind, Orson Welles's health was the antithesis of what you want to experience as you get older," says Michael Klaper, M.D., director of the Institute of Nutrition Education and Research in Manhattan Beach, California. "I would rather be a lean older person than an obese one because when it comes to heart disease, stroke, and cancer, it's clear that being overweight puts you at high risk for these diseases," Dr. Klaper says. "Overweight people in their sixties or seventies concern me because they're really setting themselves up for many of the same problems that Welles had."

While most of us don't overindulge as much as Welles did, the pounds do seem to creep up on us and threaten to erode our health as we age. But it doesn't have to be this way. "Even if you go into your sixties a bit overweight and inactive, you definitely haven't written yourself a death sentence," Dr. Klaper says. "I've seen some people at these ages who have made dramatic turnabouts in their weights. If you begin eating a good diet and become leaner and more active in your sixties or seventies, there's a good chance that you'll still be that way when you hit 90 or even 100."

Where Do These Extra Pounds Come From?

As you stride toward 60, the amount of muscle in your body naturally drops, and fat begins to account for a greater percentage of weight. Even if you don't gain a pound, you will still have more body fat at age 70 than you did at age 30.

Your Healthy Weight Changes as You Age

For years, height and weight charts were based on the assumption that one size fits all, no matter what your age. But researchers are finding that "slim and trim" takes on a whole new meaning after age 60, says Reubin Andres, M.D., clinical director of the National Institute on Aging Gerontology Research Center in Baltimore.

As we age, a greater percentage of our body weight is fat, and that is something that most height and weight charts don't make allowances for, according to Dr. Andres. Using the body mass index (BMI), a calculation of body fat based on height and weight, Dr. Andres has found that people older than 60 have lower death rates at slightly higher BMIs than those who are younger. In other words, even if you are carrying around a few more pounds than you used to, you may still be at a healthy weight for your age.

Based on his calculations, Dr. Andres believes the following weight ranges are healthy for men and women in their sixties. Although researchers haven't calculated the optimal weight after age 69, these weight ranges are probably reasonable for people in their seventies and eighties as well, says William Hazzard, M.D., chairman of the Department of Internal Medicine at Bowman Gray School of Medicine of Wake Forest University in Winston-Salem, North Carolina.

Height	Weight	Height	Weight
4'10"	115–142	5'8"	158–196
4'11"	119–147	5'9"	162–201
5'0"	123–152	5'10"	167–207
5'1"	127–157	5'11"	172–213
5'2"	131–163	6'0"	177–219
5'3"	135–168	6'1"	182–225
5'4"	140–173	6'2"	187–232
5'5"	144–179	6'3"	192–238
5'6"	148–184	6'4"	197–244
5'7"	153–190		

At the same time, your metabolism—the rate at which your body burns calories—slows down. You may also get less exercise as you age, while you continue eating the same amount of food as you did when you were younger. The result is more pounds. The fact is, many people gain about a pound each year after age 35.

By age 60, roughly 40 percent of American men and women are overweight. After age 75, the number dips to 30 percent for a sad reason—many people who were extremely overweight have died. Most of us who survive into our eighties naturally begin shedding pounds because of diminished appetites, says Artemis Simopoulos, M.D., president of the Center for Genetics, Nutrition, and Health in Washington, D.C.

Although excess weight is recognized as one of the primary causes of premature death after age 60, how much of an impact being overweight has on your risk of stroke, heart disease, and

Overweight? The Shadow Knows

Scientists rely on sophisticated formulas and tests to determine if you're overweight. But Sharon Emmons, R.D., a clinical dietitian and geriatric nutrition specialist at the University of South Alabama College of Medicine in Mobile, often uses a more down-to-earth approach.

"I tell my clients to stand out in the sun and look at their shadows. For men, if your shadow resembles Alfred Hitchcock—your belly protruding out beyond your chest—then you might want to lose a few pounds. For women, if your shadow looks more like a rectangle than an hourglass, then it may be time to lose weight as well," says Emmons.

For a more precise measure, however, Emmons and other weight-control experts turn to body mass index, or BMI—a calculation that takes into account both your height and weight—which has proven to be an excellent predictor of a person's susceptibility to certain diseases like stroke, heart disease, and cancer.

To figure your BMI, multiply your weight in pounds by 700. Divide that number by your height in inches. Then divide by your height again. The result is your BMI. For example, if you weigh 150 pounds, multiple that by 700. Then divide that number by your height—let's say 66 inches—twice. The result is 24. A healthy BMI for a man or woman over age 60 is below 29, says Jose Morais, M.D., a gerontologist and nutritionist at Royal Victoria Hospital in Montreal. If your BMI is higher, try some of the weight-loss strategies suggested in this chapter or ask your physician during your next checkup about ways to control your weight.

cancer in these years is a riddle that scientists are just beginning to probe. "It's a darn good question that we don't fully have an answer for yet," says Edward Saltzman, M.D., a scientist at the U.S. Department of Agriculture Human Nutrition Research Center on Aging at Tufts University in Boston. "In the past, the diseases associated with being extremely overweight would have precluded many people from living into their sixties or seventies. Now that medical technology is getting better at extending life, we're seeing more people who are overweight living longer. So many of the data for these people are relatively new."

The bulk of the emerging evidence suggests that too much body fat—whether it is caused by overeating, a sedentary lifestyle, or the natural reduction of muscle and buildup of fat as humans age—is just as harmful now as it was when you were 40 or 50, says Walter Willett, M.D., Dr.P.H.,

professor of epidemiology and nutrition, and chairman of the Department of Nutrition at the Harvard School of Public Health in Boston. Researchers believe that excessive body fat at any age increases the production of sex hormones, such as estrogen, that promote colon, breast, and endometrial cancer. Increased body fat also drives up blood pressure, forces the heart to work harder, and raises the level of low-density lipoprotein (LDL)—the bad cholesterol that contributes to the clogging of arteries and increases your risk of stroke and heart disease.

Losing Weight Isn't As Hard As You Think

Fortunately, losing weight after age 60 is easier than you might suspect. In fact, one study has shown that people in their sixties and seventies who enrolled in a weight-control program were twice as successful in their efforts to lose weight and make lifestyle changes than younger men and women, says Eileen Rosen-dahl, Ph.D., a geriatric psychologist and assistant professor at the Albert Einstein College of Medicine of Yeshiva University in New York City.

That is because you probably have more time to devote to the effort than you did when you were younger, and fat cells on the abdomen, the type that is really harmful, melt away more quickly than fat on the buttocks and thighs, says Lodovico Balducci, M.D., program leader of the senior adult oncology program at the University of South Florida College of Medicine in Tampa.

Losing a Little Makes a Big Difference

You don't have to get down to an ideal body weight to get the benefits of intentional weight loss. I'm starting to believe that losing just a few pounds may be very good for you," says David F. Williamson, Ph.D., a researcher at the Centers for Disease Control and Prevention in Atlanta. One way for an older person to lose those pounds is by improving his/her level of physical activity, he says.

If you're overweight, losing just 10 or 15 pounds (depending on your height) can reduce your risk of life-threatening diseases and improve your overall health. But if you don't make an effort to get your weight under control, you'll be more vulnerable to the big three killers (heart disease, stroke, and cancer), Dr. Klaper says.

How Can Losing Weight Help You?

Scientists have developed persuasive arguments for shedding modest amounts of weight (and keeping it off) after you reach age 60. Here's how trimming down can help you:

■ **Weight Loss Promotes Longevity.** In a study of 15,069 overweight women, Dr. Williamson found that those women who had lost 20 pounds in the year before the study began were 25 percent less likely to die of heart disease or cancer in the next 12 years than overweight women who didn't lose weight. These women also reduced their overall risk of dying by 20 percent and slashed in half their chances of succumbing to weight-related cancer of the breast, cervix, ovary, and others. They also reduced their risk of dying with diabetes.

Researchers traced the lives of 19,000 male Harvard University alumni for up to 26 years. Those who weighed 20 percent less than the U.S. average for men of similar age and height had the lowest rates of death.

■ **Weight Loss Protects the Heart.** In the Framingham Heart Study—an ongoing assessment of the health habits of 5,200 people in Massachusetts—researchers found that men and women in their sixties and seventies who weighed 30 percent more than what is considered a healthy weight were at least twice as likely to develop heart disease.

"I strongly feel that an overweight person who is age 60-plus should lose weight. Excess weight magnifies the risk factors of hypertension, diabetes, and high cholesterol levels that are associated with heart disease. Developing diabetes, for example, increases cardiac risk by more than 100 percent. But all these things are reversible to some extent if you lose those extra pounds," according to Robert Di Bianco, M.D., a cardiologist and associate clinical professor at Georgetown University School of Medicine in Washington, D.C.

■ **Weight Loss Slashes the Risk of Stroke.** In another ongoing phase of the Framingham study, researchers have been tracking the weights and blood pressures of men and women up to age 94 for 30 years. Every pound of excess weight, says William Kannel, M.D., professor of medicine and public health at

Body Fat: Where You Have It Matters

Apples are a food to admire. You just don't want to be shaped like one. Doctors have long known that people who have extra weight around their bellies (apple-shaped bodies) are at greater risk of heart disease, stroke, and cancer than those who are trimmer. The danger increases after age 60 because that's when more men and women develop the apple shape.

"Body shape—fat distribution—becomes more important as we age because weight, which reflects both muscle and fat mass, becomes a less reliable guide to fat stores after age 60," says Walter Willett, M.D., Dr.P.H., professor of epidemiology and nutrition and chairman of the Department of Nutrition at the Harvard School of Public Health in Boston.

If you're shaped like a pear—with more fat on your hips and thighs—you have an increased risk of developing these diseases, but not as much as an apple-shaped man or woman, according to David V. Schapira, M.D., director of the Stanley S. Scott Cancer Center at Louisiana State University Medical Center in New Orleans.

To assess your body fat distribution, measure your waist at its narrowest point and your hips at the widest point (over the buttocks). Then divide your waist measurement by your hip measurement. If you're a woman, a number higher than 0.75 suggests that you are at greater risk for health problems. For men, a number higher than 1 is a warning sign.

The best way to diminish an apple shape is through exercise. Even walking as little as 30 minutes a day, three times a week, can be an important beginning, Dr. Willett says.

Boston University Medical Center, causes you to retain more sodium in your bloodstream, increases your risk of diabetes, and drives your systolic blood pressure (the top number in a blood pressure reading) up 4.5 millimeters. Combined, these weight-related risk factors may quadruple your chances of a heart attack or stroke, Dr. Kannel says.

"Weight control is very important for preventing stroke," says Philip Wolf, M.D., professor of neurology at Boston University School of Medicine. "Being overweight doesn't seem to be an independent risk factor for stroke. But if you look at the main risk factors for stroke—high blood pressure, high blood sugar, and high cholesterol levels—losing weight will lower every one of them."

■ **Weight Loss Decreases the Risk of Cancer.** Although scientists believe that carrying extra pounds has more impact on heart disease than on cancer risk, slimming down may also decrease the possibility that you'll develop certain tumors, says Rachel Ballard-Barbash, M.D., an epidemiologist at the National Cancer Institute in Bethesda, Maryland.

Specifically, avoiding midlife weight gain may help you cut down risk for the following:

Breast and endometrial cancer—Dr. Ballard-Barbash has found that women who have more upper-body fat, the so-called apple-shaped bodies, are at 70 to 100 percent greater risk of developing breast cancer than women whose fat is on their lower bodies—the so-called pear shape in which fat settles around the hips and thighs.

Other studies of women up to age 83 found that the heaviest women who were apple-shaped had a five to six times greater risk of developing breast cancer and had 15 times greater incidence of endometrial cancer than thinner women, says David V. Schapira, M.D.,

Quiz: Do You Use Food to Feel Better?

Loneliness, frustration, boredom, anger, grief, anxiety, guilt, and other emotions are savage beasts. If you regularly soothe them with food, like many people over 60 do, you may be packing on pounds without really solving the underlying problem. Here is a simple test, developed by Stephen P. Gullo, Ph.D., author of *Thin Tastes Better,* that will help you analyze how emotions affect your eating habits and determine what to do about it. Rate each of the following statements on a scale of 1 (rarely true) to 5 (always true). Scoring follows.

1. There is no problem that can't be solved by chocolate.

2. I like to treat myself to a nice dinner or some other food treat to celebrate accomplishments.

3. On previous diets I've sometimes cheated because I just felt that I deserved a little treat.

4. When I'm stressed or upset, I feel better after I've eaten.

5. I have a favorite restaurant where my friends and I go to celebrate or just get together.

6. I have a particular food that I always crave when I'm under stress.

7. I always gain weight when I'm under pressure.

8. Whenever I've gone off a diet plan, there was something unpleasant going on in my life.

9. I always overeat when my children or grandchildren visit me.

10. I always overeat after I fight with friends or family.

Scoring: Add up your total. If you scored 21 or less, you're doing pretty well—you may occasionally turn to food for solace, but it isn't your first line of defense. If you scored 22 to 36, you may be using food to pacify your emotions, but you're just as likely to use other ways of dealing with feelings—such as talking it out with friends, taking a bath, or exercising—that are less fattening. If you scored 37 or more, you may be relying too much on food to cope with stress.

Here are alternatives to help relieve emotional strain without resorting to food:

1. Think, then act. Before you open the refrigerator, ask yourself if eating is really going to relieve your anger, boredom, depression, or other emotional need, says Eileen Rosendahl, Ph.D., a geriatric psychologist and assistant professor at the Albert Einstein College of Medicine of Yeshiva University in New York City. Try to find something else to do—take a walk, garden, or visit an ill friend—that will make you feel gratified or happy instead of guilty.

2. Beware the "comfort" trap. "I often tell groups of older people, 'Maybe you've lost someone recently and are seeking comfort in food. But keep in mind that your loved ones are at peace and watching over you. So please don't let them down. They only want what is best for you, and being overweight simply isn't healthy,'" says Maria Simonson, Sc.D., Ph.D., director of the Health, Weight, and Stress Clinic at the Johns Hopkins Medical Institutions in Baltimore.

3. Sneak in a nap instead of a snack. When you're tired, emotions can overwhelm you and tempt you to seek comfort from food, says Edith Howard Hogan, R.D., a spokeswoman for the American Dietetic Association in Washington, D.C. Get at least six hours of sleep a day. If you feel an urge to splurge, lie down, close your eyes for a few minutes, and the emotional tug to chow down should pass.

director of the Stanley S. Scott Cancer Center at Louisiana State University Medical Center in New Orleans. "Theoretically, breast cancer risk can be reduced by 45 percent just by losing 10 to 15 pounds," Dr. Schapira says.

In addition, if a woman who weighs 25 percent or more over her ideal weight develops breast cancer, she is 60 percent more likely to have a recurrence of the disease in the next 10 years than does a woman who has her weight under control at diagnosis.

"Weight control is one of the few modifiable lifestyle behaviors that may reduce a woman's risk of diagnosis and death due to breast cancer," says Ruby Senie, Ph.D., associate attending epidemiologist at Memorial Sloan-Kettering Cancer Center in New York City.

Why does excess weight elevate the risk for these cancers? Doctors suspect that excessive body fat sparks increased production of sex hormones like estrogen and testosterone that are thought to promote breast and endometrial cancer. At the same time, high amounts of body fat lower the levels of a protein that binds to these sex hormones and deactivates them. The result is a greater risk of developing these cancers, Dr. Schapira says.

Cancer of the esophagus—Men in their sixties who are 20 percent over their recommended healthy weight are at three times greater risk of developing adenocarcenoma, a cancer of the esophagus, than men who tip the scales right on their recommended weight, according to researchers at National Cancer Institute who studied 174 men who had the disease and 750 who didn't.

Extra weight also triggers gastric reflux, which bathes the esophagus with excessive amounts of acid that may promote precancerous growths, says Linda Morris Brown, an epidemi-

ologist at the National Cancer Institute in Bethesda, Maryland.

Colon cancer—In a six-year follow-up study of 47,723 male dentists, pharmacists, and other health professionals up to age 74, Harvard University researchers found that men who had waist circumferences of 43 inches or more were 2½ times more likely to develop colon cancer than those whose waists measured less than 35 inches.

Researchers are not certain how excess weight contributes to cancer of the colon. They do know, however, that some of the same things that cause excess weight—high-fat foods and lack of exercise—also increase the risk of colon cancer. So being overweight may not directly cause colon cancer, but it could be a potent warning that other aspects of your lifestyle are endangering your health, says Tim Byers, M.D., professor of preventive medicine at the University of Colorado School of Medicine in Denver.

Weight Loss Can Make a Big Difference Now

For many of us, controlling weight has been about as easy as trying to catch a live trout with our bare hands. But making another effort even after age 60 can have an immense impact on your health and well-being.

There are many advantages to being thin and maintaining a healthy weight. According to George Blackburn, M.D., Ph.D., associate professor of surgery at Harvard Medical School and chief of the nutrition/metabolism laboratory in the Cancer Research Institute at Beth Israel Deaconess Medical Center West in Boston, "There are 300,000 excess deaths in the non-thin population each year, and we spend $100 billion a year to treat diseases like heart disease, stroke, and cancer that are related to not being thin."

In most cases, diet alone won't do the job for you. Your best bet is to use dietary changes as part of a comprehensive effort that includes exercise, Dr. Balducci says. You also need to think more positively about weight control so that you can achieve your goal and permanently reduce your risk of stroke, heart disease, and cancer.

Feed Your Head First

Weight control begins in the mind. "I don't think that you'll seriously be able to get your weight under control without considering what is going on between your ears," says Maurice Larocque, M.D., a bariatric physician in Montreal and author of *Slim Within*, a 21-day weight-loss program. "The thoughts that you plant in your mind will determine if you succeed or fail."

Here's how to get the motivation you need to control your weight:

■ **Find new reasons to like yourself.** "We know that 80 percent of people who are overweight don't like themselves. They can't find any pleasure within themselves that would encourage them to care for their bodies. So you need to learn to love yourself before you can make any progress toward slimness," Dr. Larocque says. Twice a day, take a moment to focus on some aspect of yourself that you like, such as your legs, nose, or eyes. As you begin to lose weight, take pride in the features that are improving. Tell yourself something like, "I'm 70, but look at me. I really like how my belly is trimming down. I'm starting to get back the shape that I had when I was 45."

■ **Write down the reasons.** Note on an index card your three most important motivators for losing weight, such as more stamina, more energy, and lessening your risk of heart disease. Read and think about what those motivators mean to you for five minutes every day when you awaken and again just before you go to bed, recommends Peter Miller, Ph.D., executive

director of the Hilton Head Health Institute in Hilton Head, South Carolina. Doing that will keep your mind locked on your goal.

■ **Take pictures.** Once a month, have a friend or spouse take pictures of you from the front, side, and back. Focus on the parts of your body where you're making progress, like your shrinking tummy or your strengthening arms and legs. Take a couple of minutes each day to imagine how much better you'll look next month, Dr. Larocque suggests.

■ **Let go.** The more relaxed you are, the more open you'll be to the positive thoughts that will help keep your weight under control, Dr. Larocque says.

Try the following relaxation exercise twice a day:

1. Get into a comfortable position—either lying or sitting—in a darkened room.

2. Close your eyes and begin breathing very slowly and deeply. Relax the muscles of your forehead and jaw. Part your lips slightly. Relax the muscles of your mouth, neck, arms, and legs. Now breathe more deeply, inhaling slowly.

3. Then push your shoulders upward until it seems as though they are touching your ears. Hold your breath for a count of five, then exhale slowly and drop your shoulders.

4. Push your shoulders up again, repeating the breathing sequence. Sense yourself beginning to feel relaxed. Your arms may feel very heavy and limp.

5. Imagine that the sun is warming your arms. They are getting warmer and warmer. Now let your legs go limp and feel the sun's warmth on them.

6. Repeat the sun imagery with your eyelids, jaw, forehead, and finally with your entire body. Feel the sun's energy inside your body.

Slow and Steady Wins Again

Remember that pounds may come off more gradually now than in the past, says Sharon Emmons, R.D., a clinical dietitian and geriatric nutrition specialist at the University of South Alabama College of Medicine in Mobile. If you lose a half-pound to a pound a week at this age, you're doing great, she says.

Usually, losing weight at a relatively slow rate means shaving only 150 calories a day from your menu, according to Dr. Blackburn. That's roughly equivalent to a slice of cheese pizza, a 12-ounce beer, a 1/2-cup serving of vanilla ice cream, or five gingersnaps.

Shoot for losing no more than 10 pounds or 5 percent of your body weight (whichever is less) in 12 weeks, Dr. Blackburn suggests. Then try to maintain that weight loss for three months before attempting to lose more weight. The human body, particularly after age 60, is willing to lose weight for about three months, Dr. Blackburn says, then it doesn't want to budge for quite a while. If you push yourself too much, you're more likely to start overeating and regain the weight that you have dropped.

7. Imagine yourself and smile. You are full of energy, and you use it. You appreciate each step that you are taking on your road to weight control.

8. Now count to three, open your eyes, and get on with your day.

■ **Learn to visualize your goals.** "Mirror, mirror on the wall…" Like the queen in *Snow White*, you can be the fairest one of all. Just use your imagination, says Barbara Morse, an imagery counselor and recreational therapist in San Diego who works with men and women over age 60.

Try the following five-minute imaging technique twice a day:

1. Imagine yourself in a hall of mirrors, each one reflecting a different image of you. Try to see as many perspectives in the mirrors as you can. One may make you look short and fat, another tall and skinny. See reflections of yourself as a child, as a person older than you are now, and as you see yourself today.

2. Now look in one of the imaginary mirrors and give yourself whatever type of body you would like. Change your hair color or style. Work

with the image in the mirror until it reflects you exactly as you would like to be.

3. Step into that mirror and become the image you have visualized. When the image fits and you feel comfortable, walk out of the hall of mirrors, taking the magic mirror with you.

4. Ask the mirror what you need to do to maintain this image. Pay attention to the directions and follow them. Wear this new image as if it were an elegant gown or suit perfectly tailored for you.

■ **Put the scale away.** Don't weigh yourself every day, says Maria Simonson, Sc.D., Ph.D., director of the Health, Weight, and Stress Clinic at the Johns Hopkins Medical Institutions in Baltimore. Instead, step onto the scale once a week at the same time of day. It will give a more accurate measure of your progress and be more encouraging than the constant ups and downs of daily weigh-ins.

■ **Lean on a buddy.** Sharing your experience with a friend or a support group can help keep you motivated and lessen your temptation to stray. "A lot of people try to lose weight alone and that's difficult, especially after age 60 because the rate of weight loss often is slower than when you were younger, and that can be discouraging," Dr. Rosendahl says.

■ **Discard all-or-nothing thinking.** "Surprisingly, a lot of people over age 60 who are overweight are perfectionists," Dr. Larocque says. "They expect to reach 105 percent of their weight goals, and if they only achieve 90 percent, then they think the whole effort is a failure."

Instead of focusing on your overall goal, set your sights on a modest weight target—like a pound a week—that you can easily achieve. If you don't reach your goal one week, try not to think of it as a failure but as a learning experience. Jot down the things that you did and didn't do that will help you make a better effort in the next seven days.

"You don't have to be perfect, you just have to keep trying," Dr. Larocque says.

■ **Take a day off.** "We encourage our patients to take what we call 'planned holidays,'" says Patrick O'Neil, Ph.D., director of the weight management center at the Medical University of South Carolina College of Medicine in Charleston. "It's a time when you decide in advance that you're going to give yourself a rest from weight control and have a do-as-you-choose day."

Taking a break about once a month helps you learn how to regain control of your eating habits after a lapse and will boost your self-confidence so that you can get back on track after an unplanned slip, Dr. O'Neil says. A day off will also give you something to look forward to as your weight-control effort progresses.

Squelch the Saboteurs

Although positive motivation can help you overcome your own worst enemy—yourself—there are still plenty of well-intentioned friends and family members who can quickly sabotage your weight-control efforts.

"Defeating the saboteurs in your life is very important, particularly after age 60. They are one of the major obstacles that you will face, and one of the main reasons that people in this age group stop losing weight," Dr. Larocque says.

Jealousy, guilt, envy, and fear are some of the underlying reasons that provoke saboteurs to derail your efforts, he says. "Often, these people are trying to defend their own reasons for staying fat by attacking you," Dr. Larocque says. "They might tell you, 'Gee, you look so old now that you've lost all that weight. Have you seen your face? It looks like you have a lot of new wrinkles. Are you sure this weight-loss thing is right for you?'"

To overcome these attacks, realize that the saboteur is probably more concerned about his own feelings than your well-being. So ask yourself, "Why is this person really saying these things or offering me fattening foods that I shouldn't eat?" Once you understand what is motivating the saboteur, it will be easier for you to ignore his temptations or criticisms and focus on the compliments of others, says Dr. Larocque.

Here is a sampling of techniques that can help you subdue these saboteurs:

■ **Let them in on it.** Sit down with your family and close friends and discuss why you want to lose weight and what they can do to help, Dr. Miller says. You could, for example, ask for their compliments and support but discourage them from tempting you with rich desserts.

If friends or relatives ignore your request, politely remind them that you're trying to make important lifestyle changes for your health and happiness. If they persist, be blunt, Dr. Miller says. Make it clear that you, and only you, will decide what you'll eat, when you'll eat it, and why you'll eat it, and you don't appreciate their attempts to undermine your efforts.

■ **Make a contract.** Ask potential saboteurs like your spouse or a close friend to sign a written agreement to support your effort, Dr. Larocque says. In writing, let the person know why you consider being overweight a threat to your health. Point out that any serious attempt to get your weight under control will require changes in habits and attitudes, including those of people close to you. Then list five ways the other person can help you, such as providing cooperation when requested, being attentive to—and praising— even the slightest achievement, not pointing out the occasional slip-up, listening without judging your feelings, and providing encouragement to persevere regardless of difficulties.

Then ask the person to sign and date two copies. Keep one for yourself and give the other one to your new "partner." Carry your copy with you and, if necessary, pull it out to remind your friend or spouse about your deal.

■ **Help them face their fears.** Sometimes friends and loved ones worry that your new weight will ruin your relationship, particularly if their own weight or ailments prevent them from being as active as you are now. Reassure your loved ones that you're still the same inside and that you will always care and be there for them, Dr. Larocque suggests.

■ **Keep binge buddies at bay.** Some saboteurs love "eatings" rather than outings. These are the people who ask you out for lunch or dessert all the time. Instead of reluctantly accepting, suggest doing an activity that doesn't involve food, like visiting a museum, says Marilyn Cerino, R.D., coordinator of the weight-management and nutrition programs at the Benjamin Franklin Center for Health in Philadelphia.

■ **Keep playing the same tune.** Keep saying no thanks without offering an explanation. "If you give saboteurs a reason, they'll find an in. If you say, 'I can't because I'm trying to lose weight,' they'll say, 'Gee, I don't think that dieting

is good for you.' They will come up with something if you let them. So become a broken record and keep saying no thank you until they get the point," says Susan Olson, Ph.D., a Seattle psychologist and weight-control expert in private practice.

Keep Moving to Keep Losing

You can slash calories to the bone and down all the magic pills, instant liquid shakes, grapefruit, cottage cheese, or diet bars you want, but you really won't get your weight under control until you do one critical thing: exercise. "I know some older people who are very virtuous eaters who are extremely frustrated with their weight. The trouble is they don't exercise, and unless you exercise, you're not going to lose weight," Dr. Rosendahl says.

In particular, exercise helps you retain muscle and fends off the natural accumulation of body fat as you age, Dr. Blackburn says. That's important because researchers believe that moderate or mild exercise stimulates the immune system. So if you try to lose weight without exercise, you're going to lose muscle as well as fat. And once weakened this way, your body will sacrifice much of its ability to destroy viruses and abnormal cells that can develop into serious illnesses, according to Robert C. Klesges, Ph.D., professor of psychology and preventive medicine at the University of Memphis in Tennessee.

Losing just a few pounds through exercise also may be a beneficial way to reduce your risk of heart disease and stroke, says Robert S. Schwartz, M.D., professor of internal medicine and gerontology at the University of Washington School of Medicine in Seattle.

In his studies of healthy older men up to age 82, Dr. Schwartz has found that a 5-pound weight loss resulting from six months of brisk walking and biking can increase levels of the good high-density lipoprotein (HDL) cholesterol and lower levels of harmful low-density lipoprotein (LDL) cholesterol as much as a 20-pound weight loss from calorie reduction alone.

"People are more likely to be successful keeping off weight by exercising. You may not lose as much weight or look very different, but metabolically I think exercise produces tremendous improvement," Dr. Schwartz says.

Exercise also is a powerful motivator that can help suppress your appetite and keep you on track for weight control. "It certainly can help people over age 60 stick with a new lifestyle. After they begin exercising, they often feel an increased sense of well-being and accomplishment and develop better self-esteem and a sense of control over their bodies. All of these things feed into helping them eat better and staying with their effort," according to Samuel Klein, M.D., director of the Center for Human Nutrition at Washington University School of Medicine in St. Louis.

(The benefits of exercise are discussed more fully in Chapter 8. Be sure to check with your doctor before beginning any exercise routine.)

Meanwhile, here are a few suggestions for exercises that can help you control your weight:

■ **Use weights.** Resistance training will not only strengthen your muscles but also help you increase your metabolism so that you burn extra fat, says Margarita Treuth, Ph.D., assistant professor at Baylor College of Medicine in Houston.

In a pair of small studies involving 15 men up to age 65 and 15 women aged 60 to 77, Dr. Treuth found that those who worked out with resistance-training equipment three times a week for 16 weeks burned an extra 50 calories a day. Over a year, these workouts—one set (12 to 15 repetitions) of several upper-body exercises like biceps curls and two sets of lower-body

strengthening exercises like leg presses—can help burn thousands of calories, she says.

"At these ages, it appears that resistance exercise can increase resting metabolism and help control weight," Dr. Treuth says.

To do a simple biceps curl, for instance, stand with your back against a wall and grasp a 1-pound food can in each of your hands. Lower your arms so that they are fully extended at your sides. Turn your palms so that they face forward. Then, keeping your elbows at your side, slowly lift the cans so that they almost touch your shoulders. Lower and repeat 10 to 12 times. (If you feel ambitious, after you lift the cans to your shoulders, pause for a count of five, then extend your arms straight up and over your head.)

Do that once a day for three weeks, then add a second set of 10 to 12 repetitions to your daily routine, says Mark Bank, an exercise physiologist at Walter O. Boswell Memorial Hospital in Sun City, Arizona, a retirement community near Phoenix. (For other easy resistance exercises, see pages 170–172.)

■ **Walk a mile toward leanness.** Just strolling a mile daily can burn 110 calories, Dr. Simonson says. That may not seem like much, but if you stick with it, you can lose up to 11 pounds a year—even if you don't go fast. "Never overdo it. Keep it safe, even if it means moving slower," she suggests.

■ **Fight hunger pangs with yoga.** "Yoga is a good exercise for older people trying to lose weight because it energizes their minds, bodies, and spirits and supplies them with a feeling of satisfaction that can replace any desire to eat," says Morse.

And you don't have to twist yourself into a knot to do yoga. In fact, you can practice many simple yoga postures while sitting in a chair. Try the yoga sequence on pages 143–144 three times a week while remembering to breathe

1. Double Shoulder Rolls: Sit tall in a straight-back chair and lift your shoulders up as far as possible toward the back of your neck. Roll your shoulders forward and then relax them down. If you do this correctly, your shoulders should move in a circular motion, Dr. Angus says. Repeat this three to five times.

2. Elbow Rolls: Put your hands on your shoulders and point each elbow out to the side. Slowly rotate your elbows in large circles. Do five rotations forward and five backward.

deeply, evenly, and continuously, suggests Carrie Angus, M.D., director of the Center for Health and Healing at the Himalayan International Institute of Yoga Science and Philosophy in Honesdale, Pennsylvania.

■ **Do a little at a time.** "You don't have to do all your exercising at once," Dr. Simonson says. "A person over 60 can easily cover a mile a day by doing errands on foot, walking around the house, cleaning up after herself, or parking a few extra spaces away from the mall."

■ **Do what you can.** Maybe you can't always play tennis, walk, or lift weights. But you can still move your body, says Dr. Simonson, who lost nearly 200 pounds in two years. Sit in a chair and kick your feet up in the air, bend over and reach for your toes, pretend you're riding a

3. Arm Reaches: Lift your right arm up as high as possible, make a fist, and look up at your hand. Hold that position for a count of five, then relax. Do this three to five times with each arm.

143

4. Arm Rotations: Extend your arms out to the sides, fingertips turned up, and palms away from your body. Slowly rotate your arms forward in circular motions, five to 10 times. To determine how wide a circle to make, start small and increase the size until you feel a gentle stretch. Your circles may be as small as 6 inches or as wide as 2 feet. Repeat the motion in the opposite direction.

5. Seated Twists: Sitting slightly forward in the chair, take your right hand and put it on your left knee. Place your left hand behind you on the chair seat. Gently twist to your left so that you're looking over your left shoulder (make sure your feet stay flat on the floor, facing forward). Hold this position, breathing gently for a slow count of 10. Relax and repeat this sequence to the right. Do this three times in each direction.

bicycle and pedal your feet up and down, or play classical music on your stereo and flail your arms like a conductor.

Every bit of activity will help you burn calories, according to Dr. Simonson. "If you don't feel like exercising, just try it for five minutes. Even that can make a difference."

Fine-Tune Your Eating Habits

After 60, some people have already given up so much—their teeth, their eyesight, their sex lives—that they don't want to make drastic changes in their diets to control weight, says Edith Howard Hogan, R.D., a spokesperson for the American Dietetic Association in Washington, D.C.

And you don't have to. "Small changes can add up to big differences in weight," Hogan says. "All it takes is a few little daily adjustments that are so easy that you really shouldn't have any problem incorporating them into a winning weight-control effort."

Beware the Bounty of the Buffet

Buffets may seem like a good deal because they offer a wide selection of foods at a reasonable price. But unless you choose wisely, you could unwittingly load your plate with harmful amounts of calories and fat.

"People who are retired adore buffets. You have to be careful, though, because you can easily eat a meal that is more than 50 percent of calories from fat, because a lot of foods at these places are fried or drenched in butter or oils. But if you have some self-control, you can do well at a buffet," says Cheryl Pingleton, R.D., a dietitian at the Grand Court Lifestyles, a retirement community in Phoenix.

Here are some smart ways to make the most of a buffet, according to Pingleton and John Foreyt, Ph.D., director of the Nutrition Research Clinic at Baylor College of Medicine in Houston:

Eat something before you go. The worst thing you can do is to skip breakfast or lunch so that you can chow down at the buffet later in the day. By the time you hit the buffet line, you'll be so hungry that you won't make wise food choices.

Keep your distance. Nab a table as far from the buffet as possible. It will lessen your temptation to graze or go back for seconds.

Serve yourself just once. It's easy to pile on food and turn your plate into a mountain at a buffet, then eat it all and go back for more. Instead, take one plate and only go through the line once. Stick with small portions, too, so that no two foods overlap on your plate.

Make the most of the salad bar. Go for gelatin or plain green salads. Stay away from fat- and calorie-laden macaroni or potato salads. If you insist on using dressing, stick with oil-based choices like Italian or French that have a bit less fat. Even then, pour no more than half a ladle full to lightly flavor the salad instead of drenching it.

Load up on grilled food. Look for baked, roasted, or grilled entrées like a fish fillet or lean roast beef. Avoid anything that is breaded or fried like fish sticks or chicken. If you must get fried chicken, remove the skin before you eat it.

Pick a soup you can see through. Soups made from clear broth will be lower in calories than the creamed soups.

Dab oil away. Try blotting off any visible oils on vegetables like green beans or corn with paper napkins. Avoid vegetables served in creamy sauces—they have more calories and fat. Vegetables that look as though they have been cooked in water can be risky, too, because they often are covered with butter. Raw veggies like tomatoes and carrot sticks are always safe.

Ask for a baked potato. Whipped potatoes are fatty because buffets usually add whole milk and butter. Put a small amount of margarine and some chives on your baked potato or eat it plain. Stay away from gravies and sour cream.

Be wary of rolls. Some buffets smear butter-flavored oil on top of their rolls. If a roll appears oily, don't eat it. Look for bread sticks, crackers, or sliced whole-wheat bread instead.

Keep dessert light. Reach for fresh fruit, sorbet, or frozen yogurt instead of ice cream, muffins, cakes, pastries, and pies.

How to Conquer Your Cravings

Cravings are a paradox. If you say no, they just keep coming back again and again. So say yes—once in a while. "If you don't give in to cravings occasionally, your weight-control effort is headed for failure, because denying yourself too often sets you up for binges," says Maria Simonson, Sc.D., Ph.D., director of the Health, Weight, and Stress Clinic at the Johns Hopkins Medical Institutions in Baltimore. "Once a month or so, let yourself have a couple of spoonfuls of the foods you love." Here's how:

Wait out the wave. Cravings surge and ebb like waves. So instead of dashing for the kitchen, Dr. Simonson suggests that you wait 10 minutes, and the craving will probably subside.

Get naked. "If you're determined to eat something that you shouldn't, take all of your clothes off and sit in front of a mirror as you eat," Dr. Simonson says. "Believe me, you will not be tempted to do it again for a very long time."

Face your tormentor. Schedule a time when you won't be interrupted for 10 to 20 minutes. Then place the food you usually crave in front of you. Look at it, think about why you want it, then eat half of it and throw the rest away, says Peter Miller, Ph.D., executive director of the Hilton Head Health Institute in Hilton Head, South Carolina. Do that three times a week, eating smaller and smaller portions each time.

Feast on imaginary doughnuts. One simple way to fight off a craving is to imagine yourself giving in to it, says Barbara Morse, an imagery counselor and recreational therapist in San Diego. Visualize a doughnut shop, grocery store, or favorite restaurant that has lots of tempting but fattening foods. Now choose one, two, or as many as you would like. Sit down with your imaginary doughnuts and eat them bit by bit, savoring each mouthful. Feel the bites going down your throat and into your stomach. Continue to eat doughnuts until you feel full.

Repeat this visualization whenever you feel a craving for your favorite food. Eventually, you should be able to think "doughnut" and immediately feel full and satisfied without having to eat any.

Here's a sampling of small but effective changes you can make in the way you eat:

▪ **Plan your meals.** Take a moment just before you go to bed or when you wake up in the morning to go over your meal strategy for the day, Dr. Miller says. Jot down when you're going to eat, where you're going to eat, what you're going to eat, and try to stick to it. Imagine yourself making the right food choices throughout the day and feeling good about yourself.

▪ **Make your kitchen convenient, not cozy.** If your kitchen is too comfortable, you'll be tempted to spend more time there, nibbling on snacks and other foods. "Some people have a television, a rocking chair, and a desk in their kitchens. It's the focal point of their homes, and if they have a weight problem, the first thing they need to do is get all of that stuff out of there," Cerino says.

▪ **Drop the clean-plate club.** A lot of us in this age group grew up with, "Oh, good for you, you cleaned all the food from your plate," says Barbara Beahm, R.D., a registered dietitian in Great Bend, Kansas, and a spokesperson for the Kansas Dietetic Association. But as we age,

Low-Calorie Treats You're Allowed to Enjoy

Here are 10 snacks—all 100 calories or less—that can satisfy your taste buds and still fit into your weight-control effort. This list was developed by Marilyn Cerino, R.D., coordinator of the weight-management and nutrition programs at the Benjamin Franklin Center for Health in Philadelphia.

3 chocolate kisses—75 calories, 4.5 grams of fat

24 fresh grapes—81 calories, 0 gram of fat

1 cup fresh strawberries with 1 tablespoon confectioner's sugar—86 calories, 0 gram of fat

1/2 cup cranberry juice over ice with club soda and an orange slice—91 calories, 0 gram of fat

5 vanilla wafers—93 calories, 3 grams of fat

19 pieces of candy corn—95 calories, 1.9 grams of fat

2 tablespoons low-fat yogurt topped with 1/2 cup cherries and 2 teaspoons sliced almonds— 96 calories, 3 grams of fat

2 cups air-popped popcorn tossed with 1 teaspoon melted margarine and 1 teaspoon honey— 97 calories, 3.8 grams of fat

1/2 cup sugar-free instant pudding made with skim milk and 1/2 teaspoon shaved semi-sweet chocolate—99 calories, 0.6 grams of fat

10 (1-inch) cubes of angel food cake topped with 1/4 cup frozen raspberries in light syrup— 100 calories, 0 gram of fat

that philosophy can make it harder to keep weight down.

"Breaking away from the clean plate club takes some effort. But one way to do it is to ask yourself, before you eat those last bits of food on your plate, what is more wasteful: To throw something away or to carry unnecessary pounds around on your waist that will add to your risk of stroke, heart disease, cancer, and other medical problems?" Beahm says.

■ **Never say never.** "When someone tells me, 'I love cheesecake, but I'm never going to eat it again,' I can guarantee you that she's either going to drop out of our weight-loss group or be one of the few who has gained weight after six weeks," Dr. Klesges says.

If you want to reach your weight goal, strive for moderation, not denial, Dr. Simonson says. Remember that even the experts cheat once in a while.

■ **Become a stove-top eater.** Instead of putting foods into serving bowls and placing them on the table, take modest portions—so that they don't overlap on your plate—right from pots and pans in the oven or on the stove, Beahm says. Then quickly wrap up any leftovers and put them away before you eat. You'll be less tempted to go back for seconds, and you'll probably end up with a spare meal in the refrigerator instead of a spare tire around your belly.

■ **Slow down and chew.** Take your time and enjoy eating, Beahm suggests. If you eat too

How I Did It: An Expert Learned the Hard Way

Unlike some weight-loss experts who have never had to shed a pound in their lives, Maria Simonson, Sc.D., Ph.D., knows all about the dieter's struggle.

"I know how easy it is to psychologically pounce onto an excuse so that you have a reason to hold on to that weight," said Dr. Simonson, former director of the Health, Weight, and Stress Clinic at the Johns Hopkins Medical Institutions in Baltimore. How does she know? Well, after a stroke at age 50 temporarily immobilized her, she ballooned up to 348 pounds.

"I could've gotten out of my wheelchair after six months, but everyone was feeling sorry for me, and I gloried in it. I only got on my feet when the wheelchair got too small," said Dr. Simonson. Then one day when she was preparing to speak about malnutrition to a group of medical interns, she overheard one of them say, "That fat tub is going to lecture about malnutrition? I bet she doesn't even know how to spell it."

That night, Dr. Simonson took off all of her clothes and stood in front of a mirror. "I thought, 'My God, I have let myself become this. I won't live another five years if I keep on this way.' I made up my mind right then to start anew," she said.

It was a struggle. In fact, she tried at least four commercial weight-loss programs without much success.

"I'd lose 4, 5, or maybe 10 pounds. Then I'd go on a working and traveling binge, eating whatever I could get my hands on," Dr. Simonson said. "Sometimes I'd go to these professional dinner meetings and I'd tell myself, 'Oh, I'm just going to have one more helping or a piece of cake.' That would just blow all of my good resolutions to hell, and the next thing I knew, my weight was back up there.

"Finally, I decided that if I really wanted to lose weight, I'd have to do it myself. Reading about it, thinking about it, being told about it were all fine. But it was up to me to follow a program and be consistent."

So Dr. Simonson and her friend, Gwen Campbell, who also was trying to lose weight, decided to develop their own program.

For weight loss, they cut back on what they ate and began walking. For motivation, Dr. Simonson began noticing other people who were overweight and told herself that, although she looked like them now, she wouldn't for much longer. And for inspiration, she prayed.

"It may sound old-fashioned, but I asked God to help me, and it made a difference," she said. "I began to realize that it's not just what you eat but how you feel that is important."

Dr. Simonson's success inspired her to co-found the weight-loss clinic at Johns Hopkins, where she continued losing weight along with her patients. Within two years she lost 190 pounds. Afterward, she maintained 158 pounds on her 5'6" frame.

"Losing that weight gave me a better sense of self-esteem. I learned how to develop self-discipline and hold on to it," Dr. Simonson said. "Of course, I still have foods that tempt me, like chocolate eclairs—I love them. But if I get a tremendous craving, I'll talk to myself. I'll say, 'Do you really want to wear a size 52 dress again?' Even when I do give in, I'll cut off about a quarter of it for myself and give the rest to my 110-pound housekeeper.

"A friend of mine keeps a reminder on her refrigerator which reads, 'You deserve the best. That means a long, healthy life with your husband, not a piece of cheesecake.' I think it's one of the most practical and self-motivating pieces of advice to remember," said Dr. Simonson. "You are worth the effort. Always bear that in mind."

fast, your stomach may be full long before the message to stop chowing down reaches your brain. To prevent overeating, allow at least 20 minutes for every meal. That is particularly true after age 60 when your digestive tract reacts more slowly to food.

While you're eating, ask yourself if you really tasted and enjoyed that previous bite of food. If the answer is no, then it's time to slow down the conveyor belt from the plate to your mouth, Beahm says.

Put down your fork between bites and chew carefully so that you have time to savor the flavors and textures of the food in your mouth, she says. Glance at the clock before you begin eating. If you're finished within 5 minutes, try to stretch that out to 8 minutes during the next meal. Gradually increase the time it takes you to eat until you reach 20 minutes, Beahm says.

■ **Try downsizing your servings.** Use salad plates and smaller serving dishes. It will squelch your appetite and shave calories off your meals, Dr. Simonson says.

In restaurants, ask for a child's portion or request that the waiter put half of the entrée into a take-home bag before serving you with the remaining portion, she suggests.

■ **Trim off the fat.** Cutting away the visible fat from meats can save you about 60 calories per meal, Hogan says. Over a year, that can add up to 21,000 calories. And that's 6½ pounds less fat that you have to worry about gaining. Omitting other fats, including cooking oils, from your recipes can make another huge dent in your weight. (For more tips on the low-fat lifestyle, see Chapter 1.)

■ **Load up on fiber.** Fibrous foods like fruits, vegetables, beans, and grains are good for weight control because they are packed with nutrients and usually have few calories. Fiber also adds bulk to your diet, so you'll feel full faster and eat less, Beahm says.

A person over age 60 should be eating 25 to 30 grams of fiber a day (one orange has about 3 grams) for weight control and to prevent heart disease and cancer, Beahm says. (For more information about eating fiber, see Chapter 2.)

■ **Drink water.** Have an 8-ounce glass of water about 10 minutes before you eat, Dr. Simonson says. That way, your stomach will already have something in it, and you won't need to eat as much to feel full.

■ **Munch on carbs first.** Kick off meals with a food rich in carbohydrates like an angel-hair pasta appetizer or bean or noodle soup, Dr. Blackburn says. That should lessen your fat craving 20 minutes into the meal, and you probably won't yearn for calorie-laden, high-fat desserts.

■ **Eat six times a day.** If you eat smaller meals more frequently, you'll be less likely to overindulge, Hogan says. Eat breakfast, then have a midmorning snack like yogurt or an apple. Eat a hearty lunch entrée like stew, baked chicken breast, or spaghetti, then have a late-afternoon snack like cheese and crackers. Finish with a small dinner, and a light evening snack like a scoop of nonfat frozen yogurt or fruit.

■ **Eat breakfast.** Skipping meals, especially breakfast, puts your body on a starvation alert, so it's more likely to conserve fat instead of shedding it, Emmons says. Eating such foods as toast, cereal, and leftover pasta early in the morning will get you off on the right caloric track for the rest of the day and help you fend off the afternoon munchies.

If you need another incentive, consider that breakfast skippers—no matter their weight—are three times more prone to develop heart disease and stroke-inducing blood clots than people who regularly stop to taste their oatmeal,

Being Underweight Can Be Just as Dangerous

Although being overweight after age 60 poses far more of a health risk than being underweight, an unwanted plunge in weight is worrisome, too, says Maurice Larocque, M.D., a bariatric doctor in Montreal.

"People who are underweight and healthy usually live longer than people who are overweight. So if a person is underweight because they're physically active and don't overeat, that's good," says Dr. Larocque.

But a sudden, unexplained weight loss should be checked out by a physician because it can seriously weaken the heart or be an early warning sign of cancer, says Dr. Larocque.

If you're not ill, but your appetite diminishes, as it often does after age 60, it's important to increase the amount of protein in your diet and keep exercising to help the body retain lean muscle and keep the heart and other muscles working efficiently, according to Dr. Larocque.

Once you lose muscle, it's harder to get it back as you get older, he says. And what takes its place? Cancer-promoting and heart-disease-inducing body fat.

So if you're eating fewer calories than usual, he recommends having at least 1 gram of protein for every 2 pounds of body weight. If you weigh 150 pounds, for instance, you need about 70 grams total from protein-rich foods like kidney beans; skim milk, low-fat cheese, yogurt, and other dairy products; lean meats like pork tenderloin; tuna fish; and potatoes, Dr. Larocque says. Read nutrition labels to find out how much protein each food contains, he suggests.

To rekindle your appetite, try these ideas:

Have a before-dinner drink. In moderation, alcohol stimulates hunger. So if you drink, have no more than a 2-ounce glass of wine or beer about 20 minutes before you're going to eat a meal to prime your digestive tract, says Marilyn Cerino, R.D., coordinator of the weight-management and nutrition programs at the Benjamin Franklin Center for Health in Philadelphia.

Appearance counts. How a meal looks matters to you, especially after age 60 when your senses of taste, smell, and other cues that trigger appetite naturally fade, according to Cerino. Use colorful plates and napkins—orange seems to spark hunger pangs best. Try to serve three foods of differing colors, textures, and temperature at each meal, she says.

Keep track of time. Carry a small pocket alarm clock, and set it to go off every three to four hours as a reminder to eat. Even if you only have a piece of bread or fruit, the alarm may help you establish regular eating times and tweak your appetite, Cerino says.

according to researchers at Memorial University of Newfoundland in St. Johns.

▪ **Brown-bag it.** Prepare your lunch the night before, even if you don't work, Dr. Larocque says. If you do it right after dinner, you'll be more thoughtful and probably select lower-calorie foods than you might otherwise choose the next day when you're famished.

▪ **Dine light at night.** Eat your smallest meal of the day for dinner, especially if you are going to be watching television, playing bingo, or doing another sedentary activity in the evening, Hogan says. Instead of a full-course dinner, try a tuna salad or lean turkey breast sandwich and a cup of soup. If you eat most of your calories early in the day when you are most active, you'll have more opportunities to burn them off before they turn into fat, she says.

■ **Keep a top-10 list.** Write down a list of 10 healthy foods, such as carrots or fig bars, on an index card and carry it with you, Dr. Miller suggests. Then when you have a craving or are tempted by a high-calorie food, you'll have a handy list of alternatives. Update your list once a week so that you'll always have a few new foods to try.

■ **Alternate veggie colors.** It's important to ensure that you're getting a sufficient amount of nutrients like vitamins A, B, and C after you begin your weight-control effort. Eat fresh, low-calorie yellow or orange vegetables like squash, pumpkin, and carrots one day, then switch to green vegetables, such as fresh spinach, turnip greens, or dark leafy lettuces, the next day, says Virginia Stoner, past president of the Dietary Managers Association and a certified dietary manager from Hampstead, Maryland.

■ **Imbibe cautiously.** Alcohol is a double-edged sword. In moderation, it seems to have a beneficial effect on the heart. But one serving of alcohol contains more than 100 calories, and it hinders your body's ability to burn fat, Hogan says.

Alcohol also can stimulate appetite and impair your judgment so that your willpower to control what you're eating collapses. When you indulge, limit yourself to one serving, Cerino suggests. That's one 12-ounce beer, 6 ounces of wine, or one cocktail containing 1 ounce of liquor a day.

■ **Control it with carbs.** "I've found in my weight-management classes that people who avoid eating complex carbohydrates like potatoes and bread—in the mistaken belief that these foods are fattening—turn instead to chocolate and sweets in the late afternoon," Beahm says. And instead of filling you up, those sugary sweets can actually stimulate your appetite, Dr. Blackburn says.

Eating at least six servings of grains, pastas, and other complex carbohydrates a day can dampen urges for candies, cakes, and other fattening snacks, Beahm says.

■ **Don't touch the finger foods.** Many people will eat more calories with their fingers than they do with a knife and fork. Avoid keeping a large stash of finger foods like nuts, chips, and cookies. If you must have them in the house, buy smaller packages and only have one open at a time, Dr. Simonson says.

■ **Pass up the peanuts.** A 2-ounce serving of salted peanuts has 328 calories. If you need to nibble on something crunchy, reach for pretzels instead—20 small ones have as little as 80 calories, and most are fat free.

■ **Plan for smaller servings.** If you insist on eating high-fat, high-calorie snacks like peanuts or potato chips, don't eat them right out of the package. Instead, divide the chips into individual servings and store them in plastic sandwich bags for later use. That way, when you reach for these snacks, you'll be less tempted to eat more than you should, Emmons says.

■ **Skip the fried shrimp.** Boiled shrimp have about 84 calories per 3-ounce serving compared with 206 calories if they're fried, Dr. Simonson says. And stay away from other fried entrées like fried chicken, too.

■ **Pick pumpkin pies.** If you love pie, stick to pumpkin or fruit types. They're lower in calories, Dr. Simonson says. Pecan pie, for instance, has about 430 calories a slice compared with 240 for pumpkin. And you cut another 100 calories if you don't eat the crust, she says.

■ **Choose Canadian bacon.** An ounce of regular bacon (slightly more than four medium cooked slices) has 163 calories. A 1-ounce slice of Canadian bacon is leaner and only has about 57 calories, Dr. Simonson says.

Prescription for Reaching a Healthy Weight

As we age, metabolism slows and fat begins to account for a greater percentage of body weight. Overall, the average person gains about a pound a year after age 35. This extra body fat can increase the production of sex hormones (such as estrogen) that promote colon, breast, and endometrial cancer. Increased body fat also drives up blood pressure, forces the heart to work harder, and raises levels of LDL—the bad cholesterol that contributes to the clogging of arteries and increases your risk of stroke and heart disease.

DO:

▶ **Write down your three most important motivators** for losing weight. Read and think for five minutes twice a day about what those motivators mean to you.

▶ **Unwind.** Practice a relaxation technique such as guided imagery twice a day. The more relaxed you are, the more open you'll be to positive thoughts that will help keep your weight under control.

▶ **Sit down with your family and close friends** and discuss why you want to lose weight and what they can do to help you.

▶ **Exercise regularly.** Try walking 30 minutes a day, three times a week.

▶ **Serve yourself directly from the stove and immediately put leftovers away.** That will help discourage overeating.

▶ **Eat six smaller meals instead of three large ones.**

▶ **Use smaller plates and chew slowly.**

DON'T:

▶ **Weigh yourself daily.** Small fluctuations can be discouraging. Step on the scale no more than once a week. The results will seem more dramatic.

▶ **Be pressured into eating something that you don't want.** Keep saying no thank you until the person tempting you gives up.

▶ **Make your kitchen too comfortable.** You'll be tempted to spend more time there nibbling on snacks and other foods.

▶ **Keep a large stash of nuts, chips, and other snacks in your house.** Buy smaller packages and only have one open at a time.

8

Exercise Programs That Boost Health and Fitness

Y ou don't want buns of steel. You just want to steel your defenses against diseases that kill. And you would like to do it without stressing those bones, joints, and muscles that need more TLC with each passing year. It's true, physical activity is good for you. But if you're like most people aged 60 and over, you bypass the exercise programs, books, and videos that shout "no pain, no gain." And if you do, you have made the smart choice. Research shows that moderate exercise gives you as much—maybe even more—protection from disease as the old grunt-and-groan-and-sweat type of workout.

"Moderate exercise can help you lower your risk of disease and carry on an active lifestyle beyond your eighties," says James M. Rippe, M.D., director of the Center for Clinical and Lifestyle Research at Tufts University School of Medicine in Boston and author of *Fit over Forty.*

A Two-Phase Program for Protection

E xperts today recommend a two-part exercise program: aerobic exercise (walking or bicycling, for example) to condition your heart and cardiovascular system, plus strength-training exercises (calisthenics and low-intensity weight lifting) to build muscle and cut fat. And to start out, you should only exercise two or three times a week. But eventually, you need to work up to at least five times a week, according to most studies.

You can ease into this routine gradually and safely. That's a big plus since "by age 60, just about everyone has some element of osteoarthritis, osteoporosis, joint irritation, or lack of flexibility," says Dr. Rippe. "Light exercise doesn't aggravate these conditions." In fact, exercise usually improves them.

If you join an exercise group or walking club, you reap even more benefits—social activity and new friends. "We like to call this recreation, not exercise," says Gerald Fletcher, M.D., professor of medicine at the Mayo Clinic in Jacksonville, Florida.

Experts note that exercisers enjoy a better quality of life. "Exercisers are more active in the rest of their lives," says Dr. Rippe. "Many of the age-related declines that we see are tied to the expectation that people become more sedentary and uninterested in things around them as they age. It is true that if you're inactive, your metabolism slows, you gain weight, and you become even more inactive. But it doesn't have to be like that."

Exercise Keeps Your Heart Young

Researchers have found that exercise can give your aging body's systems the capacity to work as well as those of someone 20 years younger. So it is not surprising that physically active people—regardless of their biological age—have lower rates of heart disease and are less vulnerable to strokes than people who are inactive.

If you haven't exercised for years, don't be put off. It is never too late to begin. "As soon as you start to exercise, your risk of cardiovascular problems drops by 25 percent," says Dr. Fletcher.

"Studies show that even if you start a regular exercise program in your sixties, you lower your risk of heart disease for the rest of your life," says Dr. Rippe. "If you're 60 years old, you may have another 25 years left, so the quality of life during those years is something to think about."

Even if you've already had a heart attack, don't hold back. "Exercise has been proven to be a great therapy," says Kenneth H. Cooper, M.D., president and founder of the Cooper Clinic and the Cooper Institute for Aerobics in Dallas (he's known as "the father of aerobics"). Studies show that people who become involved in an exercise program after their first heart attacks are 20 to 40 percent more likely to be alive seven years later than those who survived a heart attack and then remained totally sedentary.

Exercise is so important that cardiologists often prescribe exercise for patients with heart disease (instead of just recommending or suggesting it), observes Alan Rozanski, M.D., director of nuclear cardiology and cardiac stress testing at St. Luke's Hospital in New York City.

Exercise can even mend a damaged heart. In one study, researchers followed 68 patients who were on a waiting list for heart transplants and who also participated in an exercise program of graded walking. After three to six months, the hearts of 30 patients had improved to the point that they no longer needed new hearts. Two years later, their hearts were still going strong.

How does aerobic exercise perform these miracles? Exercise helps the body get rid of triglycerides, a type of fat in the blood linked to an increased risk of heart attacks, generalized atherosclerosis (hardening of the arteries), and other medical problems. Researchers think that exercise enhances an enzyme in the blood and muscles that plucks triglycerides out of the bloodstream.

Exercise also makes your heart pump more vigorously to carry extra blood and oxygen to hardworking muscles. Over time, the demands of exercise make your heart physically fit—stronger and more efficient. "The heart becomes a bigger, stronger pump that pumps more blood with each beat," says Bryant Stamford, Ph.D., professor of exercise physiology and director of the Health Promotion Center at the University of Louisville in Kentucky.

You get practical payoffs as well: The well-exercised heart doesn't have to beat as fast when you do something demanding. Even though your body is stressed, your heart isn't. For instance, when nonexercisers shovel the sidewalk after a snowstorm, their likelihood of a heart attack jumps to 107 times their normal risk. The likelihood for someone who exercises five times a week is only 2.4 times his or her normal risk.

Exercise Drives Down High Blood Pressure

Heart attacks and strokes don't come out of the blue. Much of the trouble that leads to these killers starts in the arteries, the tubes that

Check With Your Doctor If...

It is always a good idea to check with your doctor before you begin an exercise program. But it is a must if you have more than two risk factors for heart disease, says Gerald Fletcher, M.D., professor of medicine at the Mayo Clinic in Jacksonville, Florida.

These risk factors are high cholesterol levels, high blood pressure, diabetes, a smoking habit, or a family history of heart disease.

If you're at risk for heart problems, your doctor may want you to take an exercise-tolerance test to check for cardiovascular irregularities. Then your doctor might custom-design an exercise program to ease you into the swing of things, and monitor your progress.

carry the blood and allow it to flow to the body's organs. High blood pressure, a condition that becomes more common with advancing years, often sets the stage for all the other problems. Exercise can help get it down.

When you have high blood pressure, the blood circulates too vigorously under too much force. The pressure erodes the artery walls, which allows the harmful low-density lipoprotein (LDL) cholesterol to attach and form plaque. Over time, this turns arteries that used to be as smooth and efficient as the interstate into the equivalent of one-lane gravel roads. "High blood pressure wouldn't be such a serious problem if it didn't do so much damage to artery walls," says Dr. Stamford.

If the blood flow gets blocked completely, which becomes more likely as the arteries narrow, you could have a heart attack (if an artery to the heart gets blocked) or stroke (if the blockage occurs in an artery leading to the brain). This happens when the platelets—the tiny disk-like structures that help the blood coagulate—stick to each other and to the artery walls to create a clot.

Exercise reduces your risk because it keeps the platelets from clustering excessively and damming the flow. When you exercise, you also protect your artery walls. Studies in Europe

suggest that a combination of diet and exercise decreases the soft plaque that gradually builds up and hardens, narrowing the artery.

The Honolulu Heart Program on Oahu, Hawaii, conducted a 22-year study of 5,362 Japanese–American men aged 55 to 68. The researchers found that nonexercisers were three to four times more likely to experience stroke when compared with more active men.

People with high blood pressure often find that exercise lowers it, which in turn allows their doctors to lower or eliminate their medications. "We think exercise lowers blood pressure because it opens up the small vessels and capillaries and helps blood flow into the working muscles that need the extra nourishment," says Dr. Stamford. An added benefit for the muscles: They become better able to absorb oxygen and glucose (blood sugar).

You also reap the benefits of exercise long after your workout, even when you are lolling in a recliner with the newspaper. That is because exercise lowers the resting heart rate, which reduces pressure on your whole cardiovascular system, Dr. Stamford says.

Exercise Builds Up the Good Cholesterol

Any time you exercise, your body ends up with more of the high-density lipoproteins, or

Exercise: All-Purpose Protection

Beyond combating heart disease, cancer, and stroke, exercise controls a lot of other health problems that increase as you age. Here are some of the ways exercise can help:

Improves balance. As you age, your risk of falling increases. Studies show that weight lifting or balance training improves overall balance. For instance, in healthy community-dwelling elders, tai chi has been shown to decrease fall rates.

Enhances sex life. Researchers have found that physical impotence often results from poor blood circulation to the penis. Since exercise improves circulation on a system-wide basis, doctors speculate that it will help reduce the problem.

Increases mental sharpness. When you work your heart, more blood goes to all parts of your body, including your brain. Those who exercise, studies show, perform better on mental tests and respond faster to stimuli.

Builds muscle. Strength training produces larger, stronger muscles. The stress of exercise probably creates microscopic tears in the muscle fibers, according to William J. Evans, Ph.D., a physiology and nutrition researcher at Pennsylvania State University in University Park. In between exercise sessions, the muscles repair and strengthen the fibers and learn to synthesize and use proteins more efficiently. The brain gets into the act, too, putting more muscle cells to work to meet the extra demands.

Elevates mood. "There is no question that exercise has been shown to improve mood and relieve anxiety and depression, although the reasons why are hard to prove in a laboratory setting," says Robert S. Brown, Sr., M.D., Ph.D., clinical professor of psychiatric medicine at the University of Virginia in Charlottesville and a longtime researcher on exercise and its effect on mental health. "I've never treated a physically fit person with a major depression." Exercise may produce physiological changes that elevate mood. "My theory is that exercise—at least to the point of sweating—raises body temperature, which speeds up the metabolism," says Dr. Brown. "That results in more oxygen going to the brain, optimizing essential chemical reactions." Exercise also releases endorphins, the so-called pleasure chemicals in the brain that can block pain and invoke feelings of well-being— the much-ballyhooed runner's high.

Controls diabetes. Exercise helps your body produce the insulin that it needs to process glucose (blood sugar) and get it out of the blood and into the cells. If glucose stays in the blood, it creates problems as it crystallizes. A microscopic sugar crystal looks like a medieval mace, a weapon consisting of a ball with spikes on it. It tears up the lining of small blood vessels, setting the stage for harmful cholesterol to attach to artery walls and balloon into atherosclerosis, or hardening of the arteries. Exercise can help prevent that.

Strengthens bone. Exercise strengthens bones weakened by osteoporosis because it increases blood flow and helps cells create new, healthier bone. A study at Tufts University in Boston followed 39 women aged 50 to 70 and found that bone mass, muscle mass, strength, and balance all improved with exercise.

Eases joint pain. Because exercise develops the muscles that support your joints, says Dr. Evans, it usually eases the pain of arthritis and other joint ailments.

Measure Your Need for More Exercise

One quick encounter with a tape measure will probably give you all the evidence you need that changes are taking place in your body that call for more activity. Researchers in England have determined that a person's fat level manifests itself in girth, not just weight. You're at the threshold of increased health risk if your waist measures over 31 inches (for most women) or over 37 inches (for most men).

HDLs. That's the so-called "good" cholesterol that grabs the harmful LDL cholesterol and carries it out of the bloodstream before it can attach to artery walls. The biggest predictor of future heart disease is an HDL reading below 35, says Dr. Cooper. (That number is a measure of milligrams per deciliter, or mg/dL.)

"We used to think that you had to exercise vigorously to raise HDL levels. But now," says Dr. Rippe, "we think that moderate amounts of low-key exercise such as walking can increase HDL levels by about 10 percent."

Researchers at Stanford University studied men and women aged 50 to 65 who exercised lightly. After two years, a check of their HDL showed that 52 percent of the exercisers had decreased their risk of heart disease by 10 percent. Another study showed that women who walked a slow 3 miles four or five times a week also increased their HDL levels. And a joint study of postmenopausal women showed that, as good cholesterol levels rose with exercise, their amounts of artery-clogging LDL cholesterol dropped.

As you get older, your arteries begin to stiffen. This stiffening increases your risk of developing atherosclerosis—unless you take steps to flex the arteries by exercising. Researchers at the Gerontology Research Center in Baltimore evaluated the arteries of 146 older men and women. The arteries of exercisers were up to one-third more flexible than those of the couch potatoes.

Exercise Strengthens Muscles to Block Disease

Strength-training exercises reverse one of the major risk factors in heart disease, cancer, and stroke—the otherwise inevitable increase of body fat. We're not talking about weight problems here, just the simple fact that as you age, you lose muscle and gain fat. Even if the weight of nonexercisers remains unchanged, they will probably greet their eightieth birthdays (assuming that they get there) with 30 percent less muscle than they had in their prime.

This alarming ratio makes you older than you have to be. As your muscle decreases, stairs feel like a vertical mountain climb. Hefting that can of beans off the kitchen shelf gets harder and harder. And a common sack of groceries feels like an Olympic barbell when you try to lift it. That's no good for your risk of cancer, heart disease, and stroke. It's certainly no good if you want to continue to live independently.

Researchers think that the changes in your body are connected to age-related alterations in your metabolism and your oxygen intake. And you can't head off the effects of time with diet alone. Exercise must be part of your defense. Fortunately, it can go a long way toward reversing the loss that leaves you weak and at risk, observes William J. Evans, Ph.D., professor of applied physiology and nutrition and director of the Noll Physiological Research Center at Pennsylvania State University in University Park.

Pay Attention to What Your Body Says

Most exercise-related injuries happen because people try to do more than their bodies can handle. If you're overloading your system, your body will let you know. After exercising, you should be:

Very energetic. Exercise should give you additional energy. "If you're exhausted when you finish exercising, you've overdone it," says fitness pioneer Jack LaLanne. "You should finish a session feeling exhilarated, yet relaxed. That way, you won't do too much and get hurt." If exercise leaves you languid, shorten your walk or lighten the weights used for your strength-training exercise. If you still haven't recuperated a half-hour after stopping exercise, check with your doctor, says Gerald Fletcher, M.D., professor of medicine at the Mayo Clinic in Jacksonville, Florida.

Clearheaded. A feeling of nausea or faintness tells you that your efforts may be too intense for your body, although these symptoms can also mean that you're not spending enough time on your cooldown exercises. Review your routine. Add or lengthen the cooldown exercises. If that doesn't make a difference, shorten your walk and reduce your weights, says Dr. Fletcher.

Breathing easily. Although your breathing rate will increase when you exercise, you should still be able to carry on a conversation. If you can't talk and walk or talk and lift at the same time, your work pace is probably too intense. Slow down and lighten your weight load, recommends Dr. Fletcher.

Pain-free. Exercise isn't supposed to hurt or leave you feeling stiff (although you may feel some next-day soreness when you begin to exercise). Devote more time to warm-up and cooldown exercises, because they prevent aches and pains, says Terri Merritt, a clinical exercise physiologist at the Preventive Medicine Research Institute in Sausalito, California. Remember that warm-up and cooldown exercises protect muscles and tendons as well as the cardiovascular system. Don't try to shorten your workout by omitting them. If problems persist, see your doctor or a fitness expert to rule out underlying problems and to make sure that you are doing the exercises correctly.

If You Are Overweight:

Your knees may not be strong enough to support you. If they hurt, then shorten (or eliminate) your walks and concentrate on strength-training sessions to build up your muscles and tendons so they can take some of the load off the joints, recommends William J. Evans, Ph.D., professor of applied physiology and nutrition and director of the Noll Physiological Research Center at Pennsylvania State University in University Park.

If You Have Spent a Lot of Time Sitting:

You may experience lower-back pain when you start to exercise. That's because your hamstring muscles have shortened. When you walk or exercise, these shortened hamstrings pull on the buttock muscles which, in turn, yank on the lower-back muscles. If your abdominal muscles aren't strong enough to help support the lower back, you'll feel it. To get rid of the pain, include abdominal-strengthening exercises with your warm-up and cooldown routine, says Merritt. It's also a good idea to add some gentle hamstring stretches to your warm-up and cooldown exercises.

Danger Signals You Must Not Ignore

When you exercise or do anything strenuous, you put an added burden on your cardio-vascular system. Gerald Fletcher, M.D., professor of medicine at the Mayo Clinic in Jacksonville, Florida, recommends that you see your doctor before you start or resume exercise if you have any of these symptoms or medical conditions:

If you get a headache, cramps, or heart palpitations or if you feel dizzy, faint, or cool while exercising. If you're in the sun, immediately get into the shade or someplace cool.

If you feel any discomfort in your upper body, including your chest, arms, neck, or jaw. You might feel aching, burning, tightness, or a sensation of fullness.

If you start to wheeze. You might become very short of breath, or your breathing may not return to normal within five minutes.

If walking gives you a cramp in one calf muscle that flares up when you walk and lessens when you rest. This could be a symptom of intermittent claudication, a condition caused by plaque buildup in the arteries of your leg. If that's the case, you may have similar deposits in your coronary arteries.

If you have a substantial infection, such as bronchitis. Put off exercise until all is normal—your temperature, white blood cell count, and cultures.

If you just have a cold or the flu. Wait until all symptoms, including fever, have been gone for two days before you exercise again.

If you have a small skin irritation. It's okay to exercise as long as your skin condition is not aggravated by the exertion or movement.

Healthy men and women aged 56 to 80 participated in a 12-week strength-training program and, on average, lost 4 pounds of body fat. Their metabolisms increased by 7 percent, which contributed to their needing 15 percent more calories a day just to maintain their weight.

Exercise Decreases Cancer Risk

Regular exercise is associated with lower rates of colon cancer, probably because exercise speeds the passage of substances moving through the gut, according to Dr. Evans. Researchers at the European Institute of Oncology in Milan concluded that exercise might reduce the risk of colon cancer in men by up to one-third.

Laboratory research gives further support to the importance of exercise as a cancer fighter. In one study, exercise appeared to increase the ability of killer cells to attack tumors in mice. Some studies also suggest that regular exercisers are less likely to develop prostate and breast cancer.

Moderate amounts of exercise may also strengthen the immune system, some researchers believe. The fact is, when you exercise, your blood platelets and white-blood-cell count go up. During moderate exercise, the body actually manufactures more natural killer cells, which help keep immunity strong and fight free radicals caused by pollutants. With those two factors on your side, your risk of cancer drops.

Researchers aren't sure how exercise affects the immune system, but Dr. Stamford speculates that "when you exercise, you stress all of your body's systems. The immune system reacts like the body's fire department to take care of the stress." The rest of the body responds to the

Warm Up for Comfort

Before you walk or do strength-training exercises, it's smart to ease into the effort by stretching your muscles to make them more flexible. If you just jump into vigorous exercise, you could get hurt. "Warm-up exercises that stretch your muscles prevent injury," says William J. Evans, Ph.D., professor of applied physiology and nutrition and director of the Noll Physiological Research Center at Pennsylvania State University in University Park.

"Count up to 30 during most stretches—from the time that you begin the stretch, stretch out, hold the stretch, and return to your normal position," says Richard Birrer, M.D., vice chairman of family medicine at the Catholic Medical Center in New York City.

Some experts recommend about five minutes of slow walking, followed by stretching. "I advise older people to go out and walk slowly for the first quarter mile or so, just to warm up their muscles a little, and then stretch," says Kenneth H. Cooper, M.D., president and founder of the Cooper Clinic and the Cooper Institute for Aerobics in Dallas.

While just about any warm-up exercise loosens tense muscles and makes you feel good, concentrate on exercises that work the muscles in your lower body. "They're the most important for mobility, so it's important to stretch, limber, and strengthen those muscles," explains Dr. Evans.

For warm-up exercises, Dr. Evans recommends the modified squats and knee extensions described in this chapter, as well as the step-ups.

physical stress of exercise by becoming stronger and better able to cope with a heightened round of demands. In the same way, it's likely that the immune system becomes a more powerful defense against disease, even those that are less serious. "We notice fewer colds, coughs, and bronchitis in people who exercise," says Dr. Fletcher.

You'll Live Easier with Exercise

Okay, you do have to make an effort to exercise, but there is a valuable trade-off. Exercise can make other aspects of your life a lot easier.

Here are some ways that exercise improves your life as it helps to battle disease:

■ **Exercise eases sleep.** "If you have a low activity level, it's normally hard to sleep," says Richard P. Allen, Ph.D., assistant professor in the Department of Neurology at the Johns Hopkins University Sleep Disorder Center in Baltimore. Without good sleep, you are less able to fight off all kinds of disease. A study conducted through Stanford University examined 43 people aged 50 to 76. Those who exercised four times a week fell asleep faster, slept better and longer, and felt more rested than those who didn't. And some studies show that exercise helps to improve the quality of slow-wave sleep, the phase of rest that produces the strongest sleep experience.

■ **Exercise trims off the pounds.** Extra body weight means extra risk for heart disease, cancer, and stroke. It can also hamper your everyday physical activities, making even small tasks harder to do.

If you just maintain your calorie intake and burn at least 700 calories more per week (the amount you'll use up if you walk for 20 minutes, three times a week), you'll lose that excess weight. Exercise also seems to help your body use the proteins in your food more efficiently.

■ **Exercise helps reduce stress.** "It's not stress that kills, per se," says Dr. Cooper. "Rather,

Any Time Is the Right Time—Except...

It is important to exercise when you can get the maximum benefit without risk. Here are some suggestions for choosing the right time to work out:

In the morning: If you're a morning person, exercise after you have been up and about for at least 10 minutes. While you sleep, fluids sometimes pool throughout your body, even in important places like the disks in the spinal column, in ligaments, and in muscles, says Richard Birrer, M.D., vice chairman of family medicine at the Catholic Medical Center in New York City. If you get up suddenly and begin to exercise, the accumulated fluids can cause major injuries, such as a herniated disk.

After meals: Exercising right after eating causes problems because both your intestinal tract and your muscles will need extra blood to function. The conflicting needs of each system may leave you with cramps or a feeling of nausea or faintness. Give your body two hours to complete its digestive chores.

If you have diabetes: Avoid injecting insulin into a muscle that will soon be used for exercise. Working muscles process insulin differently than nonworking muscles.

it's the way we handle it. And exercise has been shown to help people handle their stress better, and thus should lower their incidence of heart disease and other health problems."

Research also suggests that exercise decreases thromboxane, a chemical in the blood that promotes clotting and encourages platelets to stick together, which can trigger heart attacks. Non-exercisers with aggressive type A personalities show the highest levels of the chemical.

■ **Exercise lowers the need for medications.** Because exercise helps the heart work better and may speed weight loss, people with heart disease, high blood pressure, or diabetes may show so much improvement that their doctors can lower the dose of their medicines or drop the pills altogether, notes Karen Douglas, M.D., director of the program in geriatric medicine at the University of California, Irvine.

Get Off to a Good Start

Beginning an exercise program can cause aches and pains if not done carefully. By taking a few precautions, you will get your aerobic and strength-training program off the ground without any problems.

Here's how you can get started safely:

■ **Get a physical.** Exercise works because it stresses your body, which grows stronger as a result. It's important to make sure that your body's systems can handle the stress, so you'll want to schedule a checkup with your doctor, says Dr. Stamford.

■ **Warm up.** Experts recommend 10 to 15 minutes of warm-up activity, which can include stretches, light calisthenics, or slow walking. As you get older, your body needs to ease into exercise more gradually, according to Richard Birrer, M.D., vice chairman of family medicine at the Catholic Medical Center in New York City. That's because by age 65 to 70, most physiological systems, such as the pulse rate, are down by about a third and take longer to warm up and cool down, he says.

■ **Break up your sessions—or don't.** Exercising more than 30 minutes at a time helps you lose weight, if you exercise three to five times

How I Did It: Life Begins at 78

A l M. started exercising at age 78, spurred on by a friend who was a fitness professional. "He kept telling me I had to exercise. I made excuses," says the California resident. Then one day his friend enrolled Al in an exercise program at a nearby gym and followed up every two weeks to make sure Al was still going. "If he hadn't, I probably would have dropped out. When I started, I could barely pick up a 5-pound barbell," he recalls. "Now I'm doing 27 pounds."

Of his pre-exercise life the retired businessman notes, "When I owned my own company, I was always the first person there and the last to leave. But after I retired, I used to just sit down and be ready to fall asleep. People would ask me to play a game of golf or go to a ball game. I'd make arrangements, but when the day arrived, I'd find an excuse not to go."

Now Al has more go than the Energizer Bunny. When asked what an average day is like, he replies, "Today, I exercised for two hours. I'm about to participate in a charity golf tournament. I'll stay at the club for dinner and a raffle. You name it, I'm ready to do it."

Although the thought of going to a gym seemed intimidating at first, Al has found one where he's comfortable because it has "a real mix of ages. Some people are older than I am. You meet all kinds of people, and there's always some funny guy with a joke or two. It certainly helps make the day go by."

a week and follow an appropriate diet, experts say. But if you don't need to lose weight, three 10-minute exercise sessions each day will be just as beneficial for disease protection, according to Dr. Stamford.

■ **Set goals.** During your first walk or exercise session, you may plan to walk for 15 minutes and do three repetitions of each exercise. But if that turns out to be too much, adjust your goals downward and then work back up. Most people don't realize how out of shape they are. "It's not unusual for someone to get halfway around the block and feel winded. You have to start exercising gradually," says Terri Merritt, a clinical exercise physiologist at the Preventive Medicine Research Institute in Sausalito, California. Merritt works closely with Dean Ornish, M.D., in his program for reversing heart disease.

■ **Don't be discouraged.** Octogenarian fitness guru and author Jack LaLanne says, "Any time you exercise, it's like putting money in the bank. If you can only start with a nickel, that's

okay. Eventually, it'll add up. Any exercise is better than no exercise."

"If you haven't walked in 25,000 years, you're going to be winded after a block or two," says comedian Sid Caesar (another octogenarian), who started exercising at age 57 to get his life moving toward good health. "But if you keep walking, in another week or two, you won't be."

Once you can easily meet your goal, increase your efforts. Lengthen your walks or vary the terrain to make the workout harder. Add more repetitions for each exercise or use weights to make the exercise more difficult. Don't get carried away, though. Even as you intensify the work, the effort should never be too taxing, according to Merritt.

■ **Schedule a regular workout.** Experts say that you'll be able to stay with your program better if you exercise at the same time each day.

■ **Play it safe.** Find a place where you can do the walking phase of your program safely. "Your neighborhood isn't safe if you don't feel

How I Did It: Caesar Conquers Addiction

Comedian Sid Caesar did not begin exercising until age 57. Over the years, the star of stage, screen, and TV had suffered from bouts with alcohol and sleeping pills that put his career in jeopardy. "I have an addictive personality," says Caesar. "Finally, I thought, 'Why are you acting like a crazy man? The only one you're hurting is yourself.'"

Caesar looked around for ways to change his life for the better by putting that addictive personality to a positive use. One change he made was to develop a regular exercise program. "I started out with a chinning bar because I could carry it with me on the road. I did sit-ups and push-ups. I probably started with 10 or so—if that—and built up little by little."

He scoffs at the no-pain, no-gain theory of exercise. "That stuff is baloney—it's for teenagers. When you're older, you have to take it a little at a time and just do what your body can manage. If it took you 50 years to get in bad shape, you're not going to get out of it in two minutes."

Caesar spent years building up from his low-key start to the iron-man routine for which he became famous. A warmup of 15 minutes of stretching is followed by a 1½-hour walk that includes the steep slopes near his house in Beverly Hills. After that comes 200 to 300 sit-ups, 40 to 50 push-ups, 20 to 40 chin-ups and, if the weather is nice, 10 to 15 laps in the pool.

What did exercise do for him? "I felt better from the moment I started—I wouldn't have kept doing it all these years if it didn't make me feel good. When you take care of your body, you have done something for yourself, and that means you have accomplished something."

safe. If that's the case, look for other locations. Drive to another neighborhood or a public area where you feel comfortable," advises Dr. Douglas.

Mall-walking programs, often operated by hospitals or health centers, provide a haven where you can walk regardless of the weather. Call local malls to find out about programs, suggests Dr. Douglas. She recalls a trip to the Midwest, where "they opened up the mall at 7:00 AM just for walkers, and the place was mobbed with people doing laps. There were so many people, they practically knocked me over."

■ **Dress for comfort.** Your body has to get rid of the heat produced by exercise, so wear loose-fitting cotton or high-tech fabrics, such as Gore-Tex, that breathe. Layers of clothing that can be removed help you to adjust your temperature and simultaneously dispel perspiration and heat. Use sweat suits only in cold weather when you need to stay warm. In hot weather and in

direct sunlight, wear light-colored clothing and a cap to avoid sunburn or overheating, says Merritt. Athletic socks made of acrylic or other breathable materials designed to wick perspiration away from your body help to pamper your feet.

■ **Check your water supply.** It's easy to become dehydrated as you exercise. Drink water or juice beforehand to make sure that your system doesn't run dry, especially if the temperature is above 70°F. Bring liquids with you as well. Some experts advise that you take a drink of water every 20 minutes. Avoid excessive coffee, alcohol, and other diuretics that will contribute to dehydration, says Dr. Fletcher.

■ **Cool down.** End your session by walking very slowly for five minutes or by stretching gently, advises Dr. Fletcher. Don't sit down immediately after exercise; slow movement is a better way to let your body cool properly. It will reduce the likelihood of muscle cramps and help the blood

How I Did It: A Comeback from Heart Attack

Alice H. began attending an exercise program in Atlanta at age 60. "I started two months after my heart attack," she says. "I had never done any organized exercise. You never believe that anything like a heart attack is going to happen to you. Now I wonder why my heart attack didn't happen earlier."

Alice's high-pressure job had taken its toll. "When I came home after long hours, I didn't feel like doing much of anything. Then after I retired, I wanted to take it easy." Yet, she had some warning signals. "Not long before my heart attack, I went on a trip to New York with some friends and was surprised at how tired I got after a day of walking around. I had thought I was in better shape."

Once Alice made the commitment to a comeback, she worried about measuring up. "When I first started exercising, I worried that I wouldn't be able to do the program," she says. The heart attack had left her exhausted, her energy level low.

She started out with stretching exercises—for instance, trying to touch her toes. She then walked a quarter mile on a track and rode on a stationary bicycle for a few minutes. She recalls that she "also met people who live right around the corner—but I had never known them."

The program gradually became more challenging, and soon she graduated to a high-powered step-aerobics program. Now she says, "I feel great. I have a lot more energy and have been doing volunteer work, helping people in my community."

circulate. Massaging muscles after your cooldown will also keep the blood moving, according to the American Medical Association.

In hot weather, wearing sweaty clothes after exercise helps your body to cool off. But in cold weather, change out of wet clothes as soon as possible to avoid cooling down too quickly. Hot showers slow the cooling process too much, so wait for about 45 minutes, until your body temperature has returned to normal, before showering.

■ **Keep tabs on medication.** Some medications, even common over-the-counter medicines such as decongestants, raise your heart rate and blood pressure. If you're taking one, Dr. Fletcher suggests that you decrease your exercise.

Walk Toward Longevity

Ideally, about half of your exercise program should consist of aerobic exercise. And to many experts, walking is the aerobic exercise of choice, especially for people age 60 and over.

That's because when you walk, the pressure on your joints never rises above 1.5 times your body weight. Jogging or dance or step aerobics can put a lot of pressure—four times your weight or more—on your bones. But you would do well to start walking slowly, and gradually increase the length and difficulty of your walks, says Dr. Rippe.

Here's how to strengthen your heart by walking, without overtaxing your system:

■ **Start by timing yourself.** If you are really out of shape, you may get too tired to make it back home. Check your watch when you start, and walk around one block over and over until you get a little tired. Glance at your watch to see how long you have walked. That's the length that your walks should be for the next week or two, explains Dr. Douglas.

"If you get tired on the way home, stop, rest, then walk some more," advises Dr. Douglas. Some days you may tire more easily or the work

Exercise Using Everyday Routines

Some experts believe that everyday activities may be just as effective as formal exercise routines—and a lot more appealing. "Older people have a commonsense view of physical activity—possibly because they've lived through the Depression, when life was more difficult and physical activity translated into something meaningful, not just sweat," says Bryant Stamford, Ph.D., professor of exercise physiology and director of the Health Promotion Center at the University of Louisville. He suggests that, while a regular exercise program will benefit you, you may be happier—and more willing to exercise—if you simply do more of the things that you enjoy.

Utilize your everyday routine. "If you like to garden, figure out a way to turn that into 30 minutes a day of vigorous activity. It'll help you ward off lethal diseases," Dr. Stamford advises. The Centers for Disease Control and Prevention in Atlanta and the American College of Sports Medicine in Indianapolis both suggest physical activities such as walking up the stairs (rather than taking the elevator), walking instead of driving short distances, doing vigorous housework, raking leaves, and dancing.

You only gain if you take the hard road. "Make things more difficult, not easier," suggests Dr. Stamford. "Usually, if you have trouble getting up the stairs, everyone suggests that you move into a one-story house. But in reality the stairs give you trouble because you have become weaker. If you stop doing stairs, soon you won't be able to get up them at all." In fact, a report issued by these groups states that your risk of coronary heart disease increases as your level of activity goes down. "Do more of what's difficult, not less," advises Dr. Stamford.

---

may seem too much. Just shorten your session that day. Once you're comfortable, you can gradually increase the length of your walks by about 10 percent every two weeks.

■ **Keep your pace constant.** Try to maintain the same level of exertion for your entire walk. That way, you'll ask your heart to work hard (but not too hard) for your entire session. Your heart gets the biggest benefit from a sustained workout.

You may want to use walking as part of your warm-up. If that's the case, make this phase of the routine slower and more relaxed, says Dr. Fletcher.

■ **Try airport aerobics.** To get the most benefit, work up to the point where you can walk briskly —imagine that you're walking through the airport to catch a plane, suggests Dr. Stamford. But don't overdo it. Start your brisk-walking program with a goal of 10 to 15 minutes, advises Dr. Douglas.

■ **Slow down on hills.** If you come to a hill, forget the heroics. Slow your pace to maintain the same level of exertion that you had on level ground.

■ **Track the temperature.** Your workout will seem harder if it's hot or humid. Adjust your speed and intensity so that you stay at the right exertion level. If the temperature soars—say, over 95°F with 80 percent humidity—don't exercise outside for more than 30 to 45 minutes, advises Dr. Fletcher. If you have heart problems, reduce your time in the heat by at least 25 percent.

Get More Health from Your Walks

Once you get into a regular walking program and can keep up a set pace, you can start to vary it. "If you do the same thing over and over, your muscles aren't challenged and they don't respond as well—and you can get bored. I

Proper Way to Take Your Pulse

You can safely take your pulse by pressing your wrist with your fingers—not your thumb, according to Dr. Fletcher. NEVER take your pulse by pressing on the artery in your neck. That can cause a stroke.

If you're taking medications, your pulse may not accurately reflect the stress of exercise to your system. Instead, talk to your doctor. You may want to make a habit of estimating your level of exertion.

change my program every three to four weeks," says LaLanne.

Here are ways to keep a little pep in your step:

■ **Shorten your steps.** Take a tip from racewalkers. They take short steps and get their speed by packing a lot of steps into each minute, says Dr. Stamford.

■ **Try weights.** Weighted belts are popular. As your condition permits, wearing a belt with two to five pounds will add resistance, according to Dr. Evans. When you walk with extra weight, you'll expend more effort. Gradually increase the weight as your fitness improves.

■ **Walk with an arm-swing.** The more you move, the more intense your workout. Try swinging your arms vigorously. Raise them and punch at the sky, first with one arm and then with the other. "You can get a great cardiovascular workout in 12 to 17 minutes if your exercise is vigorous," says LaLanne.

Strength Exercises Beef Up Your Body–Muscle Ratio

Ever want to feel like a kid again? Well, maybe you remember calisthenics from grade school—those exercises that use the body's own weight to build and tone muscles. They're not complicated, and they require no special equipment.

Strengthening exercises such as calisthenics aren't just an exercise in vanity. When you build muscle, the ratio of body muscle to body fat shifts. Increasing your lean muscle lowers your risk of cancer, heart disease, and stroke.

Here's how to get started with a calisthenics program, in which you use your body's own weight to work your muscles. You'll need to work some muscle groups with light weight-lifting exercises using weights that you make or buy.

Use these basic guidelines to get the most benefit from strengthening exercises:

■ **Keep it slow.** Perform all exercises slowly. Unless otherwise noted, spend two seconds in the lifting phase of each exercise and four to six seconds in the lowering part. If you move too quickly, you won't get the muscle-strengthening benefits of the exercise and you could hurt yourself.

■ **Remember to keep breathing.** Always inhale before you lift, exhale as you lift, and inhale as you lower the weight for maximum benefit.

■ **Choose just a few exercises.** Pick several exercises for your upper body and several for your lower body from the resistance and weight-lifting categories. You can switch to different exercises anytime you feel like it.

■ **Up the ante.** Unless otherwise noted, work up to the point where you can do three sets of each exercise, with five to 15 repetitions of the exercise in each set. Don't rest within the sets.

Step-Ups: For this exercise you will need a step stool (or the first step of a stairway), roughly 8 to 10 inches high. Stand with both feet on the floor. Slowly raise your right leg and place your foot on the stool. Using the muscles in your right leg, lift yourself to a standing position on the stool. Hold on to something for support if you have balance problems. Then reverse that motion: Step off the stool, making sure that your right leg does all the work. Repeat 10 to 15 times. Then perform the exercise with the left leg.

You can rest briefly between each set. As the work becomes easy, add weights or increase the number of repetitions you do.

■ **Use music.** If you have trouble establishing a rhythm to your exercise routine so that you perform each repetition within a set with the same gusto, Dr. Evans suggests that you listen to triumphal march music as you exercise.

■ **Stay clear of cramps.** You're just strolling merrily along the sidewalk, when suddenly—ouch!—a muscle cramp cripples one of your legs. To avoid cramps, stretch and strengthen your leg muscles with the three exercises on page 169 recommended by Gary Gordon, D.P.M., director of the Running and Walking Clinic at the Joseph Torg Sports Medicine Center at Allegheny University of the Health Sciences in Philadelphia.

Be Sweet to Your Feet

The condition of your feet is all-important to an exercise regimen. Exercise in shoes that are designed for the job—otherwise, you issue an open invitation to aches, pains, and even stress fractures in your feet and legs. "A lot of people just put on any old shoe—and they get hurt," notes Dr. Gordon.

Here's how to stay well-shod:

■ **Pick the right kind of shoe.**

Walking or running shoes: They absorb the shock of your stride, thanks to a slightly elevated heel that also helps prevent injuries to the legs' muscles and tendons.

Tennis shoes and other types of athletic shoes: They absorb the impact of sideways movement and quick turns. (Women who normally wear high heels should avoid flat tennis-type shoes because the sudden shift in foot position may cause a strain, says Dr. Gordon.)

■ **Buy new shoes often.** Although shoes may last for years, their shock absorption lasts for only a few months. If you walk fewer than 25 miles a week, Dr. Gordon suggests that you get a new pair every four to six months. If you walk more than 25 miles a week, replace shoes every two to three months. If you already have a pair of shoes made for walking or running, examine the tread. Get a new pair if the bottom tread has

Bent-Knee Push-Ups: Lie on the floor facedown, feet together, knees and palms against the floor. Keeping your knees against the floor, push your body up with your arms. Keep your back as flat as possible. Return to the starting position. Repeat five times.

Calf Raises: Use a chair or wall for support, if necessary. Stand with the balls of your feet on a 2-inch-thick book or board, your heels off the edge. Push yourself up onto your toes, then slowly lower your heels as far as you can. Repeat five times.

Modified Squats: Stand behind a chair, holding the back of the chair for support. With your feet flat on the floor, point your toes outward. Bend your knees slightly while keeping your back straight and feet on the floor. Return to starting position. Repeat five times.

worn off, which means there has been enough wear to interfere with shock absorption.(You can use the castoffs for working around the house.)

■ **Examine the patterns.** Bring a well-worn pair of everyday shoes with you when you shop for walking shoes. Your wear patterns, particularly in the heels, may help the salesperson pick

out the best pair for your feet, advises Merritt.

■ **Insure the right fit.** To get the best fit when choosing new athletic shoes, wear the same kind of socks that you'll exercise in. Shop in the afternoon in case your feet swell during the day. Plan to try on lots of shoes to identify the ones that are the most comfortable.

Leg Lifts: Lie on the floor. Tighten the thigh muscles of one leg and then lift it 12 inches off the ground without bending your knee. Hold your leg in this position for 10 seconds. Then lower the leg and repeat with the opposite leg. Repeat the exercise five times, alternating legs. Work up to the point where you can do 30 lifts with each leg. When this becomes easy, strap on leg weights to add 1 to 2 pounds to each ankle and work your way up to 30 lifts again.

Calf Stretches: Stand with your heels apart and toes pointing in, with your arms straight out in front of you, palms touching a wall. Keep your back straight and bend your arms, then move your chest toward the wall. You should feel a stretch through the backs of your calves. If you don't, move farther away from the wall and try again. If your calves hurt, move closer to the wall. Hold the stretch for 10 to 30 seconds. Repeat five times.

Knee and Ankle Bends: Stand with your feet about 6 inches apart. With your back straight and your feet on the ground, slowly bend your ankles and knees, lowering your body as far as is comfortable. As you descend, try to point your knees out over your toes, rather than letting them point inward. Keep your hands on your thighs for support. The movement should be coming from your knees, not your back. Hold the pose for 10 to 30 seconds. Repeat five times.

Military Presses: Sit in a chair with your feet flat on the floor. Use a barbell or weighted milk jugs that have been secured to each end of a broomstick. Hold the bar behind your head with your arms bent. Slowly raise your arms up until they are straight. Return to the starting position. Repeat five times.

Shoulder Raises: Sit in a chair with your feet flat on the floor. Hold a weight in one hand with your arm resting at your side, palm facing in. Keep your elbow straight but not locked as you slowly bring your arm forward and up, until it is extended above your head. Return to starting position. Repeat five times, then switch to the opposite side.

■ **Test for toe room.** There is enough toe room if, when you stand, you can fit the tip of your thumb (about a $1/2$-inch) in the space between the end of your big toe and the front end of the shoe, says Dr. Gordon. If you have a thick thumb, of course, stick to the $1/2$-inch rule.

■ **Check the width.** A shoe is too wide if the eyelets meet when you lace them up. Your foot will slip around inside the shoe, and you won't get enough support. You may end up with blisters, says Dr. Gordon. A too-narrow shoe will be hard to tie because the eyelets are too far apart.

Lift Your Defenses with Strength Exercises

You'll need some weights for the weight-lifting exercises in this chapter. But you don't have to work out like a professional body-builder. Even a little weightlifting provides a mighty defense.

Either buy free weights—dumbbells or barbells—or use plastic bottles or milk jugs filled with water or sand. For your ankles, you'll probably want to buy inexpensive weights on Velcro bands.

Finding the best weight for you takes trial and error. The weights should be heavy enough that your muscles benefit, but not so heavy that your muscles can't handle the stress. Find the heaviest weight that you can lift five times and work with that weight.

Start by doing one set of each exercise, and work up to three. The goal is to eventually complete three sets of five repetitions of each exercise. Choose two or three exercises for your upper body and two or three for your lower body. Increase the weight when three sets of five repetitions becomes easy.

Triceps Extensions: Sit in a straight-back chair, feet flat on the floor, parallel but not touching. Hold a weight in each hand and raise both arms over your head. Bend your elbow and lower one hand behind your head, then raise it back overhead. Repeat five times, then switch to the opposite arm.

Some people think they need to wear a wide shoe because their little toe flares out. If that is the case, ask for a normal-width, curve-lasted model that won't give your little toe a pinched-in feeling, advises Jim Stewart, a registered professional shoe fitter and owner of the Finish Line Running Store, a store specializing in athletic footwear in Allentown, Pennsylvania.

■ **Keep your heel upright.** Put on the shoe and have someone look at it from behind, recommends Stewart. The heel counter—the extra-firm section of the shoe that cradles your heel—should be perpendicular to the ground. If it isn't, you're not getting the heel support that you need from the shoe.

■ **Get enough stiffness in the sole.** In some shoe models, the shock-absorbing layer of the sole is rigid; in others, it is more pliable. If you weigh more than 190 pounds, you need the rigid model just to get enough shock absorption, says Dr. Gordon. If you weigh 100 pounds or less, the

Biceps Curls:

Sit in a chair with your legs apart, feet flat on the floor, resting one hand on your thigh. Holding a weight in your other hand, extend that arm straight down, while resting your elbow against your inner thigh.

Flex one arm and slowly curl the weight to shoulder level. Return that arm to the original position. Repeat five times, then switch to the other arm.

Knee Extensions: Sit on a chair, with a weight strapped to the ankle of one leg, foot on the floor. Slowly straighten the leg. (Don't point your toe—keep your foot at about a 90-degree angle to your leg.) Then lower the leg to the starting position. Repeat five times, then switch sides.

rigid construction may make your foot work too hard, straining the arch or calf muscles. If you are between 100 and 190 pounds, you may wear a shoe that has either a rigid or pliable sole. Unfortunately, you can't easily tell the difference. Ask salespeople at quality athletic-shoe stores for recommendations.

■ **Add an insert.** You can get additional shock absorption through over-the-counter shoe inserts such as Spenco (which also prevents friction and blisters). This won't help your shoes last longer but will increase your shock-absorption protection, says Dr. Gordon.

Leave Inactivity Behind

The exercise clothes are ready to go. The new pair of shoes waits by the door. Weights, present and accounted for. But, if you're like most people, it is still hard to take that final step and, as they say in the ad, "Just do it."

Knee Flexions: Strap a weight to the ankle of one leg. Stand and hold on to the back of a chair for support. Slowly lift your heel toward your buttock. Lower your leg to the starting position. Repeat five times, then switch sides.

Odds are, this isn't the first time that you've tried to set up an exercise routine. You know how important it is to silence that little voice from within that says, "I'll 'just do it'—tomorrow."

Here's how to get on the fast track to disease prevention:

■ **Company helps.** "Get someone to go with you," advises Merritt. "You may not want to walk or do strength-training exercises because it's too cold or you just feel lazy. When you depend on someone and they depend on you, it makes it easier for both of you." In fact, a study conducted by the University of Southern California showed that people who exercise with friends at a health club and socialize with them outside the club work out more frequently and enjoy it more.

Adds LaLanne, "When people work out together, they encourage each other and make sure that they are doing the exercises correctly. They also get competitive and, as a result, they both get a more intense workout than they'd get if they worked alone."

■ **Plug in for pleasure.** Some experts recommend listening to music to help energize your workouts. Try picking something with a faster tempo for your actual workout and then something slower for your warm-up and cooldown. Choose a rhythm that's comfortable for you, Merritt advises. But listen to your body, not the music, to lessen the risk of overexertion.

■ **Keep a record.** If you measure your progress, you'll find it easier to stay motivated. Write down in a calendar or a notebook the number of minutes you walk and the number of exercises you do. You'll be surprised at how quickly you're able to do more.

Prescription for Easing Into Exercise

A two-part exercise program protects you from cancer, heart disease, and stroke. Aerobic exercise (walking or bicycling, for example) conditions your heart and cardiovascular system, while strength-training exercises (calisthenics and weight lifting) build muscle and cut fat to reduce your cancer risk.

DO:

▶ **Warm up** with stretches, light calisthenics, or slow walking before you exercise.

▶ **Exercise for more than 30 minutes** per session if you want to lose weight. Otherwise, three 10-minute sessions per day will protect against disease.

▶ **Wear loose-fitting clothing that breathes.** Use layers of clothing to stay warm and, simultaneously, dispel perspiration and heat. Wear athletic socks that are designed to wick perspiration away from your feet. Make sure your shoes fit and support your feet properly.

▶ **Cool down with slow walking or gentle stretches.**

DON'T:

▶ **Become dehydrated.**

▶ **Drink coffee, alcohol, or other diuretics before or while you exercise.**

▶ **Exercise so vigorously that you can't talk and exercise at the same time.**

9

Healthy Attitude: A Gift to Your Immune System

Maud Morgan beat the odds. The legendary Boston oil painter, whose works adorn galleries nationwide, including the Metropolitan Museum of Art in New York City, lived into her late nineties, and until the end of her life was spry, mentally alert, and eager to begin each day.

Good genes? Maybe. Healthy diet? Perhaps. Optimism? Absolutely.

"I've always instinctively seen the optimistic side of everything, and I think that helps keep me healthy," Morgan was quoted as saying. "When you're optimistic, that usually leads to action, and anything that keeps you alive and active increases your health."

If you don't believe it, just ask George Blackburn, M.D., Ph.D., associate professor of surgery at Harvard Medical School and chief of the nutrition/metabolism laboratory in the Cancer Research Institute at Beth Israel Deaconess Medical Center West in Boston. He knew Morgan for years.

"Without a shadow of a doubt, her philosophy of life had an impact on her survival. When you look at her risk factors from a statistical standpoint, she should have been gone long before. She confounded all predictions because, like many in her generation, she abused cigarettes and everything else that we now know isn't good for you," says Dr. Blackburn, who owns a dozen of Morgan's paintings. "There is no Western medicine that I practice that can explain her."

Attitude Matters

As with the fabled Fountain of Youth and mythical Atlantis, the search for a connection between mind and body has been an elusive one. But researchers are finding that the link between positive feelings and health is neither a fable nor a myth. Compelling research is beginning to show that a positive outlook on life can magnify the health-protecting powers of diet and exercise and can help diminish a multitude of ailments, including heart disease, stroke, and cancer. Even if you develop one of these three diseases, experts say joy, hope, and optimism can improve the quality of your life and enhance your chances of recovery.

"Most illnesses have a lot of psychological underpinnings. A person's lifestyle, character, and the way they cope with life have a big influence on what diseases they get, how long they live, and how they survive in their older years," says Roger Thies, Ph.D., professor of physiology at the University of Oklahoma Health Sciences Center in Oklahoma City.

Unraveling the Mystery

Although physicians and researchers had long suspected that negative emotions influenced our health, it was the late Norman Cousins, the former editor of the *Saturday Review,* who created a sensation when he claimed that laughter helped him overcome a heart attack and a rare life-threatening collagen disease—an illness of the fibrous tissue that binds cells together.

"A patient's attitude is very important," Cousins said. "If he approaches the illness with confidence and purpose—if he remains committed to a high quality of life—then he can enhance the effects of his medical treatment."

What's going on? No one is quite sure yet. In fact, your doctor probably would have an easier time explaining why your golf partner insists on wearing a polka-dot shirt, plaid pants, and fluorescent orange shoes than describing precisely how emotions affect your health. "Positive moods, optimism, and good mental health are underrated and under-studied as a helpful factor in health, particularly in terms of cancer prevention and treatment," says Karl Goodkin, M.D., Ph.D., associate professor of psychiatry, neurology, and psychology at the University of Miami School of Medicine.

Many researchers believe that an optimistic outlook indirectly helps to prevent heart disease, stroke, and cancer. Healthy people in their sixties, seventies, and eighties who are optimists are likely to have taken better care of their bodies when they were younger, says Christopher Peterson, Ph.D., professor of psychology at the University of Michigan in Ann Arbor and author of *Health and Optimism.* And those optimists usually continue to exercise regularly, eat a balanced, low-fat diet, avoid smoking, and drink moderately.

How the Mind Heals

The physiological aspects of emotions themselves—beyond prompting people to be more active—have not yet been identified. Some researchers suspect that a small portion of the brain called the insular cortex may be the key. The insular cortex regulates the autonomic nervous system, which controls such automatic functions as breathing, heartbeat, and blood pressure. But it also has a role in higher functions of the brain and helps process emotions like anger, fear, joy, happiness, and sexual arousal.

Could this be where emotions merge with the body's physiology and ultimately affect health? Maybe, says Stephen Oppenheimer, M.D., assistant professor of neurology and cardiology at Johns Hopkins University School of Medicine in Baltimore. In a long-running series of experiments on rats, Dr. Oppenheimer determined that stimulating the insular cortex for hours at a time causes a kind of damage to the heart muscle that is strikingly similar to that found in people who succumb to sudden cardiac death.

In other experiments involving people with epilepsy who were undergoing brain surgery that exposed the insular cortex, Dr. Oppenheimer found that stimulating the area with mild electrical pulses changed the person's heart rate and blood pressure.

This is why years (or decades) of persistent sorrow, hostility, and other negative emotions may cause a malfunction of the insular cortex. Such malfunction, Dr. Oppenheimer speculates,

Quiz: How Optimistic Are You?

"Cheer up," a wit said in the 1920s. "The worst is yet to come."
An optimist? A pessimist? Maybe a little of both?

It depends on what he said next, says Christopher Peterson, Ph.D., professor of psychology at the University of Michigan in Ann Arbor and author of *Health and Optimism*.

Generally, optimists have a better sense of control over their lives—at any age—than pessimists, Dr. Peterson says. "An optimist would say, 'I expect good things to happen in the future because I can make them happen,' while a pessimist might say, 'I expect bad things to happen in the future because I'm powerless to do anything about them happening,' " he says.

Unlike pessimists, optimists seem to have an internal brake that somehow helps them stop worrying about what they can't change (like cold weather) and focus on what they can do (build a fire to keep the house warm, for instance), Dr. Peterson says.

So which are you? To find out, answer the following questions on a scale of 1 (I agree a lot) to 5 (I disagree a lot) as honestly and accurately as you can. Remember that there are no correct or incorrect answers and that this is merely a rough estimate of your optimism or pessimism. Scoring follows.

1. In uncertain times, I usually expect the best.

2. If something can go wrong for me, it will.

3. I always look on the bright side of things.

4. I'm always optimistic about my future.

5. I hardly ever expect things to go my way.

6. Things never work out the way I expect them.

7. I'm a believer that every cloud has a silver lining.

8. I rarely count on good things happening to me.

9. Overall, I expect more good things to happen to me than bad.

Add up your score on group A—questions 1, 3, 4, 7, and 9—and group B—questions 2, 5, 6, and 8—separately. Low scores in group A (5 to 10) and high scores in group B (16 to 20) suggest that you are nurturing a healthy optimism. Conversely, if you have high scores in group A (16 or more) and low scores in group B (less than 6), you may want to find more reasons to let a smile be your umbrella.

This profile was developed by Charles Carver, Ph.D., professor of psychology at the University of Miami in Coral Gables, Florida, and Michael Scheier, Ph.D., professor of psychology at Carnegie Mellon University in Pittsburgh.

may subject an aging body to a steady stream of stress hormones, such as cortisol and norepinephrine, that constrict blood vessels, raise blood pressure, and suppress the immune system. These changes cause an increased vulnerability to stroke, heart disease, and cancer.

But whatever happens in the brain, many doctors believe that optimism, glee, laughter, love, and other positive emotions can counteract many of these harmful effects—even in your sixties, seventies, and eighties. Good humor seems to trigger the release of hormones, including endorphins, which relax the cardiovascular system, and cytokines, which help to alert the immune system to be more vigilant in detecting abnormalities like cancer cells.

"We don't know for a fact that what I call 'born-again optimism' will help keep you healthy in your later years, but there is every reason to believe that would be the case," Dr. Peterson says. "It certainly wouldn't hurt and will clearly improve the quality, if not the quantity, of the years you have left."

But it's important to remember that positive feelings are just one of many factors that hinder the development of cancer, stroke, and heart disease. If you rarely exercise and are overweight, smoke, drink heavily, or eat high-fat foods, your risk of these three diseases will still be considerable, no matter how optimistic or hopeful you are, Dr. Peterson warns.

Depression's Effect on Heart Disease and Stroke

We face down death by daring to hope, according to poet Maya Angelou. And, in fact, several studies suggest that people who cling to faith, optimism, and hope—particularly after age 60—may be less susceptible to the big three killers than those who feel hopeless, pessimistic, or depressed.

After analyzing the moods of 2,400 Finnish men ranging in age from 42 to 60, for instance, and following their health for the next six years, researchers at the Western Consortium for Public Health in Berkeley, California, found that men who were frequently depressed were twice as prone to heart attacks as those who said they were hopeful. In Canada, researchers at the Montreal Heart Institute tracked 222 men and women aged 24 to 88 who had had heart attacks. They found that those who had the most symptoms of depression during hospitalization, such as sadness, apathy, and appetite and sleep disturbances, were at greater risk of dying of heart problems.

"I can't say that depression or hopelessness causes heart disease. But evidence is accumulating that suggests something is going on," says Robert Anda, M.D., a medical epidemiologist at the Centers for Disease Control and Prevention in Atlanta.

Depression may increase the likelihood that heart-damaging clots will form in the arteries, speculates Nancy Frasure-Smith, Ph.D., associate professor of psychiatry at McGill University in Montreal. It's also possible that depressed people are less motivated to stick with preventive treatments. "They may be more inclined to go back to smoking and avoid making other lifestyle changes," she says.

Depression's Effect on Cancer

The blues also may be linked to cancer. In a study of the same group of 2,400 Finnish men mentioned earlier, those who strongly agreed with the statements, "The future seems hopeless to me, and I can't believe it will change for the better" and "I feel that it is impossible to reach the goals that I would like to strive for," were about 2½ times more likely to die of cancer than men who were upbeat.

Johns Hopkins University epidemiologists, in a study that included 360 men and women age 65 and older, found that nonsmokers who were relatively cheerful were 2½ to 4½ times less likely to develop cancer than depressed people who smoked more than 15 cigarettes a day. "Although further research needs to be done to confirm this finding, it makes sense that both quitting smoking and getting out of your depression would be good for you," says George W. Comstock, M.D., professor of epidemiology at Johns Hopkins University School of Hygiene and Public Health in Baltimore, and co-author of the study.

Among a group of 208 women up to age 65 at the University of Miami School of Medicine, researchers found that the women who felt hopeful and optimistic or coped well with stressful situations like divorce, retirement, or unemployment were almost two times less likely to have precancerous growths in the cervix than those who felt stressed out or hopeless. Stress, depression, pessimism, and hopelessness also may promote several types of leukemia and other lymphatic cancers, malignant melanomas, and breast and prostate cancer among men and women who are over age 60, Dr. Goodkin says.

Smile When You Say Longevity

Other positive emotions also may contribute to disease resistance and longevity. Since 1921, for example, researchers at the University of California, Riverside, have been following the aging process of 1,528 people who were preteens when the study began. Among those study subjects, the researchers concluded, such positive attributes as dependability, trust, agreeableness, and open-mindedness were associated with a two- to four-year increase in life expectancy.

"Although common wisdom might argue that a selfish, self-indulgent boor may prosper by stepping on others, this does not seem to be the case. Nor do we find a triumph of the lazy, pampered dropout. In terms of the rush toward death, the encouraging news may be that good guys finish last," according to Howard Friedman, Ph.D., professor of psychology at the university.

How Can You Keep Up Your Spirits?

Optimistic feelings can really lower your risk of developing disease. What's more, you may be able to nurture those positive emotions in yourself and tame the negative ones.

Here are some tips for cultivating a happier vision of the world:

■ **Listen to yourself.** Perhaps you have habitually put yourself down since childhood. Over a lifetime, those negative messages can turn you into a pessimist and ultimately may affect your health, says Mike Magee, M.D., a motivational speaker and professor of surgery at Jefferson Medical College of Thomas Jefferson University in Philadelphia.

For a week, write down the phrases that you say to yourself like, "I'm too old to do that anymore," or "I'm such a jerk." You'll probably end up with a list of five to 10 phrases that you repeat over and over again. Now practice stopping those thoughts and replacing them with something more positive. So, if you find yourself saying, "I'm too old to dance like that anymore," cut off that thought and replace it with something like, "I'm older now, but I can still dance if I allow for plenty of rest between songs."

■ **Write a letter to yourself.** Writing about how you feel can help resolve problems and subdue negative feelings, says James Pennebaker, Ph.D., psychology professor at Southern Methodist University in Dallas. "If the issue isn't resolved, your body is essentially reliving that experience every time you think about it," Dr. Pennebaker says. "That's very stressful on the body because it constricts blood vessels, raises blood pressure, depresses the immune system, and could exacerbate your risk of stroke, heart disease, and cancer."

Set aside 20 minutes a day for four days and write about how you feel. Don't worry about grammar or spelling. Once you begin writing, don't stop until time is up. That will encourage you to have a free flow of thoughts and feelings. If you like, throw out the paper at the end of each day, Dr. Pennebaker says.

How I Did It: Keeping the Faith

Luther H. wanted to pray, but he couldn't remember how to do it. Luther was in his forties when he had a stroke while undergoing coronary bypass surgery. The stroke paralyzed his right arm and leg. For weeks, he lay mumbling incoherently in the hospital.

The stroke also destroyed his ability to pray. "I was very despondent. I couldn't pray because I had lost the words," he said. "I sat there looking at the cross, and I just cried. That was my religion, but I couldn't get it out. It seemed hopeless."

Luther suffered so much brain damage that the doctors didn't think he would ever walk or talk again. But hope and faith would help him through the next few years.

Luther began physical and speech therapy. At first, the speech therapists told him they could only understand three of every ten words he spoke. The rest were unintelligible. But by Christmas that year he could call his wife, Kate, "Mommy." On Easter Sunday, he managed to utter a three-word prayer.

"I got up, looked at the cross and said, 'God.' Then I looked at my wife and said, 'Mommy.' Then I said, 'Amen.' That was my first prayer," Luther said.

Luther's speech improved, and he gradually regained some use of his right arm. He also learned how to walk and even drive a car. He still has difficulty reading and writing—it sometimes takes him more than 30 minutes to jot three to four sentences in his journal each day.

"I attribute all of my recovery to my faith and determination. God, my wife, and family mean everything to me," Luther said. "My advice to others is be an optimist, have faith, ask for help if you need it, and keep trying different ways of doing things if something doesn't work out for you."

"Writing will help you organize your thoughts and help you get them out of your system," he says. "By the end of the fourth day, most people feel a lot better about themselves."

■ **Watch for a miracle.** Religious texts are filled with miraculous feats, but there are plenty in modern life to ignite your hope, says Alan Epstein, Ph.D., a relationship counselor in Rome, Italy, and author of *How to Be Happier Day by Day*. Dr. Epstein, for instance, lost a valued ring on three separate occasions six years apart, only to find it each time when it seemed certain to vanish forever.

Investigate something that has happened in your lifetime that seems to defy logic and piques your interest, such as a man falling off a 100-foot cliff without breaking a bone. Write down the story and carry it with you in your purse or wallet.

When you feel despair, pull it out and look at it for inspiration, Dr. Epstein says.

■ **Seek new challenges.** "I have new projects ahead of me all of the time," said Margaret Rawson, a Frederick, Maryland, educator and an internationally recognized dyslexia researcher who lived to be 102. She took up flying at age 72, learned to use a computer at 80, and published her third book on dyslexia in her 90s.

"I'm not my age, I'm myself," Rawson always told people. "If you have a negative attitude, you're apt to say, 'No, I can't do that.' But if you have a positive attitude, you say, 'This is something that interests me, and I really want to try it. How can I do it?'"

■ **Avoid the same old rut.** Try to do one new thing every week or month. Wander through

How I Did It: Using Humor to Stare Down Death

When Richard B. found out he had lung cancer, he didn't dwell on death and taxes. He clung to hope. Given 90 days to live, Richard decided to fight back.

"The doctor took my hope away, and for five days I lived without hope. It was the worst week of my life, but I wasn't about to quit," Richard said.

Nearly 20 years later, the retired businessman credited much of his recovery to his attitude. He sought out a second opinion, began radiation and chemotherapy, and never gave up on life. "Terminal is a place where you go to catch a bus," he said. "I had too much to live for to die."

In addition to traditional cancer treatments, Richard practiced deep breathing and other relaxation techniques. He also used visual imagery to picture his body fighting off the cancer. Humor helped, too.

"Laughter has always been a big part of my life, and I had heard that humor helps activate the immune system. So while I was receiving treatment, I watched funny videos and listened to recordings of old radio programs like 'Fibber McGee and Molly,' " Richard said.

Within two months his "inoperable" tumor had shrunk enough that it could be surgically removed. Throughout the ordeal, Richard's wife, Ann, kept him focused on the future. "She was always planning something for us to do—vacations with the kids, going out to dinner," he said. "Doctors don't cure cancer; patients cure themselves with the help of their doctors. That I believe in fully," Richard said. "You can't cure a person of cancer who believes that he's going to die."

a museum, sneak into a lecture at a local college, eat at a new restaurant, or walk through a different neighborhood.

The bottom line is that monotony destroys optimism and your health, according to David Bouda, M.D., assistant professor of oncology at the University of Nebraska College of Medicine in Omaha. "If you don't use your brain and body in different ways occasionally, then you will get old very quickly," Dr. Bouda says.

■ **Look for the end of the rainbow.** Spend a moment each day to take a fresh look at something in nature and marvel at it. For instance, what happens when you look at a rainbow, Dr. Bouda asks. "I've never heard anyone say, 'Gee, I wish it had more blue and a little less red.'" Observing nature will help you get in touch with your spirituality—your being part of a larger whole—and can spark hope for the future.

■ **Find the hope within you.** Meditation or prayer can help you release from your body the anxiety, hopelessness, depression, and other negative emotions associated with heart disease, stroke, and cancer, says Patricia Norris, Ph.D., a psychophysiologic psychotherapist at the Life Sciences Institute of Mind-Body Health in Topeka, Kansas.

To try a simple meditation, sit in a comfortable chair and take several deep breaths to help you relax, Dr. Norris says. When you feel serene, close your eyes and slowly repeat, "Let my heart be like the sun and shine without judgment on everyone." And be sure to include yourself in that freedom from judgment. "The sun is a symbol. When you go outside, the sun doesn't ask, 'Are you good enough to receive my light today?' It just shines on everyone no matter who you are or how you feel. That's how I think we should envision ourselves," Dr. Norris says.

If your mind starts to wander off to concerns, like whether your Social Security check will arrive today, focus your concentrations back on the phrase. Do that for five minutes at least twice a day, or at times when you feel bitter, angry, or sad. Instead of allowing you to repress the sadness, this mental exercise will hold it out to the sun's healing light, according to Dr. Norris.

■ **Discover an abundance of happiness.** Keep a journal and write down at least 50 wonderful things that happen to you every day, says Susan Jeffers, Ph.D., a 60-year-old Los Angeles–based psychologist and author of *End the Struggle and Dance with Life.* Include even small things like finding a quarter on the sidewalk or watching a gorgeous sunset. "Make the ordinary extraordinary. After awhile, you'll realize that most things that happen are positive and you don't have to dwell on the negative," says Dr. Jeffers. She credits positive thinking with helping her to survive breast cancer.

■ **Plant hopes in growing things.** Houseplants make people feel calmer and more optimistic, says Bruno Cortis, M.D., a Chicago cardiologist in private practice and author of *Heart and Soul,* a psychological and spiritual guide to preventing and healing heart disease. In addition, Dr. Cortis says that at least one study has shown that hospital patients whose windows faced a garden recovered more quickly than those who faced a wall. So starting a garden or tending to a houseplant may help you forget problems and improve your health, he says.

■ **Pamper a pet.** "For many people over 60, a cat, dog, or other pet truly can mean the difference between life and death. Studies show that people in this age group who have pets live longer and have stronger immune systems. There is always some animal that people can connect with," says Dennis Gersten, M.D., a San Diego psychiatrist in private practice and publisher of *Atlantis: The Imagery Newsletter.*

■ **Cherish those compliments.** If someone shows appreciation for you, don't let go of it. Take a 3"x 5" card, write down the date, who the person was, and what they said about you. Put the card in a place, like the bathroom mirror, where you'll see it at least once a day. It will help you fend off negative feelings about yourself, Dr. Magee says. You also may want to keep a list of inspirational quotes—from famous people like Abraham Lincoln, Will Rogers, or Helen Keller—that are meaningful to you.

■ **Go ahead, gripe.** Surprisingly, an optimist may be the loudest complainer you know. "If you passively go along with everything, you have absolutely no sense of control, and that would foster pessimism. The person who is moaning, complaining, and demanding might not be very pleasant to be around, but they may be optimistic," Dr. Peterson says. "They believe that everything they are saying is going to make a difference, and it probably does have an effect since they probably get attention."

If you feel strongly about a problem and truly believe that complaining will make a difference, don't hold your feelings in—let someone know about it, Dr. Peterson urges.

■ **Imagine your joy.** Use your imagination to stimulate your inner-healing resources. Your imagination can help boost your self-esteem, happiness, and cancer-fighting immunity, says Dr. Gersten. This process, called guided imagery, is a powerful tool that helps to prevent and alleviate many diseases, Dr. Gersten says.

To try guided imagery, take a couple of deep breaths, then picture yourself as the spiritual elder of a clan or tribe. You are revered by all of your fellow tribe people for your knowledge and life experiences. You are useful and have a great deal to give to your tribe and the world. See yourself as being much happier now than you have been at any other time of your life because you can share your wisdom and joy with others. Use your guided imagery once or twice a day for five minutes, Dr. Gersten suggests.

■ **Eat smart.** It's hard to keep your emotions in balance if you're not eating right, Dr. Gersten says. Although no specific foods will boost your mood, he recommends eating a balanced diet that includes at least six servings of fruits and vegetables and five servings of grains each day to help fend off depression and other unwanted emotions.

Give In to Laughter

He who laughs, lasts. "You don't stop laughing because you grow old. You grow old because you stop laughing. It's that simple," says Lila Green, speaker, author of *Making Sense of Humor,* and a guest lecturer at the University of Michigan Medical School in Ann Arbor. She speaks on the topic of lighthearted physician-patient communication styles.

Although the evidence isn't conclusive, scientists are discovering that Green may be right: Laughter may well be the best medicine, particularly after age 60. For example, when 33 men and women aged 66 to 101 were asked to compare their senses of humor with those of siblings who had died of natural causes, researchers at the University of Akron found that the survivors recalled laughing more in their youth than their deceased brothers and sisters.

"It doesn't hurt to laugh. This study supports the prevailing consensus that people who enjoy humor and get a kick out of things may live longer," says Richard Haude, Ph.D., associate professor of psychology at the University of Akron in Ohio.

Laughter strengthens the immune system, decreases the production of stress-related hormones, relaxes tense muscles, keeps your mind engaged, and boosts oxygen flow and blood circulation to all parts of the body, says psychiatrist William Fry, M.D., associate clinical professor emeritus at Stanford University School of Medicine. "The relationship between humor and cancer, stroke, and heart disease is still questionable, but all indications are that they must be linked somehow," Dr. Fry says.

Here are four quick ways to make humor work for you:

■ **Make farce a habit.** Mundane routines can kill laughter, but doing something wildly different can be joyous, Green says. Sit in the bath the opposite way that you normally would, reverse the way you hang toilet paper, wear a funny mask to a friend's house, or serve dessert first at dinner. "You can't cope with change in this fast-paced world unless you're a little bit silly or zany. This will help you do that," she says.

■ **Create a humorous spot.** Instead of cluttering your refrigerator or bulletin board with reminders of doctor's appointments and meetings, reserve a spot for cartoons, funny pictures, or witty sayings, Green suggests.

■ **Think like a comic.** If you have had a particularly rough day, imagine how your favorite comedian would describe it, Green says. It will help you laugh it off.

■ **Learn to laugh at yourself.** "When you laugh at yourself, you don't break—you bend," Green says. "It gives you new perspectives about yourself. It helps keep your mind flexible and prevents what I call 'hardening of the attitudes.'" Instead of getting angry or embarrassed, laugh with others, and you'll probably feel better about yourself.

Learn the Right Way to Relax

Relaxation is one of many very valuable skills that you can use to deal with grief," says Arlene Houldin, R.N., Ph.D., associate professor of psychosocial oncology at the University of Pennsylvania School of Nursing. Practice the following technique at least three times a day, 10 to 15 minutes a session, she suggests.

1. Get into a comfortable position, close your eyes, and concentrate on the rhythmic and natural flow of your breathing.

2. Inhale and exhale slowly, feeling yourself becoming more and more calm and relaxed. Gradually allow yourself to become aware of the muscles in your forehead and scalp. Feel the muscle fibers uncoil and relax, more deeply and fully with each breath.

3. Slowly let that relaxation flow down from your forehead across your temples, through your eyelids, cheeks, nose, lips, chin, and jaw. As the relaxation gently drifts through the rest of your body, follow the same instructions for your neck, arms, elbows, hands, lungs, heart, thighs, calves, feet, and toes.

4. With your eyes still closed, say slowly to yourself five times, "I am alert, refreshed, yet deeply relaxed."

5. Slowly count to five, open your eyes, and take a couple of deep breaths before resuming your day.

Grief: Let It Out, But Don't Let It Linger

Grief is a totally normal part of life. It's as important to survival as eating and breathing," Dr. Gersten says. "If you block dealing with a death, your emotional life dies, and that can affect your physical well-being. So don't run away from the pain of grief. Realize that it is okay to be sad. You don't have to tough it out. In fact, if you try to fight it off, your grief may last forever."

Some acutely bereaved people over age 60 who lost a loved one 35 years ago have levels of complicated grief that are as high as a person who lost someone two months ago, says Holly Prigerson, Ph.D., a researcher and assistant professor of psychiatry at the University of Pittsburgh School of Medicine. In her studies, Dr. Prigerson has discovered that the grief of loss can result in considerable health problems.

For two years, she tracked the health of 150 men and women in their sixties, seventies, and eighties after the death of a spouse. Dr. Prigerson concluded that those who mourned the most severely were more susceptible to nightmares, insomnia, feelings of profound guilt, hallucinations involving the deceased, and other lingering symptoms similar to post-traumatic stress disorder—a condition that often affects soldiers, firefighters, and police officers after a catastrophe.

Significantly, these men and women were up to seven times more prone to develop cancer and five times more likely to have heart problems. Although only two people had strokes, Dr. Prigerson suspects deeply rooted grief may be a contributing factor to that disease as well.

"Most people who have these complicated grief reactions describe their marriages as wonderful. We suspect that part of the problem is that they may have been overly dependent on their spouses," Dr. Prigerson says. "So they need to start thinking about their own personal needs apart from the spouse and begin to establish a new life."

Here are some ways to mourn your loss and re-establish a positive and healthy lifestyle:

■ **Take time to relax.** Progressive relaxation and other relaxation techniques, such as deep breathing, may help to elevate your mood and give your immune system a vital boost while you are coping with grief, according to researchers at the University of Pennsylvania School of Nursing in Philadelphia. (The technique described in the box on page 183 is recommended.)

In a preliminary study of nine grieving widows up to 70 years old whose husbands had died in the previous two months, researchers found that the women who practiced progressive relaxation consistently three or four times a day for four weeks had increases in their immune cell activity, which may be beneficial in maintaining long-term health.

■ **Keep grief at arm's length.** Try this exercise: Close one eye and hold an arm out in front of you. Then slowly move your thumb toward your open eye. What happens? The thumb dominates your view and you can't see around it. The same thing can happen with grief. If you become overly consumed by grief, you'll stop seeing the joys of life, says Michael A. Zevon, Ph.D., a psychologist at the Roswell Park Cancer Institute in Buffalo, New York.

"People who can still find meaning and joy in life when they are grieving do better than those who focus all of their attention on their loss," Dr. Zevon says. Get back into your normal routine as soon as it feels comfortable and give yourself a break from your grief every day, he suggests. Spend time doing things you enjoy, like playing with your grandchildren, working in the garden, or walking in a park just marveling at the beauty around you.

■ **Talk it out.** Sharing your feelings will help you accept the loss, says Mark Berman,

Ph.D., a Phoenix psychologist in private practice who specializes in issues of the aging. It also will give others a chance to reassure you that your reactions are normal or suggest that you seek grief counseling.

■ **Get some help.** After six months, if you are still grieving, consult a psychiatrist, grief counselor, or other mental health care professional, recommends Dr. Gersten. Signs that you could use help include: a noticeable deterioration of personal hygiene, depression, chronic fatigue, insomnia, weight loss, or withdrawal or isolation.

Alleviate Anger, Heal Hostility, Curb Cynicism

Most of us have heard of the type-A personality—someone who is driven, fast-talking, competitive, distrustful, impatient, aggressive. For a long time, researchers thought that this combination of traits would increase the risk of heart disease and other killers. Although those characteristics aren't particularly charming, scientists now consider most of them fairly harmless. Instead, researchers are zeroing in on what may be the real dangers of being type A: hostility and anger.

"We know that people, including those over 60, who have negative feelings in their relationships are less healthy. In terms of the killers like heart disease, stroke, and cancer, the mortality rates are higher among those who say that they get angry frequently," says Redford Williams, M.D., director of the Behavioral Medicine Research Center at Duke University Medical Center in Durham, North Carolina, and author of *Anger Kills.*

In fact, it is becoming clearer that comedian Woody Allen was brushing up against the truth when his character in the movie *Manhattan* quipped, "I can't get angry...I grow a tumor instead."

Wise Words for a Brighter Day

The power of positive words can be significant. Here are some uplifting quotes to help you start your own list of inspirational sayings:

"Nothing is worth more than this day."
—Johann Wolfgang von Goethe, author

"My hopes are not always realized, but I always hope."
—Ovid, poet

"Although the world is full of suffering, it is also full of overcoming it."
—Helen Keller

"No matter what happens, keep on beginning and failing. Each time you fail, start all over again, and you will grow stronger until you find that you have accomplished a purpose—not the one you began with, perhaps, but one you will be glad to remember."
—Anne Sullivan, teacher of Helen Keller

"A clown is like aspirin, only he works twice as fast."
—Groucho Marx, comedian

"Frame your mind to mirth and merriment, which bar a thousand harms and lengthen life."
—William Shakespeare, poet and playwright

"To laugh often and much, to win the respect of intelligent people and the affection of children...to leave the world a bit better...to know one life breathed easier because you have lived, that is to have succeeded."
—Ralph Waldo Emerson, essayist and poet

"It is something to be able to paint a particular picture or to carve a statue...but it is far more glorious to carve and paint the very atmosphere and medium through which we look, which we morally can do. To affect the quality of the day, that is the highest of the arts."
—Henry David Thoreau, philosopher

"I keep my ideals, because in spite of everything I still believe that people are really good at heart."
—Anne Frank, from *Anne Frank: The Diary of a Young Girl*

In a preliminary study, for instance, researchers at the Institute of HeartMath in Boulder Creek, California, a biomedical research center that examines mind-body connections, asked 30 men and women to think for five minutes of either a compassionate moment in their lives or a time when they were upset or angry. "We found that simply recalling one episode of anger depresses the immune system for up to seven hours—and that's pretty interesting, considering how many times the average person gets upset in a typical day. But one episode of feeling compassion or caring enhances the immune system for about the same amount of time," says Jerry Kaiser, the Institute's director of health services. Since the immune system is the body's first line of defense against emerging cancers, this discovery may be an important step toward understanding the

Reach Out and Touch Someone

Sharing your thoughts with others may have a positive impact on quality of life and your chances of survival, says Elizabeth Maunsell, Ph.D., an epidemiologist at Hôpital du Saint-Sacrement in Quebec City.

In her study of 224 women with breast cancer—the majority over age 50—Dr. Maunsell found that those who confided in one or more people within three months of treatment were 40 percent less likely to die in the next seven years.

Ask yourself a few questions such as: Who would listen to me no matter what? Who notices my health? Who would come to me in the middle of the night just to talk? If you're not satisfied with those answers, you may need to seek out more social contact, says Bruno Cortis, M.D., a Chicago cardiologist in private practice and author of the book, *Heart and Soul*.

"It's important for 60-plus people to know that they can dare to connect, because there are a lot of others in the same situation," says Susan Jeffers, Ph.D., a Los Angeles–based psychologist and author of *End the Struggle and Dance with Life*.

At a party, recreation center, or other gathering place, focus on making other people feel good about themselves. Introduce yourself to someone and consciously make an effort to keep the conversation focused on that person's interests. The result? You'll probably feel better about yourself and may make a new friend, Dr. Jeffers says.

Note: If you have difficulty getting out of your house, call your local geriatric social service agency and ask for a list of others who are interested in developing a network of phone pals.

possible role of the mind-body connection in the development of tumors, Dr. Williams says.

At Cedars-Sinai Medical Center in Los Angeles, researchers examined 70 men and women in their sixties and seventies. Researchers concluded that not only were those people who had high levels of hostility, anger, and frustration also more likely to have myocardial ischemia (reduced blood flow to the heart that can cause angina or a heart attack), but also, their episodes lasted longer than in people who were less easily provoked.

Japanese researchers who examined negative emotions in 34 men and women concluded that anger and aggression were associated with stroke because these hostile characteristics lead to increased plaque formation and narrowing of the carotid artery, the main artery leading to the brain.

In some cases, the tendencies toward anger and hostility that are associated with type-A personality naturally diminish somewhat after age 60, but they still can be a problem for many people, according to Bart Sparagon, M.D., director of the Meyer Friedman Institute, a type-A treatment center in San Francisco.

Cynicism—an angry negativism toward daily life—seems to provoke an unhealthy physiological response similar to that of anger and hostility. After studying 1,871 male employees at Western Electric Company in Chicago for over 25 years —until the youngest of the men were age 65— researchers concluded that cynicism can elevate the risk of heart disease by 40 to 60 percent, says Richard Shekelle, Ph.D., former professor of epidemiology at the University of Texas Health Sciences Center in Houston and co-author of the study.

Simply suppressing angry feelings instead of releasing them can also create havoc in your body. After following 972 medical students for up to 40 years—until many were in their sixties and seventies—researchers at Johns Hopkins University found that those students who were considered loners and who suppressed their emotions beneath a bland exterior were 16 times more likely to develop cancer than subjects who vented their feelings.

Here's how some of the experts suggest you handle anger, hostility, and cynicism:

■ **Make this your best day.** Pretend that the world will end tomorrow. What would you do? Get angry and seek revenge against your enemies? "I know of no one who has ever done this exercise who said they'd go out and do nasty things," Dr. Williams says. "People usually say they'd go out and smell the roses or get in touch with family and friends. It's always something positive and upbeat."

Now take it a step further by writing down what you would do, and then *do it*. You'll probably accomplish something constructive with your day, be more tolerant of others, and have a more hopeful outlook on life, Dr. Williams says.

■ **Talk yourself out of a mood.** Listen to what you're telling yourself about a situation. If, for instance, the guy at the front of the buffet line seems to be holding up everyone else, is your inner voice allowing you to objectively analyze the facts—he must be hungry—or is it leading you to jump to conclusions—he's doing this on purpose? Reason with yourself, Dr. Williams says, even if you think your anger is justified. Ask yourself why you are making a big deal out of a short delay. After all, there is still plenty of food left. Once you take control of your feelings, your anger will probably subside.

■ **Counter your mood with curiosity.** If you're in a situation that normally triggers rage,

like standing in a long line at the grocery store, take a time-out. Observe other people or read a magazine rather than focusing on your anger. Also, try to recollect a very pleasant event that made you feel calm or peaceful, Dr. Sparagon suggests.

■ **Make time a friend.** Each week, write down the most precious thing you want to accomplish in the next seven days. That way, if you accomplish nothing else, you can feel good that you did one important thing. You'll also be less apt to see time as an enemy and get upset that you didn't complete everything that you set out to do, says Meyer Friedman, M.D., a pioneering researcher of type-A behavior and founder of the Meyer Friedman Institute.

Be Your Own Best Friend

Although experts can suggest many paths to happiness, ultimately, hope and optimism come from within you, says Frosty Westering, Ed.D., an educational psychologist and legendary head football coach at Pacific Lutheran University in Tacoma, Washington.

"The biggest opponent you have in life is yourself. You're either your own opponent or your own friend," says Dr. Westering, author of *Make the Big Time Where You Are*. "So be the best friend that you can be to yourself. So many people put themselves down. They're constantly telling themselves what they can't do.

"After games, for instance, we never talk about what we didn't do as a team. We always talk about the things that are good about this team. So win or lose, we leave the field feeling upbeat. That's a lesson we all can learn at any age. It is what's inside that counts. If you feel good about yourself, if you feel young at heart, if you feel as if you're the best you can be every day, then that can make all the difference in your mental and physical well-being."

Prescription for Gaining a Good Attitude

Joy, hope, and optimism can improve the quality of your life at any age, doctors say. Intriguing research indicates that positive feelings can enhance the health-protective powers of diet and exercise and can help suppress many diseases, including heart disease, cancer, and stroke.

DO:

▶ **Jot down at least 50 terrific things** that happen to you each day.

▶ **Laugh often.** It heals both the mind and the body.

▶ **Find one new challenge each month.** Try new projects and hobbies. Fulfill a lifelong ambition.

▶ **Meditate for five minutes, twice a day.** It will help you purge depression, anxiety, and other negative feelings from your body.

DON'T:

▶ **Dwell on negative thoughts.** If your mind is saturated with glum feelings, write down those feelings and find positive thoughts to replace them.

▶ **Neglect good foods.** Your emotions can spiral downward if you don't eat right. Eating a well-balanced diet that includes at least six servings of fruits and vegetables, like apples and carrots, can help fend off depression and other unwanted emotions.

10

Is It Too Late to Quit Smoking?

Long before all the illusions about tobacco evaporated like stale smoke, lighting up was the stylish thing to do. Joltin' Joe DiMaggio, who became the pride of the New York Yankees in the 1930s, encouraged young baseball fans to smoke cigarettes. "They don't get your wind," he said, claiming they were "so mild, athletes smoke as many as they please." Stars like Betty Grable, the popular World War II pinup girl and the highest paid female in 1940s' Hollywood, was one of a bevy of stars who showed movie audiences how alluring it was to light up. In the 1950s, a cigarette dangling from James Dean's lips defined coolness for an entirely new generation.

Smoking was not just considered glamorous during the mid-twentieth century—cigarette manufacturers actually claimed that it was healthy, too. Smoking steadied the nerves, they said, as it increased energy and suppressed appetite.

In fact, for several years one tobacco company proclaimed that more doctors smoked its brand than any other. Most doctors didn't object when attractive young women from tobacco firms regularly replenished supplies of free cigarettes in their waiting rooms.

So when you may have been enticed to start puffing—along with a lot of other unsuspecting young men and women—the powerfully addictive nature of tobacco and the devastating effects of smoking on the body were virtually unknown. But now you know better.

If you are like the typical male smoker in his sixties or seventies, you began at age 17 and have smoked about 27 cigarettes a day for 51 years. If you are a woman in the same age range, you probably first lit up at about age 24 and have been smoking 20 cigarettes a day for 45 years.

And, like about 80 percent of people who smoke, you have probably tried at least once to quit.

Will Quitting Now Really Make a Difference?

Can quitting at this point in your life change anything? Even after you've been smoking for decades? You bet it can. The evidence is unimpeachable: Stamping out your last cigarette as late as age 60, 70, or even 80 can halt many of the worst effects of smoking.

What If I Switch to Light Cigarettes?

Switching to low-tar, low-nicotine cigarettes may seem like a logical way to slash your risk of debilitating diseases, but doctors say it doesn't help. "Light" and "ultra-light" cigarettes still contain dangerous amounts of nicotine, carbon monoxide, and tar.

"Smoking a low-tar cigarette is like jumping off a 20-story building instead of a 30-story one. There simply is no such thing as a safe, safer, or safest cigarette," says Alan Blum, M.D., assistant professor of family medicine at Baylor College of Medicine in Houston.

"Quitting will significantly reduce your risk of stroke, heart disease, and cancer regardless of your age, and it will improve your quality of life," says Thomas Brandon, Ph.D., associate professor of psychology at the State University of New York at Binghamton and a smoking-cessation expert.

Yet an astounding 46 percent of older smokers still don't believe that smoking is very harmful, or that the benefits of quitting are really worthwhile.

If you're among those doubters, ponder these facts:

■ Within eight hours of quitting, your pulse rate and blood pressure drop, and oxygen levels in your body rise.

■ Within 24 hours of quitting, your risk of a heart attack decreases.

■ After one month, your circulation improves, your energy levels surge, and your lung function expands by up to 30 percent.

■ After one year, your risk of heart disease is half that of someone who continues to smoke.

■ After five years, your risk of having a stroke begins to decline.

■ After 10 years, your chances of developing lung cancer are the same as that of someone who has never smoked.

"To know that your risk of sudden death from smoking-related heart disease has dramatically decreased is tremendous," says Alan Blum, M.D., assistant professor of family medicine at Baylor College of Medicine in Houston.

Each Puff Is Harmful

With each puff, a smoker inhales more than 4,700 chemicals that have been shown to have a wide-reaching effect throughout the body. Some of the milder effects include:

Accelerated wrinkling of the skin
Yellowing of the teeth and fingers
Slow wound healing

Then there are the dangerous downsides of smoking, including increases in the risk of devastating disabilities such as:

Osteoporosis
Hip fractures
Cataracts
Diabetes
Tooth loss
Emphysema

Finally, smoking causes fatal complications. Every year, more than 400,000 Americans die of smoking-related causes. That adds up to more than 1,000 a day, making smoking the most preventable cause of death in the United States. Some 50 percent of those deaths are caused by cardiovascular disease and 30 percent by lung cancer.

Here's a quick look at how smoking magnifies the impact of cardiovascular disease and cancer, and how quitting can slash your risk of developing these conditions:

■ **Smoking hurts your heart.** The chemicals in tobacco smoke, including nicotine and carbon monoxide—yes, the same poisonous gas that's found in automobile exhaust—raise blood pressure, constrict blood vessels, and starve the heart of oxygen, forcing it to work harder. At the same time, smoking increases the stickiness of blood platelets so that they are more likely to form dangerous blood clots. It also raises total and low-density lipoprotein (the so-called bad cholesterol), lowers levels of high-density lipoprotein (the good cholesterol), and accelerates the accumulation of plaque in arteries that causes atherosclerosis (hardening of the arteries).

People age 64 and over who smoke have arteries clogged with about the same levels of plaque as people a decade older who have never smoked, according to researchers at Bowman Gray School of Medicine of Wake Forest University in Winston-Salem, North Carolina.

The bottom line: A person who smokes is three times more likely to develop heart disease and is four times more likely to have a stroke as a nonsmoker. In addition, one in every four deaths is linked to smoking.

If you quit: Your risk of a heart attack is slashed by 50 percent in one year, and after about five years your chances of having a stroke are virtually the same as for someone who never smoked.

■ **Smoking tops the list of cancer risks.** Smoking is linked to one in three cancer deaths and nearly 90 percent of all lung cancers. Smoking is associated with cancer of the mouth, throat, esophagus, bladder, pancreas, and kidneys. "If it weren't for smoking, these cancers would barely exist," says Andrea LaCroix, Ph.D., associate professor of epidemiology at the University of Washington School of Public Health and Community Medicine in Seattle. Smoking also appears to contribute to 30 percent of cervical cancer cases.

Tobacco smoke contains at least 43 cancer-causing substances that can scramble a cell's genetic code, causing it to reproduce abnormally. Constant exposure to the toxic compounds in smoke can cause these abnormal cells to gradually transform into cancer.

If you quit: Even at age 65, your risk of developing lung cancer by age 75 is less than half that of someone who continues to smoke, according to researchers at the University of Michigan. The risk of developing many other cancers—including those affecting the mouth, kidney, and pancreas—begins to diminish within 10 years of quitting.

"The time to quit smoking is when you still feel fine, because by the time you develop cancer and it is detected, it may be too late to cure it," says Teresa Hayes, M.D., an oncologist at Baylor College of Medicine in Houston. "If you quit smoking, not only will you stop adding to your risk, but if you do develop cancer, your chances of survival will be better because your body will be in better shape."

Can You Still Quit?

Like four of every five smokers, you may want to quit and may already have tried several times, only to be lured back to tobacco. But don't blame yourself. It's not a sign of weakness, according to smoking-cessation experts. Nicotine, the prime ingredient in tobacco, is one of the most addictive drugs known. Once you're in its grasp, it takes a determined effort to break free, particularly if you have been smoking for many years. But you can do it.

What Exactly Are You Smoking?

When tobacco giant Philip Morris announced an unprecedented recall of 8 billion defective cigarettes in 1995, a young woman smoking in New York told a newspaper reporter, "At least it's not cyanide."

Wrong.

Not only does tobacco smoke contain hydrogen cyanide—a deadly poison used in prison gas chambers—it also harbors 4,700 other chemicals and toxins, including at least 43 cancer-causing substances. Here's just a sampling of what a typical smoker inhales with each puff. The common description for each chemical is also listed below.

Chemicals in Cigarette Smoke	Common Description
Acetone	paint stripper
Ammonia	floor cleaner
Arsenic	ant poison
Butane	lighter fluid
Cadmium	car-battery component
Carbon monoxide	car exhaust
Formaldehyde	morgue preservative
Methanol	antifreeze
Naphthalene	mothballs
Nicotine	insecticide
Polonium 210	radioactive substance

"Many older people have smoked for so long that they don't think they can overcome it. But I've helped people who have smoked for 50 years quit successfully," says Gary DeNelsky, Ph.D., director of the smoking-cessation program at the Cleveland Clinic. "Quitting isn't easy, but it isn't like climbing Mount Everest either."

In fact, of those people over age 65 who have smoked, 77 percent have stopped, according to the Office of Smoking and Health at the Centers for Disease Control and Prevention in Atlanta. But that still leaves nearly 16 million people who continue to smoke after age 65.

About 1.3 million Americans each year break free of tobacco's hold and become nonsmokers. Most quit using a variety of techniques, ranging from Nicotine Anonymous to stress management to improved nutrition.

How to Become Smoke-Free

Everybody needs to find his own way to quit. That's the key. You have to be motivated to quit and be creative in finding ways to not smoke," says Mitchell Nides, Ph.D., a psychologist at the University of California, Los Angeles.

But no matter how you choose to quit, smoking-cessation experts suggest you keep these points in mind:

■ **Set a quit date.** People who designate a definite day to quit and stick to it are more likely to stop smoking than those who don't, Dr. Brandon says. Avoid picking stressful

How We Did It: Douse That Deadly Habit

Tracy G. doesn't remember smoking his last cigarette. But neither he nor his wife, Bernice, will ever forget what happened next.

A two-pack-a-day smoker since his teens, Tracy had just lit a cigarette after an ocean swim. Seconds later, his heart stopped beating, and he slumped over in his beach chair. For the next 11 minutes lifeguards, volunteer firefighters, and paramedics desperately performed cardiopulmonary resuscitation and administered electroshocks to his heart. In the hospital emergency room, his heart was shocked more than 14 times to keep it beating. After Tracy regained consciousness, he couldn't recall much of that eventful day.

"My heart failure was caused by hardening of the arteries due to smoking and a fast-food diet," said the former gas station owner. "I had always enjoyed smoking and never really gave much thought to quitting until after that day. But having something like that happen was like going through a very advanced stop-smoking clinic. I've never really had a desire for a cigarette again. I feel better, I breathe better, food tastes better, my clothes don't stink. I'm very thankful to be alive."

For Bernice, watching her husband's near-death experience was enough to make her ditch her own two-pack-a-day habit. On the day Tracy came home from the hospital, she got rid of her favorite lighter and all the remaining cigarettes.

"I didn't want to tempt him," said Bernice. He wasn't tempted, but she was. "My toughest times were after I ate meals because I was used to having a cigarette then," she said.

Her solution? Bernice changed her routine. "I sat in a different spot at the table than I normally would," she said. "After I was finished eating, I would get right up and start doing the dishes. Sometimes when I was doing the dishes, I'd scream, 'I need a cigarette! I need a cigarette!' But everyone would realize that I was just releasing tension and ignore me. After about 30 seconds of that, the urge would pass."

Within a couple of months, her desire to smoke was entirely gone. The couple also started walking three miles a day and eating a low-fat, high-fiber diet. And they never lit up again.

"Our kids tell me, 'Mom, you don't look like a smoker anymore.' And I really don't feel like a smoker," Bernice said. "It's great."

holidays like New Year's Day or Thanksgiving. Also, don't select a date that is weeks or months away. Chances are that your resolve to quit will melt away by then. Instead, once you decide to stop, choose a day that falls within the next two weeks.

■ **Go cold turkey.** President Dwight D. Eisenhower began smoking when he was a cadet at West Point. By World War II, Ike was up to four packs a day. In 1949, doctors advised that he should cut back. After a few days, he decided

that rationing his cigarettes was worse than not smoking at all. So he quit cold turkey and never had another cigarette in his life, according to late historian Stephen E. Ambrose, Ph.D., author of *Eisenhower: Soldier and President.*

All that he did was put smoking out of his mind. He developed "a scornful attitude toward those weaklings who did not have the willpower to break their enslavement to nicotine," Ambrose wrote.

It worked for Ike, and it can work for you.

"If you quit cold turkey, you'll probably have a week to 10 days of withdrawal, but then you'll be almost over it. Most people find it a lot easier to quit cold turkey than to gradually reduce their smoking," Dr. Brandon says.

■ **Toss 'em overboard.** On your quit date, throw away all of your tobacco products. Don't hold back. Anything hidden in sweaters, pockets, or glove compartments should be tossed as well, advises C. Tracy Orleans, Ph.D., director of Tobacco Control Research at Fox Chase Cancer Center in Philadelphia and principal creator of Clear Horizons, a self-help smoking-cessation program for people aged 50 and older. Get rid of your lighters, matches, and ashtrays, too.

■ **Banish the booze.** Alcohol dissolves your resolve and makes it easier for you to light up again, says Thomas Cooper, D.D.S., a nicotine-dependency researcher and professor of oral health sciences at the University of Kentucky College of Dentistry in Lexington. He recommends that you avoid drinking alcohol for at least a month after you quit smoking.

■ **Prepare to fight the urge.** The first seven to 10 days of any effort to quit smoking are the toughest, Dr. Brandon says. As your body adjusts to the lack of nicotine, you'll go through at least some of these withdrawal symptoms:

> *Upset stomach*
>
> *Difficulty concentrating*
>
> *Drowsiness*
>
> *Insomnia*
>
> *Irritability*

Once the nicotine is flushed out of your body, your withdrawal symptoms—and your cravings—should gradually subside. But you still may be occasionally tempted to smoke for months or even years afterward. Eleven years after he quit, President Eisenhower scribbled, "God, I wish I

had a cigarette," on a memo pad during a tense meeting with Soviet Premier Nikita Khrushchev. Still, the longer you go without smoking, the more likely you'll be able to resist the urge.

■ **One is never enough.** Nicotine is a life-long addiction, so smoking just one cigarette—even after years of abstinence—can often lead to another and another.

"'Smoking one won't hurt me,' has probably been the downfall of more smokers who are trying to quit than any other single thing," says Dr. Cooper. He smoked for 36 years before he finally quit.

Psychologically, smoking just one cigarette often makes people who have quit feel bad about themselves. And to cope with those bad feelings, they smoke more cigarettes and quickly tumble back into the habit, Dr. Nides says.

If you're severely tempted, get away from the situation or call a supportive friend who can help talk you out of it, Dr. Nides suggests.

Making the Change Permanent

When you wake up, you smoke. Take out the garbage, you smoke. Go bowling, you smoke. The urge to have a cigarette is often triggered by everyday tasks and routines. But if you change your habits, you can become a non-smoker, doctors say.

These self-help techniques, used alone or in combination, will help keep you from starting to smoke again:

■ **Keep a record.** Whenever you smoke, jot down the time of day and what you were doing. Then describe in detail the step-by-step process of lighting up. A description of an after-dinner cigarette, for example, might read: "I push my chair back from the table. I take a deep breath. I reach into my pocket and grab the package. I tap the package on the table. I slip out a cigarette

The Hardest Smoke to Give Up

All cigarettes aren't created equal. If you smoke, you probably have one special time of day when lighting up gives you the greatest pleasure.

In a survey of 5,051 men and women who smoke, 44 percent said that they would miss an after-dinner cigarette the most if they quit smoking, according to researchers at Stanford University and the West Los Angeles Veterans Affairs Hospital. One in three said that the first cigarette in the morning would be the hardest to forgo, followed by the last one of the day and lighting up when drinking alcoholic beverages.

"For most smokers, the after-dinner cigarette seems to be almost irresistible," says Murray Jarvik, M.D., professor of psychiatry at the University of California, Los Angeles, School of Medicine. Why? Eating a big meal like dinner slightly reduces the amount of nicotine in the blood, and that may trigger physical cravings. You also can develop a strong psychological urge to smoke if you associate finishing a meal with lighting up an after-dinner cigarette.

But no matter when you are used to smoking your favorite cigarette, a key part of quitting is getting past that particular moment without taking a puff. The best strategy is changing your routine, says Michael Cummings, Ph.D., senior research scientist and director of the smoking cessation clinic at Roswell Park Cancer Institute in Buffalo, New York.

Instead of smoking after a meal, go for a walk or do the dishes immediately. Try munching on a low-fat dessert like fresh fruit in a room where you normally don't eat. Avoid eating any food that seems to bolster your craving for tobacco.

Instead of smoking first thing in the morning, distract yourself. Get up and shower, dress, eat breakfast, and then vigorously plunge into your daily activities. To ensure that you'll have a busy morning, Dr. Cummings suggests that you make appointments for early in the day, then stay in bed for an extra few minutes so that you must rush to get ready and won't have time to smoke.

Instead of smoking during the day, keep a distractive device nearby—a small ball, a pencil, a pen, chewing gum, or hard candies. Then you will have something to do with your hands and mouth.

and twiddle it in my right hand. I put the cigarette in my mouth and reach for my lighter. I light the cigarette and take my first puff."

This record-keeping is an important starting point for making changes, because it helps you become aware of your smoking patterns and the complex rituals that you may have created for lighting up, says Dennis Gersten, M.D., a San Diego psychiatrist.

■ **Change your rituals.** Once you are aware of your smoking routines, try to break them up somehow. It can be as simple as switch-

ing the hand that holds the cigarette. "I find that switching hands makes people very uncomfortable, which turns out to be a good thing," Dr. Gersten says. "I had one patient who had been smoking for 40 years. He simply switched from smoking with his right hand to his left, and that was the end of his smoking. It broke the pattern right on the spot."

■ **Short-circuit stress.** "A lot of people smoke to cope with stress. So when you quit, you have to come up with some new coping devices," says Michael Cummings, Ph.D., senior research

Tobacco: There's No Safety Valve

Pipes, cigars, and chewing tobacco can be just as deadly as cigarettes. Here's why:

- Pipe and cigar smoke contains the same number of toxic compounds as cigarette smoke.

- If you smoke a pipe or cigars and don't inhale, you still have a higher risk for developing cancers of the mouth and lips than a nonsmoker.

- A former cigarette smoker is more likely to inhale when smoking a pipe or cigar. If you do inhale, you have the same risk of developing lung cancer and heart disease as a regular cigarette smoker.

- A person who uses chewing tobacco can achieve blood nicotine levels comparable with someone who smokes cigarettes.

- Nitrosamine, a potent cancer-causing agent, is present in chewing tobacco products at levels up to 100 times higher than those allowed in bacon, beer, and certain other foods.

- Users of chewing tobacco are twice as likely to die of heart disease than those who don't smoke or chew. The constant flow of nicotine from this type of tobacco product increases a person's heart rate and blood pressure and can lead to an increased risk of stroke.

Chemicals in Chewing Tobacco	Common Description
Arsenic	ant poison
Benzene	toxic gasoline ingredient
Cadmium	car-battery component
Cyanide	poison
Formaldehyde	morgue preservative
Lead	nerve poison
Nicotine	insecticide
N-Nitrosamine	cancer-causing agent
Polonium 210	radioactive substance

scientist and director of the smoking-cessation clinic at Roswell Park Cancer Institute in Buffalo, New York. Try deep breathing, meditation, exercise, squeezing a rubber ball, or just pushing your tongue into the roof of your mouth for 10 to 15 seconds.

■ **Quit early in the week.** "We suggest that our patients try to quit on a Monday or a Tuesday of a busy week," Dr. Cooper says. "You don't want to quit smoking when you have a lot of time on your hands to think about it."

■ **Stay in a smoke-free world.** Plan out your day so that you'll be less tempted to smoke. Browse in a smoke-free shopping mall, eat in a smoke-free restaurant, or go to a movie or museum where smoking is prohibited, suggests Dr. Nides.

■ **Give yourself daily pep talks.** Every morning and at bedtime, write down all the reasons why you want to quit. It will reinforce your resolve to stop smoking. "It's easy to forget why you're trying to quit when you're going through nicotine withdrawal. So reminders are

Medical Advances Make It Easy to Quit

It's only a few inches around and doesn't look very impressive, but the transdermal nicotine patch is rapidly becoming a formidable weapon in the struggle to quit smoking. When worn on the skin, the patch releases tiny amounts of nicotine into the bloodstream for up to 24 hours. The nicotine eases withdrawal symptoms and makes it easier for you to quit. Over several weeks, the dosage of each successive patch is gradually reduced to wean you off the drug.

Of 1,070 male and female patch users aged 65 to 74, nearly 30 percent were still smoke-free six months later, says C. Tracy Orleans, Ph.D., director of Tobacco Control Research at Fox Chase Cancer Center in Philadelphia. Most of those who had tried to quit before said that the patch made quitting easier. "The patch is state of the art," he says. "It increases quit rates by two to three times. We're recommending it for anyone who has had trouble dealing with withdrawal symptoms in the past."

Nicotine gum, another form of nicotine replacement, also has helped many people quit. Both the patch and gum are readily available over the counter.

Warning: Be sure to check with your doctor to see if nicotine gum or the patch would be appropriate for you.

---

an important way to keep yourself on track," Dr. Brandon says.

You also might try jotting down something you did that day—such as walking a mile—that you weren't able to do when you smoked, Dr. Nides says.

■ **Make a deal.** Sign a contract with yourself, Dr. Brandon suggests. Every day that you go without a cigarette, reward yourself—buy a magazine, sleep in for an extra 30 minutes or take a long stroll.

If you smoke, punish yourself with an activity you detest, like cleaning the refrigerator or washing out the gutters, Dr. Brandon says.

■ **Save those dollars.** Put the money that you would normally spend on cigarettes into a clear container so that you can see it add up. After six months, use that money for a big reward, like a vacation, Dr. Brandon suggests.

■ **Stall for time.** When an urge hits, if you can delay lighting up for just a minute or two the feeling may pass, Dr. Cummings says. Carry a photo of your grandchildren or other loved ones

and pull it out every time an urge strikes. Or write down the reasons why you want to quit and keep the list handy for when you're stalling.

Stay Smoke-Free by Eating Well

Smokers who begin eating a nonsmoker's typical diet are more likely to be smoke-free a year later than those who attempt to quit without dietary changes, says Dr. William McCarthy, Ph.D., director of science at the Pritikin Longevity Center in Santa Monica, California. "Dietary changes are a way of moving away from the smoker lifestyle," he says. "If you simply extinguish the cigarette and do nothing else about your lifestyle habits, you will still be acting and living like a typical smoker."

Smokers tend to eat more meat, drink more coffee and alcohol, eat fewer fruits and vegetables, consume fewer cereals and grains. No wonder smokers are more likely than nonsmokers to be deficient in vitamins A, C, E, and minerals like calcium, selenium, and zinc.

Diet First, Then Quit Smoking

It may be too difficult to make major changes in your diet at the same time that you have to cope with nicotine withdrawal. Some nutritionists suggest that if you need to lose significant weight, you should adjust your diet first. Then, when you feel comfortable with your new eating habits, proceed with your plans to quit smoking.

Dietary changes—particularly cutting fats and adding fruits and vegetables like oranges, apricots, carrots, and sweet potatoes, which are loaded with antioxidants—can help offset the ill effects of smoking and reduce your risk of stroke, heart disease, and cancer, says James Scala, Ph.D., a nutritional biochemist and author of *If You Can't/Won't Stop Smoking*. Antioxidants like vitamin C help block or reverse some of the harm done by free radicals, which are unstable molecules that damage cells and tissues. "Research indicates that it is sensible to take up to 1,000 milligrams of vitamin C daily and about 400 international units of vitamin E to reverse some of the bad influences of smoking," says Dr. Scala.

A good diet also will help you counteract weight gain, according to Dr. Scala. Fear of gaining weight is an imposing barrier for many smokers who are trying to quit. In a survey of 1,234 people who smoked, aged 50 to 74, nearly half believed that gaining 20 pounds is more harmful than smoking. "Actually, you would probably have to gain at least 100 pounds to equal the health risks of continued smoking," says Robert C. Klesges, Ph.D., professor of psychology and preventive medicine at the University of Memphis in Tennessee.

In reality, about half of all people who quit smoking don't gain weight, and those who do put on about 10 pounds. The weight gain only occurs shortly after you quit smoking, and you

do not continue to gain weight any faster than someone who had never smoked.

Here are some ways you can use food as an ally to help you keep from smoking:

■ **Balance the pyramid.** If you follow the guidelines of the basic U.S. Department of Agriculture food pyramid, you'll be eating more like a nonsmoker and may be less tempted to light up again, Dr. McCarthy says. That means two to four servings of fruits a day; three to five servings of vegetables; two to three servings of dairy products, like milk and cheese; six to 11 servings of breads, rice, and cereals; and no more than one 3-ounce serving of meat, poultry, or fish or two to three servings of beans, egg whites, and nuts.

■ **Sip on OJ.** Tobacco smoke destroys vitamin C. Replenish your supply by drinking two 8-ounce glasses of orange juice daily, particularly in the first few days after you quit, Dr. Scala says.

Orange juice will also help flush nicotine out of your body and help you become nicotine-free faster, Dr. Cooper says. (Avoid orange juice, however, if you're using the nicotine patch or gum, because you want that nicotine to stay in your body to help avoid withdrawal symptoms.)

■ **Cut down on caffeine.** Laying off tobacco increases the stimulating effects of caffeine. So if you drink coffee, you may feel more jittery and might start craving a smoke, Dr. Brandon says. Switch to decaffeinated coffee and drink no more than two 8-ounce cups a day, he suggests.

Nicotine Anonymous: No Names, but Lots of Support

Nicotine Anonymous, a 12-step program similar to Alcoholics Anonymous, offers support to those who want to be nicotine-free. The organization, founded in 1982, has about 500 chapters worldwide. Members acknowledge that nicotine is an addictive drug and they cannot control their use of it. They say that the meetings support them as they strive to stay smoke-free. The only requirement for membership is the desire to abstain from nicotine.

"I heard things in meetings from others who had quit before me, and I thought, 'Oh my God, I'm going through that, too.' I just realized that what I was experiencing was normal," says Lynn H., a Chicago woman who smoked for 34 years before quitting in her sixties.

"There is something in those meetings that grabs you. There is a lot of caring, friendship, and support," she says. "I still go to remind myself what it was like because it's so easy to forget. And I know that if I forget and decide I can smoke socially, I'll end up right back where I started."

For more information, send a stamped, self-addressed envelope to: Nicotine Anonymous World Service Office, Department R, P. O. Box 591777, San Francisco, CA 94159-1777.

■ **Stay hydrated.** Carry a bottle of water around with you. Whenever you feel the urge for a smoke, take a swig of water instead, Dr. Cummings says. Water helps flush nicotine and other tobacco toxins out of the body and speeds withdrawal. In addition to the normal amount that you drink, he recommends having another six to eight glasses daily when you're trying to quit.

■ **Eat breakfast.** People who smoke often use a cigarette to elevate blood sugars and suppress appetite, Dr. Cooper says. It's important to replace your early-morning smoke with an energizing low-fat breakfast like a bran muffin and a glass of apple juice.

■ **Become a Johnny Appleseed.** Snacking on an apple twice daily for the first 90 days after you quit will help get you past the mid-morning and midafternoon slumps without reaching for a cigarette, Dr. Cooper says.

■ **Try new foods.** Avoid eating or drinking any foods that you link with smoking, Dr. Brandon says. So if you have always had a cup of coffee and a muffin for breakfast followed by a cigarette, try a glass of milk and a piece of raisin toast instead. The change in foods may dampen your urge to smoke.

■ **Make food work for you.** In the first few days after quitting, keep healthy, low-fat foods like breadsticks, crackers, carrots, celery, and popcorn handy to snack on whenever you feel the urge to smoke.

■ **Play with your food.** If you need something to do with your hands, try eating foods that require peeling, such as oranges, sunflower seeds, tangerines, nuts in the shell, or artichokes, suggests C. Barr Taylor, M.D., professor of psychiatry at Stanford University School of Medicine and author of *The Facts About Smoking*.

■ **Indulge your sweet tooth.** If eating a sweet will prevent you from smoking, do it, Dr. Taylor says. If possible, avoid high-fat sweets like cake, ice cream, and chocolate. Instead, pick low-fat alternatives like jelly beans, sherbets, or hard candies, or fruits like grapes, bananas, or dates.

Fight the Stress with Meditation

The average person has about 15,000 thoughts a day. If you're trying to quit, it can seem like

Fight the Urge with Relaxation Techniques

If you want to use the calming effect of physical exertion to combat the urge to smoke, try the exercise regimens described in Chapter 8. Simple relaxation and meditation techniques that can be used at your desk or your kitchen table can be found below on this page, in the box on page 183, and in Chapter 7 on weight control, pages 143–144.

every one of those thoughts is the same: *Smoke!* But meditation can help you dampen that mental noise and help you become a nonsmoker, says Dr. Gersten.

Meditation is a form of concentration that allows you to focus your mind internally and step back from your thoughts and feelings, Dr. Gersten says. In its simpler forms, meditation uses pictures, words (mantras), objects (such as a candle flame), or sensations (such as breathing) to focus the mind. If your mind begins to drift, you refocus your attention on your chosen image or word.

Studies have shown that meditation can help reduce the severity of many medical conditions, including anxiety, asthma, migraines, high blood pressure, and chronic pain. And it can help you quit smoking, Dr. Gersten says.

Every time you feel an urge to smoke, try this meditation technique:

1. Each time you inhale, say the word "peace."

2. As you exhale, say "love."

3. Repeat for five minutes. By then the urge to smoke may have passed or subsided to the point that you can resist it.

4. If your mind begins to wander, refocus it on the words.

"This meditation will help you deal with the craving. You're not saying that the urge to smoke isn't there," Dr. Gersten says. "You're acknowledging that the urge exists, but you don't have to do anything about it. You just turn your mind back to your mantra."

If You Must, Let Go Slowly

Although going cold turkey is your best bet, there is a gradual alternative that works for some people, says Dr. Orleans.

The process is known as nicotine fading, and Dr. Orleans calls it a form of "cool turkey" because it prepares you both physically and psychologically for the day when you finally quit altogether.

"Quitting abruptly on a target date is the best way to go," Dr. Orleans says. "But nothing says that you shouldn't prepare yourself for your quit date. Nicotine fading is one of the ways you can do that." By making small weekly drops in nicotine, you avoid strong withdrawal symptoms when you quit, particularly if you smoke a high- or medium-nicotine brand.

High-nicotine brands include unfiltered cigarettes and any filtered brand that isn't labeled with the words "mild," "light," or "ultra-light." Medium-nicotine brands are labeled "mild" or "light." Low-nicotine cigarettes bear words like "extra mild," "ultra," and "ultra-light."

The nicotine-fading program allows two weeks to complete the process if you smoke a high-nicotine brand, and one week for medium- or low-nicotine brands.

Here's how you can proceed:

■ **Step down your nicotine dose.** If you smoke a high-nicotine brand, switch to medium for one week, and then to a low brand for another week before you quit. That way, you will cut the dose of nicotine you get by $1/3$ each week. If you smoke mediums, switch to lows for a week before you quit.

■ **Don't drop too quickly.** Avoid going directly from a high-nicotine brand to a low one, Dr. Orleans says. If the nicotine in your body drops too rapidly, it can cause cravings and withdrawal symptoms, which will defeat the purpose of fading.

■ **Don't kid yourself.** Keep your cigarette use on an even keel. Dr. Orleans warns that if you switch to lower-nicotine cigarettes but smoke more of them, you risk getting the same dose of nicotine that you were getting before. Avoid inhaling more often or deeply than you have in the past, and try not to cover the tiny airholes near the bottom of the filter with your fingers or lips.

■ **Stick to your quit date.** Having an absolute quit date is a must with nicotine fading, Dr. Orleans says. Without it, you may be tempted to think that cutting back on nicotine is good enough. It isn't. For the sake of your health, you need to shake the habit completely.

(For more information on the Clear Horizons program, write to: Fox Chase Cancer Center, 510 Township Line Road, Cheltenham, PA 19012.)

Prescription for Quitting Smoking

Quitting smoking is the most important thing that a person can do to slash the risk of stroke, cancer, and heart disease. Even if you have smoked for years, quitting at age 60, 70, or 80 can reverse many of the worst effects of smoking and improve the quality of your life.

DO:

▶ **Set a quit date and stick to it.**

▶ **Throw out all of your tobacco products** on your quit date.

▶ **Quit cold turkey.**

▶ **Plan out your day so that you'll be less tempted to smoke.** Window shop in a smoke-free shopping mall, for example.

▶ **Eat like a nonsmoker.** A balanced diet that includes at least five servings of fruits and vegetables like apples and carrots can help reduce your urge to smoke.

▶ **Drink at least two 8-ounce glasses of orange juice daily.** It will help flush nicotine out of your body. Orange juice, however, is not recommended if you are using the nicotine patch or gum.

▶ **Persevere.** Nicotine, a prime ingredient in tobacco, is one of the most addictive substances in the world. It may take several attempts to quit. But if you keep trying, you will become a nonsmoker.

DON'T:

▶ **Drink alcohol for at least 30 days** after you quit smoking.

▶ **Drink caffeinated beverages like coffee, tea, or colas.** Caffeine can increase your urge to smoke.

▶ **Let stress defeat your effort to quit.** Practice relaxation techniques like meditation.

11

Is Drinking Alcohol
Good or Bad?

hink Mediterranean: blue skies, white beaches, and the to-die-for Mediterranean diet, full of vegetables, fruits, pastas and olive oil that's oh-so-healthy. Add to this idyllic picture an unexpected bonus—a glass of red wine with dinner. Sound too good to be true? Well, it may not be just a fantasy. Such a diet—complete with wine—may lower your risk of heart disease and stroke. It may even help fight cancer.

Lifting a wine glass at the dinner table may be part of the reason that people in Mediterranean countries can eat heavy foods and still have low rates of heart disease. In fact, part of the reason for a phenomenon known as "the French paradox"—the fact that French people can eat super-rich cuisine, yet they have an unexpectedly low risk of heart disease—could lie in their vineyards, researchers believe. Or, more precisely, in ethanol, the main ingredient in alcoholic beverages—the very stuff that can make you light-headed.

As for protection from cancer, scientists have found that some of the plant chemicals in wine shield your system from disease. While you're enjoying a glass, wine goes to work blocking the formation of harmful low-density lipoprotein (LDL) cholesterol and warding off cancer.

Keep It Light

Light to moderate drinking—a serving or two of alcohol per day—may help you live longer, says J. Michael Gaziano, M.D., director of cardiovascular epidemiology at Brigham and Women's Hospital in Boston. "People who drink light to moderate amounts of alcohol have the lowest mortality—even lower than nondrinkers."

"In some instances, the risk of heart attack is 20 percent to 30 percent lower in light drinkers than in people who don't drink," says Arthur Klatsky, M.D., senior consultant in cardiology for the Kaiser-Permanente Medical Center in Oakland, California. When researchers at the Harvard School of Public Health studied 85,709 women over a 12-year period, they found that those who were light to moderate drinkers had the lowest risk of fatal heart disease—even if they already had other risk factors for heart disease.

Who Benefits Most from Alcohol?

Drinking alcohol may sound like a merry way to protect your health, but it's actually a serious, complex issue. No two people share identical risk for developing health problems or alcohol addiction, says Arthur Klatsky, M.D., senior consultant in cardiology for the Kaiser-Permanente Medical Center in Oakland, California. But Dr. Klatsky suggests these sample scenarios to help you make an informed choice about whether drinking is for you:

You have had a cardiac episode. You don't have a history of alcohol abuse. You have given up smoking and followed your doctor's instructions to the letter. In this scenario, you're probably not at risk for alcohol addiction. Alcohol may help lower your risk of further heart problems. Check with your doctor—he or she will probably give you the go-ahead to drink a glass a day.

You have no history of alcohol abuse. You drink occasionally, maybe once every few weeks. Ask your doctor how much to drink to protect your heart.

Your parents died of heart attacks. You have high cholesterol, and you've never abused alcohol. In this case, your doctor may advise you to have one drink a day at the most to reduce your risk of cardiovascular problems.

Your parents lived into their nineties. You have never had a drinking problem. You don't have heart disease, you don't smoke, and you have low cholesterol. In this scenario, your heart disease risk is likely to be quite low. You probably don't need the protection of alcohol.

Make a Toast to the Health of Your Heart

Dr. Gaziano's research shows that you will get similar protective effects from wine, beer, or liquor. "The cardiovascular benefits of alcohol come from the alcohol itself, no matter what drink it's in," he says. Ethanol raises the levels of HDL cholesterol, which helps to keep your arteries from filling up with plaque, thereby reducing your risk of heart disease.

Alcohol may help your circulatory system in other ways, too. Some data suggest that it reduces the blood's tendency to clot, and it may help keep the blood vessels more flexible. Furthermore, it's possible that a drink a day relieves stress. All of this could lead to lower risks of heart attack and possibly stroke.

"We know that the phytochemicals in wine are potent antioxidants that may help keep blood from clotting," explains Andrew Waterhouse, Ph.D., a researcher in the Department of Viticulture and Enology at the University of California, Davis. Wine is rich in a group of phytochemicals known as flavonoids, which are what shield you from cancer and prevent LDL cholesterol from oxidizing. In one of his studies, Dr. Waterhouse tested the effect of California wines on the oxidation of the harmful LDL form of human cholesterol. Both red and white wines blocked LDL formation by 46 to 100 percent—but you may want to stick with the reds, because they produce three times as much of the healthful effects.

Just a Little Protects Your Heart

Alcohol is a bit like jalapeño pepper. A pinch adds spicy flavor, but any more than that seems to set your system on fire. "Luckily, light drinking doesn't affect blood pressure. But more

Caution: If You Can't Stop Drinking...

Alcohol is a double-edged sword. Small amounts protect you, but more than that will actually damage your health, increasing your risk of heart disease, cancer, and stroke as well as an assortment of other health problems. If you find that you can't stop after just one drink, you should stop drinking altogether. Here's how you can do that, according to Arthur Klatsky, M.D., senior consultant in cardiology for the Kaiser-Permanente Medical Center in Oakland, California:

Get help. Ask your doctor to assist you in making contact with an alcohol-treatment program. Or, if you want to handle it yourself, write to Alcoholics Anonymous, P. O. Box 459, Grand Central Station, New York, NY 10163. You may also find a local chapter of the organization by checking your phone book.

Go public. Some experts think that it is easier to quit if you tell your friends and family that you have a problem and want to solve it. While you're at it, ask loved ones to help you avoid temptation by not drinking alcohol in your presence.

Tell it like it is. If someone offers you alcohol at a social gathering, just say, "I don't drink," and ask for something nonalcoholic.

than two drinks a day may make your blood pressure go up," says Dr. Gaziano.

It's not completely understood why a little alcohol is good for you while a lot can do big-time damage. But the fact is, heavy drinkers—people who put away three or more drinks a day—significantly increase their risk of a variety of problems, including heart disease, stroke, esophageal cancer, and liver disease.

That's not all. In a study of more than 15,000 women up to age 74, researchers found that moderate drinking greatly increases the risk of breast cancer. And a lifetime average of even one drink a day increases that risk.

Still, "For most people, light drinking is associated with a lower chance of prematurely dying because the benefits in terms of lower rates of heart disease outweigh any small risk of cancer," says Dr. Gaziano.

Get Maximum Protection

For some folks, the best approach to alcohol is not approaching it at all. Drinking should be off-limits to anyone who might abuse it. The advantages of alcohol are not so great that a non-drinker should take up the habit, given the risks of addiction. But for many other people, a moderate amount can do a lot of good.

Get the Benefits Without the Buzz

Some research suggests that you can get the same antioxidant protection from nonalcoholic foods such as grape juice, and plenty of other fruits and vegetables. Following that route will help you steer clear of the risks of alcohol, including addiction, traffic accidents, and citations for driving under the influence.

If you do drink, here is how you can get the most protection from alcohol:

- **A little goes a long way.** Alcohol concentrates in lean body tissue such as muscle, not fat. As you age, lean body mass decreases and fat increases. This means that you are more likely to feel the effects of alcohol when you're older, and it is more likely to do damage to your system if you overindulge. "There's absolutely no reason for anyone, especially older people, to have more than a drink or two a day," says Dr. Gaziano.

- **Women should drink less.** Because women tend to have less lean body mass than men, along with a slightly different liver metabolism, they should have no more than a half to one serving of alcohol per day.

- **Spread it out.** "One reason that French and Italian drinkers have lower heart attack rates might be because they have a little wine each day with meals, while northern Europeans drink large amounts on weekend nights," says Dr. Gaziano. "You wouldn't take all your cholesterol medicine on Saturday—you take it in very small doses every day."

- **Wine and dine.** Having your drink with a meal is a doubly good idea. For one thing, consuming large meals promotes blood clotting, which increases your risk of stroke, says Dr. Klatsky. Drinking wine—either red or white—may help prevent that. "But wine's biggest benefit may be that it encourages people to eat more slowly, which also reduces risk," he says.

- **Imbibe in the evening.** Have your drink (or part of it) with your evening meal. Beyond the digestive benefits, you will cut down on other types of risk as well. After dinner, "You're less likely to climb ladders, drive cars, and do other activities that increase risk," says Dr. Klatsky.

- **Consider it a food.** In some cultures, people consume alcohol primarily in small amounts with meals. That keeps consumption within safe limits and may explain why there is less alcoholism in those countries. "In Mediterranean countries, such as Greece and Italy, people think of alcohol as a food rather than something that you consume on the weekends for its mind-numbing effect," says Dr. Gaziano.

- **Switch to red.** Because red wine is richer in flavonoids, some people are choosing red over white for protection. So should you switch? It's true that the more intense the wine's color, the greater its antioxidant content. Red wine contains skins, seeds, and stems. All of this ferments, giving red wine its rich color and flavor. Dr. Klatsky notes that the darker the wine, the greater the concentration of flavonoids.

White wine also contains healthy flavonoids and other antioxidants, although in far lesser amounts than red. If you can't stand chianti but you would still like to drink wine, chardonnay or another white variety will give you at least some of the same benefits.

Prescription for Getting the Most from Alcohol

Just a little alcohol helps protect against heart disease and heart attacks. But a bit too much can do major damage to your heart and other vital organs. It can also increase your risk of cancer. As you get older, your body stores alcohol somewhat differently, making it especially important to keep consumption low.

DO:

▶ **Discuss your drinking habits with your doctor.** If he or she feels it is safe for you to drink alcohol, limit yourself to just one or two drinks per day (for men) and $1/2$ or one drink per day (for women).

▶ **Drink a little every day for maximum protection,** if your drinking is approved by your doctor. Drink alcohol with a meal to lower the risk of blood clots.

DON'T:

▶ **Drink more than two drinks a day for men and one drink a day for women,** because it will increase your risk of cancer, heart disease, and stroke. (Women should consider cutting back to half a drink per day if they have risk factors for breast cancer.)

▶ **Drink if you have ever had a problem with alcohol addiction.**

▶ **Drive or operate any heavy machinery if you've had any alcohol to drink.**

12

How Can Aspirin Protect You from Disease?

Once, it was just a ho-hum over-the-counter remedy for aches and pains. But during the last few years, aspirin has been transformed into a superstar drug, touted for its tantalizing promise to prevent heart attacks, fend off recurrent strokes, and possibly deter digestive cancers.

Can it help some people prevent the three big killers? Probably. Can everyone benefit from it? Nobody knows yet. Most researchers are cautious, but several aspirin advocates say that the existing evidence is compelling enough for broad recommendations. Even so, before you rush to your medicine cabinet, you should realize that researchers still have a lot of questions about this powerful—and potentially toxic—"wonder" drug.

"The real controversy with aspirin has been whether someone who isn't at high risk for these diseases should take it. In my estimation, the medical establishment has been a bit too conservative about aspirin," says Tim Byers, M.D., professor of preventive medicine at the University of Colorado School of Medicine in Denver. "The risks of low doses of aspirin are fairly minimal, and the benefits may be high. I know I'm going to start taking aspirin regularly when I reach age 50. I think it's a reasonable choice to make for most people who are 50 and above."

Is Aspirin a Boon to Cardiovascular Health?

Ironically, when aspirin was first developed in the late 1890s, it was rarely used because doctors feared that it would weaken the heart. Now many physicians and scientists consider it to be a simple, cheap deterrent to cardiovascular disease.

In the landmark Physicians' Health Study, for instance, 22,000 healthy male doctors up to age 84 took either a standard 325-milligram aspirin or a placebo every other day. (A placebo is a look-alike tablet that has no medical effects.) After five years, those who had been taking the aspirin instead of the placebo had a 44 percent lower risk of suffering a first heart attack.

Warning: Limit Over-the-Counter Drugs That Contain Aspirin

If you're taking aspirin, avoid using other over-the-counter medications that contain the drug. These products can increase your risk of overdosing. Read the list of ingredients carefully. Look for words like aspirin, acetylsalicylic acid (aspirin's chemical name), or other salicylic acids like bismuth subsalicylate, which can interact with aspirin and cause many of the same side effects, says W. Steven Pray, R.Ph., Ph.D., professor of nonprescription products at Southwestern Oklahoma State University in Weatherford.

Some common brand-name products to avoid if you're already taking aspirin:

Alka-Seltzer	Aspergum
BC Powder	Cope
Ecotrin	Goody's Headache Powders
Halfprin	Momentum
Stanback Powders	Vanquish
Pepto-Bismol	

Taking one of the pink antidiarrheal products can be particularly tricky, Dr. Pray warns, because it's often not obvious from the label that it contains a salicylate. "So people who have upset stomachs, hangovers, or diarrhea may take one of them without realizing that it contains a salicylate. Then they'll take a couple of aspirin for their headache. So they're actually doubling their dosage of salicylates. That sort of thing can be very troublesome," he says.

When the results of 25 similar studies of people who had previous heart attacks and strokes were pooled together, researchers found that those who took aspirin regularly had a 32 percent lower rate of subsequent nonfatal heart attacks. They also had 27 percent fewer nonfatal strokes and had a 15 percent reduction in death from cardiovascular diseases.

"I think what we know for sure right now is that, in healthy people, aspirin will prevent a first heart attack," says Charles Hennekens, M.D., Dr.P.H., professor of medicine at Harvard Medical School in Boston. "If you've had a prior heart attack, stroke, or unstable angina—the kind that occurs even when you're not exerting yourself—

we know conclusively that aspirin will prevent a recurrence of all of those events and lower the death rate."

Whether aspirin can help reduce the risk of a first stroke is still open to debate. Researchers simply don't have enough information yet, Dr. Hennekens says.

Researchers do know that aspirin protects the heart in a couple ways, says W. Steven Pray, R.Ph., Ph.D., professor of nonprescription products at Southwestern Oklahoma State University in Weatherford and a columnist for *U.S. Pharmacist* magazine. First, the drug prevents blood platelets from sticking together and forming blood clots. Second, it may suppress the secretion of

Aspirin Allergy: Rare, but Potentially Lethal

Like all drugs, aspirin isn't for everyone. About three of every 1,000 people develop allergic reactions to aspirin. By age 60, most people who are allergic to aspirin know it because they have had at least one adverse reaction. But the allergy can develop at any age.

"It's like a bee sting. At any time, your body can develop an allergic reaction to aspirin even if you have never had a problem in the past," says W. Steven Pray, R.Ph., Ph.D., professor of nonprescription products at Southwestern Oklahoma State University in Weatherford and a columnist for *U.S. Pharmacist* magazine. "Many people develop hives or rashes, but it can be life-threatening. If you're allergic to aspirin, your airways can shut down so that you can't breathe."

People over age 60 who have asthma should be particularly cautious about aspirin use, since they are 10 times more prone to serious allergic reactions than those who don't have asthma, Dr. Pray says. If you have hay fever, you are five times more likely to be aspirin-sensitive.

If you take aspirin and develop hives or a rash, stop using the drug and see an allergist or your family doctor as soon as possible. Seek emergency medical attention immediately if you have difficulty breathing after taking aspirin.

chemicals in the blood that contribute to the formation of atherosclerosis, hardening of the arteries, according to Dr. Pray.

Can an Aspirin a Day Keep Cancer Away?

Researchers also are excited about aspirin's potential to squelch digestive tumors. In an analysis of 662,000 white men and women, American Cancer Society researchers found that those subjects who took aspirin 16 or more times a month for a year had 40 percent lower rates of esophageal, stomach, colon, and rectal cancer than those who didn't use the drug.

Harvard University researchers found a 37 percent reduction of colon cancer risk after 10 years of regular aspirin use among 90,000 nurses up to age 72. The most effective dose appeared to be four to six aspirin tablets a week. A similar Harvard study of 48,000 male health professionals up to age 75 found that those men who took two or more aspirin a week had a 32 percent lower risk of colon cancer.

Other studies have shown that, at least in animals and in people who have a rare genetic predisposition to polyps, aspirin helps block the formation of precancerous polyps in the colon, according to Michael Thun, M.D., director of analytic epidemiology at the American Cancer Society in Atlanta.

How aspirin protects the digestive tract isn't clear. The drug may inhibit the production of prostaglandins, hormonelike substances that may cause cancer cells to grow more rapidly. Another possibility is that aspirin boosts the body's immune system so that the body is better able to fight off tumors.

More studies are needed, however, before researchers can endorse aspirin as a preventive measure for digestive cancers, Dr. Thun says. "Basically, there are good reasons to think that aspirin may have some role in the prevention of colorectal cancer," he says. "The catch is that we haven't proven it."

Should You Try Taking Aspirin?

Because aspirin will help some people and harm others, it's difficult to recommend its

First Aid in Case of Heart Attack

If you are having a heart attack, take a 325-milligram aspirin while you wait for the paramedics to arrive—this may reduce the severity of the attack and save your life, according to Charles Hennekens, M.D., Dr.P.H., professor of medicine at Harvard Medical School in Boston.

"The benefits of aspirin are enormous in that situation," Dr. Hennekens says. "If it's a heart attack, aspirin will reduce the death rate by 23 percent if it is taken within 24 hours of onset and continued daily for 30 days. That alone could save 10,000 lives in the United States a year."

broad, regular use in the general population, Dr. Thun says. In some people, even one adult aspirin (325 milligrams) daily can cause stomach bleeding or strokes from bleeding. There is still no certainty that these risks are outweighed by the potential benefit, except possibly in people who are at high risk of heart attacks or strokes from clotting.

Dr. Byers believes that it is only a matter of time before more doctors advise people to use aspirin to stave off cancer and cardiovascular diseases. "The only questions that really remain are what is the proper dose and how often should you take it," he says.

Making It Work for You

Because researchers do suggest such a wide range of doses—varying from 81 milligrams every other day to 325 milligrams daily—consult your doctor before you begin taking aspirin routinely, advises Dr. Hennekens. Your doctor will help you determine if taking the drug is a worthwhile step for you, and he can recommend a proper dosage.

Here are other suggestions about how to take aspirin:

■ **Scope out your medicine cabinet.** Check with your doctor or pharmacist before taking aspirin if you are using any other drugs, whether they are prescription or over-the-counter, Dr. Pray says. Ibuprofen and other anti-inflammatory drugs, for instance, add to the adverse effects of aspirin.

■ **Sit up.** After age 60, it often becomes harder to swallow aspirin and other tablets. Stand or sit up when swallowing your aspirin. Take the drug with an 8-ounce glass of water at least an hour before bedtime or lying down, says Jacob Karsh, M.D., a rheumatologist and professor of medicine at the University of Ottawa in Ontario, Canada.

■ **Munch on something.** Aspirin is less likely to cause stomach pain, nausea, or other digestive upsets if you take it with food, Dr. Byers says. So have the drug with a meal or snack.

■ **Protect your stomach.** Some aspirins are easier on your digestive tract because they have special coatings that allow them to pass through the stomach and digest in your small intestine, Dr. Byers says. Look for brands that are buffered or enteric-coated.

■ **Go beyond aspirin.** As promising as aspirin appears to be in preventing certain diseases, it still needs your help, Dr. Hennekens says. Lifestyle factors such as eating a low-fat diet, exercising regularly, and not smoking have more impact on your risk of disease than any drug.

Prescription for Getting the Most from Aspirin

While doctors remain reluctant to recommend that everyone take aspirin on a daily basis, a growing stack of evidence suggests that this reliable drug may be more than just a remedy for muscle soreness and headaches. When used in combination with other healthy habits, such as regular exercise and low-fat eating, aspirin may offer a powerful preventive action against stroke, heart disease, and cancer for people over age 60.

DO:

▶ **Check with your doctor** before taking aspirin on a regular basis.

▶ **Take coated aspirin** with food to protect your stomach.

▶ **Take your aspirin with 8 ounces of water at least an hour before bedtime** or before you lie down for a nap.

DON'T:

▶ **Take aspirin without checking your other medications.** Some prescription medications like Percodan and over-the-counter drugs like Alka-Seltzer contain aspirin (also called acetyl-salicylic acid) or other salicylic acids like bismuth subsalicylate. If you're already taking aspirin, the additional aspirin in these products can cause adverse reactions. Ibuprofen may also be problematic when combined with aspirin. Read product labels carefully and check with your doctor before taking aspirin or any new medication.

13

How Important Are Screenings and Self-Exams?

L et's rephrase that question. What is the most important thing in your life? Your spouse? Your grandchildren? That little sports car you just bought? (Just because you are over age 60 doesn't mean that you have to slow down.) Well, medical screenings and self-exams are equally important. They protect you from cancer, heart disease, and stroke—and make it possible for you to enjoy all those good things in your life.

But you don't want to walk into your doctor's office and ask for every test in the book. Some tests just aren't worth taking. Here is a rundown of what you do and don't need.

Blood-Pressure Screening

H igh blood pressure damages artery walls and dramatically increases your risk of heart disease and stroke. "Testing for high blood pressure is at the top of the list of needed tests," says Timothy A. McAfee, M.D., associate director of preventive care at the nation's oldest and largest consumer-governed health maintenance organization (HMO), the Group Health Cooperative of Puget Sound in Seattle.

It is easy enough to get a reading on the machine at the drugstore or take your own reading at home, but this test also is part of just about any visit to your doctor's office. Your doctor or an assistant will place an inflatable cuff on your upper arm. When the cuff tightens, the doctor will get a reading of how forcefully your blood is being pumped by your heart. According to recent findings by the American Heart Association, acceptable blood pressure falls within a range rather than a set number. For most adults, a reading that is less than 120/80 millimeters of mercury (mmHg) is acceptable. Talk to your doctor about what is a healthy blood-pressure range for you.

Blood pressure goes up and down over the course of the day, so a random reading may not be accurate. Lawrence LaPalio, M.D., medical director of geriatrics at Columbia La Grange Memorial Hospital in La Grange, Illinois, recommends that you take some care in preparing for your blood-pressure screening, so that you can be sure you get a reading that is correct. Your activities, your mood, and even the drinks you indulge in may affect the results of the screening. It could be necessary to

Get Yourself Covered

Many health insurance programs cover preventive care, such as health screenings, so check your policy or call your agent about the tests you need. If you are age 65 or older and/or have a disability, you probably use Medicare. During the past few years, the number of screening tests covered by Medicare have been expanded.

Medicare doesn't cover routine checkups. "But if you visit the doctor because something's wrong—if you have a symptom—Medicare will cover the visit," states an official of the Health Care Administration in Baltimore. "It covers tests your doctor then decides that you need."

Here are the screening tests and other preventive services covered by Medicare:

Screenings for breast, cervical, vaginal, colorectal, and prostate cancer

Testing for loss of bone mass, which causes osteoporosis

Diabetes monitoring and self-management

Flu, pneumonia, and Hepatitis B vaccinations

For more information, order the Medicare handbook, *Medicare and You*, by calling 800-MEDICARE (800-633-4227).

take your pressure several times to obtain a clear picture of any problem that may exist.

Here's how you can get the most accurate reading:

■ **Control your consumption.** Avoid certain stimulants that speed up your heart rate, such as coffee or alcohol, before you have a blood-pressure test. Even a drink the night before can interfere with a blood-pressure reading.

■ **Get comfortable.** Five minutes before the test, sit in a comfortable, relaxed position with your arm at heart-height. Rest quietly.

■ **Take an average.** Ask your doctor to take several readings and average them. Then get another reading before you head home—you may be more relaxed. Or average the readings taken over several office visits.

■ **Forget the "white-coat" syndrome.** You may have heard that, for some people, just being in the doctor's office causes their nerves to surge and blood pressure to rise. "Unfortunately," says Dr. La Palio, "if your blood pressure rises because of stress in the doctor's office, it may also

rise in response to everyday events. If it goes up every time you drive in traffic or go to a new place, it should be treated."

■ **Get the full picture.** For high blood pressure, go for treatment immediately, says Dr. LaPalio. If you have mild to moderate blood pressure readings, get the true picture by monitoring your own blood pressure for a month or so. Dr. LaPalio recommends the following routine:

Check it morning, noon, and night. Measure your blood pressure at different times of the day.

Track your moods. Measure when you are stressed, relaxed, happy, depressed, and active.

Keep a diary. Write down the readings, the time, and other relevant factors—what you ate and drank, if you exercised, if you took medications, and what you were doing when you took the measurement.

Breast Examination and Mammography

You may have heard about the controversy over whether mammograms can help prevent breast cancer mortality. Many health professionals still insist on them. Joseph Aisner, M.D., director of clinical sciences at the Cancer Institute of New Jersey in New Brunswick, has said, "A yearly mammogram and professional breast examination plus a monthly self-examination can reduce your risk of breast cancer death by a third. Every woman age 50 and over should have an annual screening."

Breast cancer is the most common cancer among American women, and statistically, your risk of breast cancer increases as you get older. Because few studies have been conducted on the over-60 population, there is some controversy as to whether screenings are needed after age 60, but "From an individual's point of view, it makes sense to continue to get mammograms," Dr. McAfee explains.

To perform a mammogram, the breast has to be compressed briefly between two plates, which may be a little uncomfortable. A low-dose X-ray records two or three images of the tissues. Your doctor should also feel for any lumps in the breast as part of your annual physical examination.

Tumors that have absorbed calcium or distorted the breast's structure often show up on a mammogram. Physical examinations—by you every month, and by your doctor every year—often may pick up what the mammogram misses. While this combination of procedures may not find all breast tumors, it generally provides earlier diagnosis.

What good can screening do? One 20-year study of breast cancer published by the American Cancer Society showed that early screening results in a survival rate of 86 percent in women diagnosed with breast cancer.

Here are some tips on how to get the best results from your examination:

■ **Check for quality.** Make sure that the facility you go to for a mammogram is accredited by the American College of Radiology. That tells you the machinery is adequate and the staff has been properly trained.

■ **Make one trip.** Use a facility that develops the pictures on the spot. That way, if there is a problem with the film, the technician can re-shoot. You don't have to return for a second test.

■ **Improve your own technique.** Ask your doctor or nurse to show you exactly how to perform a self-exam. Or ask for a referral to a class, especially one where you can learn by using a "phantom," a silicone model in which several tumorlike BBs have been implanted. That way, you can learn how to recognize potential problems in your own breasts.

Cervical Screening

Pap smears have reduced death from cervical cancer by more than 95 percent in the past 35 to 40 years," notes Dr. Aisner. Yet, a lot of women stop getting this important test as they get older—which is not a good idea.

In this relatively painless test, your doctor inserts a speculum into the vagina, opens it to reveal the cervix, and takes a small sample of cells from the vagina and the cervix. The cells are examined for cancer.

Unless you have had a full or partial hysterectomy, your doctor should get samples both from the vagina and from the endocervix, which is the cervix at its opening, advises Dr. Aisner. In premenopausal and menopausal women, an endocervical sample is necessary. A vaginal Pap smear isn't always enough because the most common site for cancer is at the opening to the cervix. (In postmenopausal women, it may not be possible to obtain an endocervical sample.)

How do you find out if you need to have a Pap smear? Ask your doctor what tests were done

Get Screened for Free

It's the best bargain around.

Some states get grants from the Centers for Disease Control and Prevention to provide screenings for breast and cervical cancer. That means you can get free mammograms and Pap smears, according to Joseph Aisner, M.D., director of clinical sciences at the Cancer Institute of New Jersey in New Brunswick.

Ask your doctor, or call the American Cancer Society or an area hospital to check on the availability of low-cost or free mammograms and Pap smears. You may also want to ask about any other low-cost or free-of-charge screenings they offer.

and what the results were in your previous three exams. If they were interpreted as adequate and normal, you may need exams only once every three years. Otherwise, Dr. Aisner suggests that you continue with annual screenings.

Cholesterol Testing

Think of cholesterol as fat that comes in two forms. Low-density lipoprotein (LDL) cholesterol latches onto artery walls and over time narrows them, thus increasing your risk of heart attack and stroke. High-density lipoprotein (HDL) cholesterol is the good stuff that keeps the LDL in check. Low levels of total cholesterol and LDL, plus high levels of HDL, will help protect you from the adverse effects of cholesterol. Low levels of total cholesterol—with a ratio of total cholesterol to HDL below 4.5—also protects you.

A long-term study completed in 1992 indicated that people with HDL levels below 35 milligrams per deciliter (mg/dL) had a risk of dying from heart disease that was three times as high as those people with levels greater than 60 mg/dL. In women, studies indicate that total cholesterol levels above 240 mg/dL increase their risk of dying from heart disease by 80 percent.

Inexpensive home test kits give you the total-cholesterol results, but not the level of important HDL cholesterol. Still, these tests may provide a starting point for you and your doctor to determine your risk, says Dr. LaPalio. If your doctor thinks that you are at risk for heart disease, more expensive cholesterol testing to determine your levels of HDL and total cholesterol will probably be covered by Medicare or other insurance. You'll need to provide just a very small blood sample for a lab test to determine your levels.

Your cholesterol level varies. Ask your doctor to give you a second test one week to two months after the first and average the results. If the difference between the two is over 30, take a third test and average the results of all three.

These procedures can help make your readings more accurate:

■ **Take a seat.** Sit down for five to 15 minutes before your test. Standing up or lying down can affect the readings.

■ **Keep it low-key.** Don't do strenuous exercise the day before your test—it will temporarily raise HDL levels, which may be misleading.

■ **Stay alcohol-free.** Stay away from alcohol for 48 hours before your test—it artificially elevates HDL levels.

Colon and Rectal Screening

Colon cancer is the third leading cause of cancer death in the United States for men

Get Your Levels in Line

Here's a scorecard to help track your progress in controlling your cholesterol levels. To lower your risk of heart disease, you generally want to have higher levels of the beneficial HDL cholesterol and lower readings for total cholesterol and the harmful LDL cholesterol. Remember, your LDL level greatly affects your risk of heart attack, and the lower your LDL level, the lower the risk.

Here is a rundown of what the cholesterol readings indicate when you get a blood test, according to the American Heart Association:

Total Cholesterol (mg/dL)	Evaluation
Less than 200	Desirable
200 to 239	Borderline high
240 and over	High
LDL Cholesterol (mg/dL)	**Evaluation**
Less than 130	Desirable
130 to 159	Borderline high
160 or more	High
HDL Cholesterol (mg/dL)	**Evaluation**
50 to 60	Desirable for an average woman
40 to 50	Desirable for an average man
Less than 35	Low

and women, despite the fact that this cancer often starts out as a benign polyp.

Screening can make a huge difference. "Screening decreases colon cancer mortality," says James E. Allison, M.D., clinical professor of medicine and assistant director of the internal medicine program at the University of California, San Francisco. The most common screening test for colon and rectal cancers is called the fecal occult-blood test.

Here's advice to consider for getting reliable screening results:

■ **Take a sample.** A fecal occult-blood test can be performed in several ways. One involves the doctor taking a smear sample as part of your physical examination. Another test can be done at home using a kit from your doctor. You just wipe a bit of stool on pieces of cardboard that are then analyzed by a laboratory.

■ **Watch what you eat.** Chemicals in the test kit react to some foods, says Dr. Allison. To get an accurate reading, change your diet a few days before the test. Your doctor should send directions with the kit, but generally you'll be asked to stay away from red meat, turnips, horseradish, broccoli, radishes, cauliflower, cantaloupes, and other melons. But do eat lots of other fresh vegetables and fruits—it will help stimulate bleeding from any lesions you may have, which helps ensure that this problem shows up on the test.

■ **Avoid confusing results.** Test results may be skewed by vitamin C supplements (which sometimes give false negatives), and aspirin and other nonsteroidal anti-inflammatory drugs (which may give false positives). Avoid medication that can cause gastrointestinal bleeding. If you have hemorrhoids that are flaring up, wait until they quiet down, too, suggests Dr. Allison.

There is a newer home test available at drugstores without a prescription that uses a specially treated pad that you drop into the toilet after a bowel movement. The manufacturer of one such test, EZ-Detect, says that there are no diet constraints and that the test results are not affected by vitamin C.

Many tests give false positives. They just look for blood in the feces, which could be caused by hemorrhoids, diverticulosis, or a host of other conditions. And no fecal occult-blood test picks up nonbleeding cancerous lesions. Still, this is a test worth taking because it is very inexpensive—under $20 for the lab work. Even if you have to pay for the test, a positive reading means that the more expensive tests that give you maximum protection will probably be covered by Medicare and other insurance.

■ **Let the doctor take a look.** Okay, now we must discuss a test that, although brief, can be slightly uncomfortable: flexible sigmoidoscopy. Both men and women should have one performed about every three to five years, says Dr. Allison. In this procedure, a thin, hollow, lighted tube is inserted into the rectum and lower colon. There, it picks up precancerous polyps and removes them before they turn dangerous (a development that usually takes several years). The device may also spot cancerous lesions.

The downside is that it views only one-third of the length of the large intestine's left side, although that is where many cancers develop, notes Dr. McAfee. But this test is less expensive than the more thorough colonoscopy.

■ **Be thorough.** "I think colonoscopy is probably the best screening examination," says Dr. McAfee. That is because the thin tube travels the entire length of your large intestine. What's more, it allows your doctor to snip off any polyps and identify any cancerous formations

right then and there. It is more comfortable than a sigmoidoscopy, because you are sedated slightly during the procedure. The only inconvenience is cleaning out the bowel prior to the procedure. But since colon cancer takes so long to develop, you may not have to repeat the colonoscopy for a long while, especially if colon cancer doesn't show up in your family history. "You're home free for five to 10 years, maybe longer," Dr. McAfee says.

Diabetes Screening

Forty percent of people over age 65 have diabetes. It is a significant risk factor for heart disease," says Dr. LaPalio. When you have diabetes, the extra sugar in your blood tears up artery walls and leaves them more vulnerable to the accumulation of fatty deposits and blockages.

How serious is one more risk factor? When you have three or four risk factors—like diabetes, high blood pressure, high cholesterol levels, lack of exercise, being overweight, being a smoker, or having a family history of heart disease—you are 15 to 20 times more likely to develop heart disease than someone who has just one risk factor.

Talk about easy—testing for diabetes only requires one drop of blood. Dr. McAfee suggests that you ask your doctor to test the levels of sugar in your blood if you show symptoms of diabetes: you are overweight, get thirsty often, urinate more frequently than you used to, or just don't feel well.

Electrocardiogram

An electrocardiogram gives a printout of your heart's activity. In short, it lets you know whether your heart is working efficiently. But you need it only if you already have heart disease or risk factors for heart disease.

"It's reasonable to have this test if you have a family history of heart disease, if you smoke, if

One Test You Don't Need

We don't recommend chest X-rays or any screening for lung cancer anymore," says Dr. McAfee. Studies show that by the time you can see a lesion on an X-ray, it has already spread too far. Also, doctors worry that clean X-rays may lull smokers into a false sense of security.

you have diabetes or are hypertensive," says Dr. McAfee. Medicare usually covers it.

Oral Cancer Screening

You're at risk for oral cancer if you have been a tobacco user or if you have a history of alcohol consumption. "I've never seen oral cancer in a patient who didn't smoke or drink," says Dr. McAfee. All the same, he notes, there is no reason not to make this part of a regular visit. Your doctor will simply perform a visual check of your mouth and throat to look for suspicious-looking growths or lesions. Your dentist also may routinely check for oral cancer at your annual visits.

Ovarian Cancer Screening

Your doctor may recommend an ultrasound examination if you have a close relative who was diagnosed with ovarian cancer, says Dr. McAfee. If your family history puts you at extra risk, your insurance will probably foot the bill.

In this test, a probe is inserted into the vagina, transmitting images of the uterus and ovaries to a monitor. Your doctor will look for any irregularities in the cells lining the ovaries.

Prostate Cancer Screening

Eighty percent of prostate cancer cases are diagnosed in men over age 65, and 40,000 men die from it every year. Testing is a simple two-part affair: Your doctor will perform a rectal exam to check the prostate. And a blood test, the prostate-specific antigen (PSA) test, will measure levels of a protein produced by the prostate.

Many doctors do not actively recommend screening for prostate cancer, however. Screening is controversial because there can be false test results, both positive and negative, and besides, the disease often develops slowly. Most men never experience any symptoms, and only one in 380 men diagnosed with prostate cancer dies of it. "Right now, we don't know that prostate surgery increases your chances of staying alive," says Dr. McAfee.

Further complicating matters, biopsied tumors that look dangerous under the microscope sometimes turn out to be slow-growing. And tumors that look easygoing can suddenly shift into high gear, says Gerald W. Chodak, M.D., director of the Prostate and Urology Center at the University of Chicago Hospitals.

Consider these factors when deciding whether to get tested for prostate cancer, and get tested if:

▪ **You can handle possible effects.** You want to minimize your risk of cancer and increase your chances of living as long as possible, regardless of the side effects from prostate surgery or radiation. (Both of these may result in impotence or incontinence.)

▪ **You are strong and in good health.** You may easily live for another 10 to 15 years.

▪ **You are patient.** You and your loved ones can handle the psychological burden of watching and waiting—one option for some slow-growing tumors.

Skin Cancer Screening

The difference between life and death is $1/8$ of an inch," says Perry Robins, M.D., president of the Skin Cancer Foundation in New York City. We're not talking about that time you almost walked in front of the fast-moving truck, but about minute changes in the moles and freckles that dot your body. Most freckling occurs when the skin gets suddenly baked by the sun. Moles are bits of malformed skin tissue. Little changes in these spots can signal the onset of malignant melanoma, a skin cancer that can be cured easily in its early stages but that quickly spreads.

You're at extra risk if you spend a lot of time indoors and then go out and get "burned and blasted" by the sun, says Dr. Robins. "It's the sudden shock or intense exposure to sun that increases your risk." Also at risk are those who had severe sunburns as children, who sunburn easily, or who have a family history of the disease.

Examine your entire body—from your scalp to the bottom of your feet—twice a year. If anything looks suspicious, consult your doctor. If you are in a high-risk group, ask your doctor to do a skin check for you, says Dr. Robins. He will be able to get a better look at hard-to-see places.

The Skin Cancer Foundation has developed a self-exam guide called "The ABCDs of Moles and Melanomas." Keep these pointers in mind when you examine any suspicious moles or freckles.

A is for asymmetry. An irregular shape is a sign of trouble.

B is for border. Beware of irregular, scalloped, or notched borders.

C is for color. Different shades of brown or black signal a problem.

D is for diameter. Anything larger than the size of a pencil eraser may indicate a melanoma.

Here are some other ways to detect trouble brewing:

■ **Keep count.** Count your moles. You're at risk if your total exceeds 100.

■ **Check for changes.** Keep a record. Use two line drawings of the human body—one of the back view and one of the front—to make a chart (or ask your doctor for illustrations you can use). On the drawings, make marks that correspond to the location of moles on your body. Draw a line from each mark and write down the size, color, and shape of each mole, along with the date of the examination. Use this chart to keep track of any changes you notice during your next self-examination.

Stroke Screening

Someone in the United States has a stroke every 60 seconds. Thirty-one percent of all stroke survivors need long-term help to care for themselves. Fortunately, many people experience warning symptoms before a stroke.

Here is what you (and your doctor) should look for:

■ **Heed the mini-stroke.** Your body does the screening for you. About 10 percent of strokes are preceded by transient ischemic attacks, or mini-strokes. Symptoms, which may last just a few minutes, include:

Blurred vision
Numbness or weakness on one side
 of the body
Slurred speech
Inability to talk
Difficulty in thinking

All these symptoms shout out that your brain isn't getting the blood supply it needs, according to Dr. McAfee.

■ **Beware the bruit.** Your doctor can use a stethoscope to listen to the carotid arteries on either side of the neck that carry blood to the brain. A soft, whooshing sound (called a bruit and pronounced *BRU-ee*) may indicate blockage in the arteries, says Dr. LaPalio. If your doctor hears this sound, he will probably do an ultrasound test, using sound waves to provide a picture of the inside of the arteries.

Okay so far? Here's the next problem: The surgery that is used to clear a blockage in the arteries may occasionally cause a stroke. And the jury is out on just how effective such surgery is. "So far, one good study has shown that screening in certain select populations and then operating on the carotid artery does lower the stroke rate, but we need to know more," says Dr. McAfee.

If surgery isn't your cup of tea, now is the time to make significant changes in your lifestyle to lower your risk of stroke. In addition to healthy eating and exercise, preventive screening tests can help.

Prescription for Getting the Proper Tests

Having the right screening tests performed early and regularly can dramatically cut your risk of developing heart disease, cancer, and stroke. They can let you know if you need to make protective changes in your lifestyle and identify small problems before they get out of control.

DO:

▶ **Get your blood pressure checked annually.**

▶ **Have yearly breast examinations and mammography screenings.**

▶ **Check your HDL and LDL cholesterol levels every year.**

▶ **Get a Pap smear every year.**

▶ **Use an inexpensive fecal occult-blood test to check for colon cancer.**

▶ **Have a sigmoidoscopy done at least every three to five years or a colonoscopy** done at least every 10 years. Your doctor may recommend more frequent colonoscopies if any of your family members have had colon cancer.

▶ **Get a simple blood test** to check for diabetes.

▶ **Check your skin for changes to freckles and moles.**

DON'T:

▶ **Automatically get every test available to you.** Discuss with your doctor the positive and negative aspects of certain tests.

14

Do Environmental Hazards Cause Disease?

Pollution is civilization's oldest companion. The ancient Greeks and Romans spewed massive amounts of toxins into the air as they extracted silver from lead ore. During the Civil War, an abandoned canal in Washington, D.C., was so clogged with animal carcasses and household waste that the stench permeated the White House.

During the second half of the twentieth century, more than 70,000 new chemical compounds—including many that cause cancer in laboratory animals—were developed and have been spread throughout the environment. So how does this affect your risk of developing cancer, heart disease, and stroke beyond age 60? In more ways than you might think.

While estimates vary, some researchers believe that up to 25 percent of all cancers could be prevented if Americans reduced their exposure to smog, pesticides, secondhand smoke, and other hazards that we breathe, drink, eat, and absorb into our bodies, says Devra Lee Davis, Ph.D., senior fellow and program director at the World Resources Institute, an environmental research center in Washington, D.C. Reducing our exposure to toxins also might prevent thousands of heart attacks and strokes each year.

"Unlike some things that have been identified as causes of cancer, stroke, and heart disease that you can't control—like family history—environmental factors are often things you can do something about," Dr. Davis says. "Even after age 60, it represents an opportunity for prevention that, in many ways, is easy to achieve."

What We're Doing to Ourselves

All of us carry the residue of a few toxins in our cells. DDT, for example, an insecticide suspected of promoting breast cancer, has been banned in the United States since 1972. Yet because traces of it can linger in food and water for more than 50 years, virtually all people in this country have some DDT in their bodies, according to Dr. Davis.

In most cases, these minute amounts of toxins probably won't harm you. Only 30 chemicals, for instance, have been proven to cause cancer in humans. But at least another 400 have been shown to

Toxic Jobs That Can Damage Your Health

Certain occupations may expose workers to substances that can increase their risk of cancer and heart disease. Max Costa, Ph.D., chairman of the Norton Nelson Institute of Environmental Medicine at New York University Medical Center, suggests that, even if you're retired, you should consult your doctor if you have worked in any industry that may have exposed you to hazardous materials.

Occupation	Hazardous Substances	Risks
Agriculture worker	Arsenic, pesticides, carbon monoxide, carbon disulfide	Lung, liver, skin cancers; increased atherosclerosis
Assembly line worker	Halogenated hydrocarbon solvents	Heart arrhythmias
Automotive mechanic	Cadmium, carbon monoxide, halogenated hydrocarbon solvents, chromium, polycyclic aromatic hydrocarbons	High blood pressure; increased atherosclerosis; arrhythmias; lung, bladder, skin cancers
Ceramics worker	Arsenic, cadmium, nickel	High blood pressure; nasal, skin, lung cancers
Construction worker	Asbestos, polycyclic aromatic hydrocarbons, halogenated hydrocarbon solvents	Lung, bladder, skin cancers; arrhythmias
Dry cleaner	Benzene, carbon disulfide, halogenated hydrocarbon solvents	Leukemia; increased atherosclerosis; high blood pressure
Dye or ink maker	Benzene, chromium, nickel, carbon disulfide	Leukemia; lung and bladder cancers; arrhythmias
Leather worker (tanner)	Benzene, chromium, arsenic, halogenated hydrocarbon solvents	Leukemia; lung cancer; high blood pressure
Textile mill worker	Arsenic, cadmium, nickel, halogenated hydrocarbon solvents, carbon disulfide	Lung, nasal, and bladder cancers; arrhythmias; increased atherosclerosis
Welder	Arsenic, benzene, nickel, chromium	Leukemia, lung and nasal cancers

cause cancer in laboratory animals and are suspected of promoting human tumors.

Here's a sample of the findings:

▪ **Pollution increases heart attack risk.** Certain automotive air pollutants, such as carbon monoxide, reduce the ability of the blood to carry oxygen and can trigger heart attacks and angina in people over age 60, according to Robert Morris, M.D., Ph.D., director of the Center for Environmental Epidemiology at the Medical College of Wisconsin in Milwaukee. Long-term exposure to carbon monoxide also may promote

Keep Your Hands Off Asbestos

Once considered safe and efficient, asbestos insulation now tops almost every list of environmental hazards in the United States. That's because asbestos fibers can cause a rare form of cancer that is both painful and deadly.

"Asbestos has been an absolute disaster. Ultimately, there will be 300,000 to 400,000 deaths in this country due to asbestos before this epidemic burns itself out in the twenty-first century," says Philip Landrigan, M.D., director of environmental and occupational medicine at the Mount Sinai School of Medicine of the City University of New York in New York City.

Mesothelioma, a cancer that starts in the linings of the chest, heart, and abdomen, affects about 2,000 people annually in the United States, says Joseph Testa, Ph.D., senior member of the Department of Medical Oncology at Fox Chase Cancer Center in Philadelphia. Construction workers and shipbuilders who have had years of exposure to asbestos are more prone to developing the disease. But people who live in homes built prior to 1972, when asbestos was phased out of use in household construction, also may be at risk.

Homeowners probably won't be able to distinguish asbestos from other types of insulation, says Pat Eiding, business manager of the Insulators and Asbestos Workers Union in Philadelphia. But if your home was built before the early 1970s, there is a 50 percent chance that it is insulated with asbestos. As long as the insulation remains sealed and intact, asbestos can't harm you.

If you live in an older home and notice a piece of tattered or worn insulation, carefully cover it with duct tape. Then seek the advice of an asbestos-removal contractor listed in the Yellow Pages of the telephone book, Dr. Landrigan says.

Trying to remove asbestos yourself can create more of a hazard than leaving it alone, according to Dr. Landrigan. If removal is done improperly, asbestos fibers can flake off the insulation, lodge in your lungs, and possibly spark a cancer into forming.

"Asbestos removal is a complex job that requires specialized skills and equipment. It's not for amateurs," Eiding says.

Professional asbestos removal is expensive, sometimes costing more than $8,000, according to Eiding. Get several bids, ask the contractor for references, and avoid letting price dictate your selection. An unusually low bid might be a sign that the contractor is more concerned about profit than your safety, he cautions.

the formation of blood clots in the arteries and possibly lead to stroke.

In his three-year study of 204,000 Medicare patients, age 65 and older, in seven American cities, Dr. Morris found close to a 30 percent increase in hospital admissions for congestive heart failure, which corresponded to rising carbon monoxide levels.

"There's a steady increase in hospital admissions as carbon monoxide goes up," Dr. Morris says. "There's no question that if you're exposed to excessive amounts of carbon monoxide, your heart is going to have to work harder to deliver oxygen to the cells. So if an older person has an underlying heart condition, carbon monoxide can push the heart to a dangerous extent."

■ **Breast cancer rates may be higher in industrial areas.** Postmenopausal women in Nassau County, New York, who live within a mile of a chemical, petroleum, rubber, or plastics facility are 60 percent more likely to develop breast cancer than postmenopausal women who lived in other parts of Long Island, according to a study by New York State Department of Health researchers.

"This study adds credibility to the suggestion that environmental exposure may be important in the development of breast cancer," says Elizabeth Lewis-Michl, Ph.D., lead author of the study and a research scientist at the Center for Environmental Health at the New York State Department of Health in Albany.

■ **Some cancers are more common among farmers who use pesticides.** In a 16-year study of 70,000 Canadian farmers, those who routinely sprayed more than 250 acres with herbicide were 2.2 times more likely to develop prostate cancer than farmers who didn't use pesticides, says Howard Morrison, Ph.D., chief of behavioral risk assessment, Cancer Bureau, at Health Canada (the equivalent of the U.S. Department of Health) in Ottawa. In another 16-year study, 143,000 herbicide-using farmers, most of whom were at least in their sixties by the end of the study, were twice as likely to develop non-Hodgkin's lymphoma, a life-threatening cancer of the lymphatic system, than their colleagues who did not spray with herbicides.

Other studies have found that farmers who work with insecticides have higher rates of leukemia, bone marrow cancer, and brain cancer. Dr. Davis points out that some of these same chemicals are used in lower doses by household gardeners.

"It's absolutely established that many herbicides are carcinogens," says Philip Landrigan, M.D., director of environmental and occupational medicine at the Mount Sinai School of Medicine of the City University of New York in New York City. "It just doesn't make any sense to expose yourself to these compounds at any age."

■ **Radon is linked to lung cancer.** Swedish researchers found that people up to age 74 who lived in homes with high levels of radon were 80 percent more susceptible to lung cancer than those who lived in houses containing little or no radon. Radon is an invisible, odorless radioactive gas that seeps into homes from the decay of underground uranium deposits.

"Radon is clearly a carcinogen, there's no doubt about it. But the degree of risk of lung cancer from residential exposure is not clear," says Aaron Blair, Ph.D., chief of the occupational studies section at the National Cancer Institute in Bethesda, Maryland.

Many Questions Remain Unanswered

Although these studies strongly suggest the powerful impact of environmental hazards, scientists are still struggling to determine the thresholds at which many of these toxins cause trouble.

"That's the $64,000 question," says Jane Koenig, Ph.D., professor of environmental health at the University of Washington in Seattle. "In a lot of cases, we don't have the answers yet."

A few substances—like carbon monoxide and asbestos, a potent carcinogen that causes a rare form of lung cancer—have no known safe exposure levels. For others, like radon, the Environmental Protection Agency (EPA) has set exposure limits. But in general, the degree of risk depends on what substance you have been exposed to, how much and how often you are exposed to it, and your age.

Certain occupations, for example, can come back to haunt you, even if you have long been retired. Workers who installed asbestos insulation in the 1940s and 1950s have tremendously high rates of lung cancer. Textile workers who were exposed to benzene-related dyes have unusually high rates of bladder cancer, according

Don't Make Yourself Sick from Making Crafts

Hobbies are fun, relaxing, and rewarding. But unless you are careful, pastimes involving ceramics, jewelry, paint remover, solders, metals, or clays can also be hazardous to your health. "Certain hobbies can expose you to solvents and dust that may contain cancer-promoting compounds," says Michael Thun, M.D., director of analytic epidemiology for the American Cancer Society in Atlanta. "So you need to use some common sense when you're working at a hobby to minimize your risk of inhaling or coming in contact with these compounds."

Here are a few safety precautions to reduce your risks:

Read labels and follow directions. Before you buy, make sure that extremely dangerous toxic chemicals aren't in the product. Avoid using art materials that contain known or suspected carcinogens, such as benzene, carbon tetrachloride, trichloroethylene, or dioxane, Dr. Thun says. Choose nontoxic art materials whenever possible. Read and understand the package directions fully before you begin using the product.

Keep air circulating. Good ventilation is a must when working with toxic or cancer-promoting substances like lead, cadmium, or nickel found in clays and metals. Work in a space that can be easily ventilated like a garage or large hobby area. Before you begin, open adjacent doors and windows. Use a large floor fan to disperse the toxins, advises Dr. Thun.

Wear protective clothing. Don a ventilation mask, heavy-duty overalls, and latex gloves, available at most hardware stores. These items will help prevent you from accidentally inhaling or coming in contact with many carcinogen-containing dusts and fumes while participating in your hobby, Dr. Thun says. When you're finished, wash your clothing in hot water, separate from other household laundry.

Mop up. Sweeping stirs up harmful dusts and toxins, Dr. Thun says. Wet mopping is a safer way to clean an area that may contain harmful substances.

to Max Costa, Ph.D., chairman of the Norton Nelson Institute of Environmental Medicine at New York University Medical Center. Furniture workers who were exposed to wood dust may be susceptible to nasal and sinus cancers for up to 40 years after their first exposure. Some hobbyists who frequently use toxic paints, solvents, and solders also are more prone to certain cancers than the general population, he says.

Toxins Carry More Clout as You Age

The damage that these hazards inflict on the body often increases as you get older. That's because as you age, your lungs, liver, kidneys, and other organs gradually lose much of their ability to rid the body of cell-damaging toxins,

says Jonathan Samet, M.D., chairman of the Department of Epidemiology at Johns Hopkins University School of Medicine in Baltimore.

Although doctors still aren't sure how these toxins trigger cancer, heart disease, or stroke, they suspect that hazardous substances may cause gradual changes in DNA, the genetic building blocks that cells use to reproduce. Over time, these changes might cause mutations in cells that spark cancerous growths and might also accelerate atherosclerosis (hardening of the arteries), according to Chris Schonwalder, Ph.D., assistant to the director of the National Institute of Environmental Health Sciences of the National Institutes of Health in Research Triangle Park, North Carolina.

Many pollutants also may weaken the immune system so that it is less capable of destroying the abnormal cells that may eventually become cancerous, says Mary Wolff, Ph.D., a toxicologist and professor of community medicine at the Mount Sinai School of Medicine of the City University of New York.

Keep Your Guard Up

Even if you have been exposed to massive amounts of environmental hazards in your lifetime, it's not too late, Dr. Landrigan says. If you eliminate an environmental hazard like pesticides from your life now, you may be able to prevent that one final exposure that would set you on a collision course with one of the big three killers (cancer, heart attack, and stroke).

"Older people need to engage in prudent avoidance and try to minimize their exposure to environmental hazards," Dr. Davis says. "That doesn't mean you have to live in a bubble. But if you pay attention to your environment—as well as exercise regularly, eat well, and don't smoke—you will be healthier."

The following pages describe four major environmental hazards that are known or suspected of causing the big three killers, and give suggestions for what you can do about them.

Smoking Is Never Passive

Tobacco smoke is one of the most dangerous and most pervasive environmental hazards. Approximately 53,000 people die of passive-smoking–related causes each year, according to Stanton Glantz, Ph.D., professor of medicine at the University of California, San Francisco, School of Medicine. That's because sidestream or secondhand smoke from burning tobacco emits virtually all of the same toxic chemicals and carcinogenic substances into the air that someone gets from taking a puff.

A nonsmoker who regularly inhales secondhand fumes has a 30 percent greater risk of developing lung cancer and heart disease and may be more likely to develop breast cancer than a nonsmoker who lives in a smoke-free home. "Passive smoking increases the need of the heart for oxygen and decreases the body's ability to use it effectively," Dr. Glantz says. "So if you already have some heart disease or atherosclerosis and then you throw in secondhand smoke, this could easily push you over the edge."

According to Dr. Glantz, studies have found that exposure to secondhand smoke thickens artery walls and promotes the formation of artery-clogging plaque. It also lowers blood levels of HDL, the "good" cholesterol that normally prevents plaque buildup in the arteries. If a heart attack occurs, exposure to sidestream smoke increases heart damage and complicates recovery.

In addition, according to the Environmental Protection Agency (EPA), there are at least 3,000 lung-related deaths among nonsmokers each year that can be attributed to their exposure to secondhand smoke.

Persuading household smokers to quit is the best way to protect nonsmokers like young grandchildren. But until that happens, everyone in your home is at risk.

Here are a few things you and your nonsmoking loved ones can do to reduce the risk from secondhand smoke:

■ **Take it outside.** Allow smokers to puff outdoors only, says C. Barr Taylor, M.D., professor of psychiatry at Stanford University School of Medicine and author of *The Facts About Smoking.* As an alternative, designate a well-ventilated room in your home (not normally used by others) where smokers can light up. Ask all guests who smoke to use the room.

Natural Way to Remove Indoor Carcinogens

You don't have to install high-tech gadgetry, rip up walls, or spend a fortune to banish certain cancer-promoting substances from the air in your home. All you may need is a green thumb. "Plants can have a vital role in clearing carcinogens and other unstable organic chemicals from household air," says B. C. "Bill" Wolverton, Ph.D., a former NASA senior scientist who has studied plants and pollution treatment for more than 20 years. "They can make a significant difference in the pollution levels in your home."

Here are a few suggestions from Dr. Wolverton to help make houseplants work most effectively for you:

Pick the right plant. Lady palm, peace lily, *Ficus alii,* golden pothos, and areca palm are easy to grow, insect-resistant, and can absorb many of the cancer-causing chemicals like benzene, arsenic, and formaldehyde found in secondhand smoke and other household pollutants, says Dr. Wolverton, author of *How to Grow Fresh Air.* Azalea, Boston fern, spider plant, chrysanthemum, philodendron, and mother-in-law's tongue also clean the air but they may require more diligent care, he says.

Plant in your breathing zone. A typical houseplant filters about six cubic feet of air—about the area of a lounge chair. Position the plant on a table or on the floor beside your bed or favorite chair to maximize the amount of clean air around you. Dr. Wolverton says, "Place those plants in your breathing zones, where you spend most of your time. Then you will have significant air-quality improvement with just one or two plants."

Keep a fan and filter nearby. Plants remove invisible chemicals like benzene from the air but do little to dissipate smoke and other visible particles, according to Dr. Wolverton. "Ideally, you would have cleaner indoor air if you used a HEPA filter in conjunction with two or three indoor plants in each room." High-efficiency particulate (HEPA) filters, available at many hardware stores, quickly remove most particulates from the air.

■ **Create a breeze.** If possible, open windows or install strong exhaust fans to quickly clear smoke out of your home, Dr. Taylor suggests.

■ **Eat in self-defense.** Eating at least seven servings a day of fruits and vegetables, such as apples, pears, carrots, and broccoli, that are rich in antioxidants may help a nonsmoker counteract some of the risks of breathing secondhand smoke, says James Scala, Ph.D., a nutritional biochemist and author of *If You Can't/Won't Stop Smoking.* Antioxidants fight off the effects of the free radicals found in tobacco smoke that rob cells of oxygen.

Dirty Air Hurts Your Heart

Inhale. Exhale. You do that about 17,000 times in an average day. And what are you breathing? Carbon monoxide, sulfates, and other dangerous pollutants that can strain your heart and lungs to the breaking point.

"Studies have consistently shown that there are increased numbers of deaths associated with increasing levels of particulate material in the air. One to three percent of the deaths that occur on days with high levels of particulate material are due to cardiac problems in people over age 65," Dr. Koenig says.

Researchers have also found that people who live in cities with high air-pollution levels die an average of 2½ years earlier than those who live in the least-polluted areas, Dr. Koenig says.

"Air pollution is similar to secondhand smoke. The more you breathe it, the more toxic effects it is going to have on your body," Dr. Koenig says. "So you should do everything you can to reduce the amount of air pollution that you breathe, particularly if you're 60 or 70 and already have an underlying heart or lung condition that could be exacerbated by breathing dirty air."

Here's how to lower your intake of air pollutants:

■ **Stick to side streets.** Regular exercise, such as walking, strengthens the heart. But avoid strolling along busy streets where carbon monoxide levels are higher. Head for a secluded park or neighborhood, Dr. Morris says.

■ **Dodge rush hour.** The more cars there are on the road, the more air pollution you are likely to encounter. Dr. Morris suggests that you try doing outdoor activities, such as walking and gardening, at off-peak times like the middle of the day so that you avoid being exposed to fumes from morning and evening rush-hour traffic.

■ **Live smoke-free.** Tobacco smoke contains large amounts of heart-damaging carbon monoxide. "Certainly, one of the biggest sources of carbon monoxide you can be exposed to is the end of a lit cigarette," says Dr. Morris. He suggests that you avoid secondhand smoke, and if you smoke, quit.

■ **Clean your air.** Even indoors you can be exposed to air pollutants that seep into your home, Dr. Koenig says. Consider getting a high-efficiency particulate (HEPA) filter. About the size of a footstool, HEPA filters collect many of the worst pollutants. They are available at most hardware or building supply stores and generally cost less than $200.

■ **Avoid problem periods.** Scan the newspaper or watch television weather reports for pollution alerts in your area. When a pollution alert is declared, stay indoors, cut back on your regular activities, and take more frequent rest breaks. This will help reduce the amount of hazardous air you breathe and avoid overexerting your heart and lungs, Dr. Koenig says.

Pesticides: Look to Natural Alternatives

A foggy mist of DDT engulfing beaches, campgrounds, and parks once was a sure sign that summer had arrived. Trucks belching out this potent concoction sometimes displayed signs proclaiming, "DDT: powerful insecticide, harmless to humans."

But far from being harmless, DDT was found to provoke cancers, Dr. Landrigan says. This chemical is now banned in the United States. Many other harmful pesticides, such as dimethoate, however, are still in use.

"You're never so old that you're immune from the effects of pesticides," Dr. Landrigan says. "My advice to people is reduce their use as much as possible. If you must, use the minimal amount necessary and integrate other, more natural approaches into your effort to control pests."

In a study by Dr. Wolff, women who had elevated blood levels of DDE, a residual component of DDT, were four times more likely to develop breast cancer than women who had lower blood concentrations of the residue.

"The older you are, the more DDT you have," Dr. Wolff says. "We're still uncertain whether DDT actually causes breast cancer. But it's something that we need to understand better because there is still plenty of it around. Although it is banned in the United States, it is widely used in Mexico and other Third World countries. So it can still get into this country."

Alternatives to the "Dirty Dozen"

Here, in order from most to least toxic, are the 12 fruits and vegetables—the "dirty dozen"—that have the highest amounts of suspected cancer-causing pesticide residues, according to the Environmental Working Group, a nonprofit environmental research organization in Washington, D.C. Since many of these foods are American favorites, the Environmental Working Group recommends limiting, rather than eliminating, consumption of these fruits and vegetables. You also may consider trying some of the nutritionally equivalent, less toxic alternatives listed. In some cases, the Environmental Working Group recommends avoiding certain fruits grown in a specific country (listed in parentheses).

Food	Alternatives
1. Strawberries	Blueberries, blackberries, oranges, kiwifruit, grapefruit
2. and 3. (tie) Spinach and bell peppers	Green peas, broccoli, romaine lettuce Broccoli, brussels sprouts, asparagus
4. Cherries (U.S.)	Oranges, blueberries, raspberries, grapefruit, kiwifruit
5. Peaches	Nectarines, U.S. cantaloupe, tangerines, watermelon
6. Cantaloupe (Mexico)	U.S. cantaloupe in season (May to December) or watermelon
7. Celery	Carrots, romaine lettuce, broccoli, radishes
8. Apples	Pears, oranges, nectarines, bananas, virtually any fruit that isn't one of the "dirty dozen"
9. Apricots	Nectarines, U.S. cantaloupe, tangerines, oranges
10. Green beans	Green peas, broccoli, cauliflower, asparagus, potatoes, brussels sprouts
11. Grapes (Chile)	U.S. grapes in season (May to December)
12. Cucumbers	Virtually any other vegetable that isn't one of the "dirty dozen"

According to Dr. Wolff, some researchers speculate that substances called xenoestrogens in DDT and other pesticides may promote breast, prostate, and other hormonally linked cancers.

These xenoestrogens may mimic sexual hormones in the body and fuel cancer development by damaging DNA or helping cancer cells form new blood vessels that are needed for tumor growth, Dr. Davis says.

Here's how you can battle pesticide poisoning:

■ **Load up on vegetables and soy.** Broccoli, cauliflower, cabbage, and soy products like tofu have compounds that may enhance the body's ability to repair damaged DNA and fend off the worst effects of xenoestrogens, Dr. Scala says. He suggests eating plenty of vegetables and soy products each day.

■ **Lay off meat.** Pesticides tend to accumulate in animal fats like those in beef, pork, and chicken. Try to eat no more than one 3-ounce serving of meat a day, Dr. Scala says.

■ **Peel it off.** Carefully wash and peel all fruits and vegetables before eating, says Dr. Schonwalder. That should eliminate most of the pesticide residues on the food.

Chlorine Is for Swimming, Not Drinking

In 1969, Neil Armstrong walked on the moon. But back on Earth, he couldn't swim in horribly polluted Lake Erie, just a few miles from his home.

We've cleaned up our act since then, and the bulk of America's water supply is safe, says James M. Symons, Sc.D., author of *Drinking Water: Refreshing Answers to All Your Questions,* and former director of the drinking water treatment program for the U.S. Environmental Protection Agency in Cincinnati. But at least one chemical—chlorine, which is used to purify tap water—may contribute to cancer, heart disease, and stroke, according to Michael Klaper, M.D., director of the Institute of Nutrition Education and Research in Manhattan Beach, California.

Chlorine is added to the public water supply to kill bacteria and other germs that are present. But it also might cause cholesterol to cling to artery walls and accelerate atherosclerosis and combine with other chemicals in drinking water to form cancer-promoting substances. "If an older person has cells on the verge of becoming cancerous, how do you know that one more glass of water containing these cancer-promoting substances won't push him over the edge?" Dr. Klaper says. "If I were an older person, I wouldn't drink chlorinated water, especially if I had a history of these three diseases."

Use bottled water instead of tap, he suggests. Bottled water is purified by a process called reverse osmosis and usually contains little or no chlorine. As an alternative, use a reverse-osmosis water filter, available at many department stores. It's an inexpensive way to rid chlorine from tap water.

■ **Keep your kitchen pesticide-free.** You may unwittingly contaminate your meals if pesticides are used on kitchen counters and other food preparation areas, Dr. Davis says. Instead, keep your kitchen clean at all times, and use pest-control methods that are less toxic, like boric acid dust, available at most hardware stores. It will slowly kill ants and cockroaches without harming you. But even boric acid dust should be used carefully and not inhaled, says Jay Feldman, executive director of the National Coalition Against the Misuse of Pesticides (NCAMP).

For more information on other natural pest-control techniques, write NCAMP, 701 E Street SE, Suite 200, Washington, D.C. 20003.

■ **Create a barrier.** Skin barriers, thin nonpenetrable solutions similar to petroleum jelly, can prevent pesticides from soaking into your skin whenever you must work with them, Dr. Schonwalder says. Used by petrochemical workers, skin barriers are available in most drugstores.

■ **Don't track in trouble.** "Most houses are so airtight these days that once a pesticide gets into your home, it's there to stay," says Dr. Schonwalder. After applying pesticides to outdoor plants, take off your shoes before entering your house. Remove all of your clothes in an entryway and wash them in hot water (separate from other laundry) as soon as possible. Then take a shower to wash away any remaining residue from your body, he suggests.

Radon: Shut Out This Cancer Culprit

When a construction engineer set off radiation detectors as he walked into a nuclear power plant in Limerick, Pennsylvania, in 1984, investigators narrowed their search for the contamination down to a startling culprit. It was radon that was seeping into the man's home, exposing his family to 50 times more than the annual level of radiation allowed for uranium miners. Although the family quickly fixed the problem, they may have an elevated risk of developing lung cancer for years or decades to follow.

"Radon isn't a small problem," says Charles T. Hess, Ph.D., professor of physics at the University of Maine at Orono, who has studied the health effects of radon for more than 20 years. "It's in the air. It's in the water. It's one of the biggest sources of radiation exposure in the United States."

Radon is a naturally occurring gas that is produced by the radioactive decay of uranium in soil and water. It is the second most common cause of lung cancer (after smoking) in the US, contributing to 10,000 deaths a year. Smoking combined with radon exposure more than doubles your risk of developing lung cancer, Dr. Landrigan says.

Because radon is a gas, it can easily slip into a home through cracks in floors and walls, construction joints, and gaps around pipes. It also is commonly found in wells or municipal water systems that use groundwater, Dr. Hess says. Up to six million homes in the United States may exceed EPA standards for radon exposure.

"If you have excessive radon in your home, it's prudent to take corrective measures to get it out, no matter what your age. It's just a gas, and you can get rid of it very easily," says Dr. Landrigan, who is also co-author of *Raising Children Toxic Free.*

Here are some tips for clearing radon from your surroundings:

■ **Ask around.** Call your county or city health department and ask if they have received any reports of high radon levels in your neighborhood, says Richard Sextro, Ph.D., a staff scientist at the Lawrence Berkeley Laboratory at the University of California, Berkeley. Ask neighbors if they have taken recent radon measurements. Since radon levels can fluctuate dramatically from house to house, this isn't a foolproof method, but at least it will give you a better idea of whether you should test.

■ **Check it out.** Get a radon detector, available at many hardware stores, and place it in the basement or lowest living areas of your home, Dr. Landrigan says. Detectors that accumulate radon for two to 90 days will give you a general idea of your risk. If the reading is high, get a detector that will measure radon levels for six to 12 months. Since radon levels can vary from day to day, a long-term test will give you a better idea of your year-round radon exposure. When the detector is ready, it must be mailed to a lab, which will analyze the contents and then send you a report.

Radon is measured in units called picocuries per liter. If your test results are greater than four picocuries per liter, the highest exposure recommended by the EPA, you should consider ways to fix the problem. In most cases, it can be done for $500 to $2,500, according to the EPA. You should also have your water supply tested for radon. Contact your state's radon office for more information.

■ **Stop those leaks.** Seal large cracks in your basement with caulk to prevent radon from pouring in, advises Dr. Hess. In basements with porous or cracked concrete, apply several layers of epoxy paint or masonry sealer to the floor and walls.

■ **Get some fresh air.** Open all of the windows in your house, particularly in the basement, and use a window fan to flush the radon out, Dr. Landrigan suggests.

■ **Take it out before it gets in.** Installing a four-inch plastic pipe through the foundation and venting it to a small fan in the roof will suck the gas away before it gets in the house, Dr. Sextro suggests. You may want to consider having this done professionally, since pipe and fan size can be dependent on house size and local codes.

■ **Bathe wisely.** If you get your household water from a well, taking a long, hot shower can make radon levels in your bathroom soar more than 28 times higher than normal, Dr. Hess says. That's because some wells and other groundwater sources are loaded with the radioactive gas.

If your water supply tests positive for radon, you must take care when you bathe or shower. Turn on the bathroom exhaust fan and the water, then leave the room while the water warms or the tub fills, Dr. Hess suggests. Shower for no more than five minutes, then grab a towel and dry off in another room. That should reduce your radon exposure to about 20 percent. Be sure to close the bathroom door while you are showering or whenever you leave the room so that the gas won't flow freely into the rest of the house. And take warm rather than hot showers—hot water releases more radon.

Prescription for Avoiding Toxins

Exposure to radon, secondhand smoke, asbestos, and other environmental toxins can increase the risk of stroke, heart disease, and certain forms of cancer, especially after age 60. But even if you have lived or worked around hazardous materials for years, you can still make lifestyle changes to cut down on your chances of getting ill.

DO:

▶ **Make your home a smoke-free zone.**

▶ **Exercise in parks or neighborhoods,** away from congested or busy streets that have high concentrations of carbon monoxide.

▶ **Get a HEPA filter.** It will eradicate many of the worst pollutants.

▶ **Carefully wash and peel all fruits and vegetables** before eating them. This should prevent you from inadvertently digesting pesticides.

▶ **Get a radon detector.** If levels of the gas in your home are high, open windows and seal all cracks in the foundation and basement flooring.

DON'T:

▶ **Exercise in morning or evening rush hours.** Pollution from traffic is highest at those times.

▶ **Use pesticides on kitchen counters.** Residues can contaminate foods.

▶ **Abuse pesticides.** In large amounts, they can poison you. Follow the label directions carefully.

15

Do Genes Contribute to Your Disease Risk?

The shape of your nose, the color of your eyes and hair, the size of your feet, and other family traits are passed on from generation to generation like newspapers rolling off a printing press. Genetics seems simple but is actually so complex that scientists are still mystified by some aspects of the process. What they do know is that genes, which are composed of millions of encoded nitrogen molecules, carry all your reproductive blueprints. And they are busy. Every day, your body's 100 trillion cells rely on genes to tell them what they are supposed to do. With such an efficient system in place, what could possibly go wrong? Plenty.

"The genetic code is a set of instructions that tells cells how to function properly. A cell follows those instructions rigorously. But if one of the instructions is wrong, it then messes up how the cell functions. These mistakes can cause disease—if they prevent the cell from carrying out important tasks or cause the cell to die," says Richard H. Myers, Ph.D., professor of neurology at Boston University School of Medicine.

Mistakes in genes are called mutations. They develop slowly over a lifetime because of aging or exposure to harmful substances like tobacco smoke. But these spontaneous mutations are seldom transmitted from one generation to the next, Dr. Myers says. Sometimes the mutation is caused by a mangled gene that is passed on to you from one or both of your parents. People who inherit these defects, which can remain dormant for decades, are more prone to certain diseases, including some types of cancer, heart disease, and stroke, researchers say.

Your Family History May Not Mean Doom

Having a mutation doesn't mean that you're absolutely going to get the disease. It should just make you more cautious about monitoring your health. If you are truly concerned about your family history, there is genetic testing and counseling available that in some cases may help ease your mind," says Glenn A. Miller, Ph.D., head of the clinical studies laboratory at Genzyme Genetics, a genetic research and testing company in Framingham, Massachusetts.

Unraveling the Mystery

Just sorting out what every gene does is an enormous task. Each one of your cells has up to 100,000 genes. Scientists have identified all of these genes only recently, and they are now developing procedures to detect how the genes can cause illness, and possibly modify those that cause the most dangerous maladies.

"This effort is a marathon, and the starting gun has just gone off," Dr. Miller says. "We're still only a couple of hundred yards down the track."

Here is a look at some of the pioneering research that may help us forestall or combat these diseases:

■ **It can be all in the family.** In ongoing research at the Framingham Heart Study, which has been tracking 5,209 Massachusetts adults, many now in their eighties and nineties, for almost 50 years, investigators found that strokes were three times more common among men and women whose parents had had heart disease.

In a second Framingham report, the researchers concluded that people were 29 percent more likely to develop heart disease if a parent also had cardiovascular ailments, says Dr. Myers, lead author of the study.

"I don't think we're going to find a single gene that causes [stroke and heart disease]. But there are a number of genes that increase blood pressure and others that affect cholesterol. So the presence of the same genes may result in heart disease in some people and stroke in others," Dr. Myers says.

■ **Genes aren't responsible for everything.** Only five percent of breast cancers are hereditary. But among women who have families with a history of breast cancer and carry either the BRCA1 or BRCA2 gene (BRCA stands for "breast cancer"), the lifetime risk of breast cancer is about 80 percent, says Raymond L. White, Ph.D., director of the Huntsman Cancer Institute at the University of Utah Medical Center in Salt Lake City.

"Women who have an inherited breast cancer gene do tend to get the disease 10 to 15 years earlier than other women. But it's also true that close to half the women who inherit the BRCA1 gene won't get their breast cancer until after age 60," Dr. White says. "Overall, the great majority of these breast cancers will develop between the ages of 50 and 70."

Other researchers have isolated genes that may be linked to melanoma and colon and ovarian cancer, Dr. White says.

It's All Relative

For most of us, the odds of developing an inherited form of cancer or heart disease is about as likely as winning the lottery and being struck by lightning on the same day.

To grasp how unlikely it is that you will inherit one of these diseases, think of your genetic risk in terms of a fire hazard, Dr. Miller says. If the house down the street is in flames, you probably wouldn't abandon your home. But if the fire is next door and flames are leaping onto your roof, it's time to take emergency measures.

"For the great majority of us, genetically predisposed cancers and heart disease are fires that are burning well down the block," Dr. Miller says. "Only a small number of individuals are at risk."

But if it appears that your family is prone to a particular disease, it may be worth taking some precautions. Dr. Myers says, "If my mother or father had died of a heart attack, or my brother died of a stroke at a young age, I'd certainly tell my doctor about it. I'd also try to make some modifications in my lifestyle such as regular exercise, eating well, and not smoking."

Before you seek genetic counseling and testing, it's important to take a look at your family history. Here's how to do it:

How to Outsmart a Dangerous Gene

Although we can't turn off genes that contribute to stroke, heart disease, and cancer, we can at least slow one of them down, according to French researchers.

A gene that causes excessive production of fibrinogen, a blood protein that contributes to heart disease and stroke, may be more active if you smoke, says François Cambien, M.D., director of research at the Institut National de la Santé et de la Recherche Medicale in Paris. This may help explain why people who smoke have more heart attacks than nonsmokers.

One in five people carried a mutation of the beta fibrinogen gene in Dr. Cambien's study of 565 men who had heart attacks and 668 healthy men up to age 64. Fibrinogen, which is present in all of our bodies, thickens blood by making blood platelets stickier. The more fibrinogen in the blood, the more likely a person is to develop atherosclerosis and form blood clots that can lead to heart attack and stroke, Dr. Cambien says.

Among people who don't smoke, the gene seems to have only a small influence on cardiovascular diseases. But if you do smoke, its impact is greater and may be just enough to trigger cardiovascular problems.

A test for this gene isn't on the horizon. But quitting smoking would significantly reduce your fibrinogen levels even if you don't carry the gene, Dr. Cambien explains. "People who smoke have elevated levels of fibrinogen anyway. So if you can quit smoking, you'll positively affect your risk of coronary disease and stroke," he says.

■ **Ask for volunteers.** The more information you have, the better. Compiling all the family history that you would want can be a big job.

"If you're looking at breast, ovarian, or other female cancers, for example, you really need to have a broad reach. So you wouldn't look only at mothers, sisters, and aunts but at first cousins, second cousins, and great-aunts," says Katherine Schneider, a genetic counselor at Dana Farber Cancer Institute in Boston. Information about fathers, uncles, and grandparents can provide vital clues, too.

Ask family members to help, Schneider suggests. Elect a family historian to compile all the pieces of information that others gather.

■ **Look forward as well as back.** Most of the health information you need may be buried deep in your family's past. But don't forget to examine the health of your children and grand-children. If they have had heart disease, cancer, or stroke, it may be time to seek genetic counseling, advises Mary Daly, M.D., director of the Family Risk Assessment Program at Fox Chase Cancer Center in Philadelphia.

"We have some families where the daughter gets breast cancer before the mother, and then the mother goes on to get it, too," Dr. Daly says. Discovering that you carry the same mutated gene as your ill children may help you consider your options, she says.

■ **Check everything out.** If you know only that your aunt died of "female" cancer or that your grandfather had "cancer all through his body when he died," that won't help you very much, Schneider says.

"A lot of family myths about death are passed on from generation to generation," Schneider says. "It could turn out that the relative had a completely different cancer than family legend claims. It could be that he didn't have cancer or heart disease at all."

Get as many official documents as you can, including a death certificate, suggests Schneider. Your best bets are local hospitals, coroners, or the state department of vital statistics in the area where the relative died.

■ **Dig deeper.** Check out diaries, letters, old photographs, anything that will give you clues about how your relatives lived. Did they smoke? What were their occupations? Where did they live? What did they eat? Were they overweight? Did they have high blood pressure? Did they have high cholesterol levels? These questions will help you figure out if lifestyle or genetics played a bigger role in their pattern of disease, Dr. Hopkins says.

"If they all developed lung cancer, but they also smoked for 20 to 30 years, you can probably bet it wasn't inherited," Schneider says.

Is Genetic Testing Worthwhile for You?

Once you compile your family history, you might notice some patterns of heart disease, stroke, and cancer that can't be accounted for by poor diet, smoking, and other risk factors. If this is the case, you may want to consider taking the next step—genetic counseling and testing. But for most of us, it is probably unnecessary, Dr. Miller says. As a general rule, these diseases are caused by lifestyle factors like smoking.

Genetic counselors are available at most major medical and cancer centers, Schneider says. A counselor can help you evaluate your family's history of disease and determine if genetic testing is appropriate.

If genetic testing is the next step, a laboratory technician will either draw some of your blood or use a small brush to swab a few cells from the inside of your mouth. Both methods will disclose the same genetic information, Dr.

Miller says. The lab would then evaluate the sample of your cells for known genetic markers of cancer and heart disease.

It takes anywhere from three weeks to six months to get your initial results, depending on what type of testing is done. Cancer markers, for example, are very complex, says Dr. Myers. Researchers have to analyze thousands of genetic patterns to find the mutation they are looking for. But once a defective gene has been detected in one family member, it usually takes only one to four weeks to check for that mutation in other relatives.

Here are a few points to keep in mind before you seek counseling and testing:

■ **Ask yourself why you are doing this.** Before seeking genetic testing, it's important to think about all of the possible emotional and economic consequences for you and your family, advises Dr. Daly.

Consider how genetic testing might affect you or your children's ability to get insurance or find employment, Dr. Daly says. Imagine how it might affect your relationship with your sister, daughter, or spouse.

Think about what you will really do with this information. Some people do nothing. Some begin getting more frequent checkups to detect these diseases early. Others opt for preventive surgery to remove cancer-prone organs, says Dr. Daly.

Imagine how you might react to positive test results. Take time to seriously contemplate these issues before making the decision to undergo testing. A certified genetic counselor will help you understand how the risks and benefits of genetic testing may affect you.

■ **Get a referral.** This process isn't cheap —up to $200 for counseling and more than $1,500 for testing. Schneider suggests asking your doctor to refer you to a genetic research project that might pay some of the costs.

Prescription for Overcoming Your Genes

Genetic defects that cause inherited forms of cancer and cardiovascular diseases are rare. Genetic testing can detect some of the mutant genes that are passed from one generation to the next. But even if you carry a mutated gene, it doesn't mean you are doomed to develop one of these diseases. A healthy lifestyle that includes not smoking may help keep these genes dormant.

DO:

▶ **Think carefully about the economic and social consequences** of genetic testing on you and your family.

▶ **Get a referral** to a genetic testing study at a major medical center.

▶ **Gather specific information** about your relatives—both ancestors and children—such as how they lived and died.

DON'T:

▶ **Panic.** The vast majority of cancers, heart attacks, and strokes are not caused by inherited genetic defects. Focus on living as healthy a life as you can.

16

What Other Ailments Affect Your Disease Risk?

You know your body's main enemies—cancer, heart attack, and stroke. But in reality, these high-profile diseases are more like the four-star generals of the opposing forces. In any army, the big brass may get all the attention, but it's the foot soldiers who lead the assault. Cancer, heart disease, and stroke couldn't wage their battles without lots of help from other medical conditions that report for duty on the front line.

Here is a rundown of some of the factors that help pave the way for the high-profile diseases to attack. The good news is that if you can control them, you may be able to outflank the big three as well.

Atherosclerosis

Atherosclerosis is just the fancy name for hardening of the arteries. And that's what happens—they get stiff and narrow. But that's not all. "Bad" low-density lipoprotein (LDL) cholesterol starts the process, attaching to artery walls and even attracting other cells to the site. The walls thicken and stiffen. Then tiny shards of bone actually form within the walls, which become inflamed. The body tries to repair the damage but ends up making plaque, the stuff that can break loose and form a clot—increasing your risk of a heart attack or stroke.

The destructive process picks up speed if you already have high blood pressure, diabetes, or elevated cholesterol levels. But you can fight the effects, says John Cantwell, M.D., director of preventive medicine and cardiac rehabilitation at Georgia Baptist Hospital in Atlanta.

Here are some ways to protect yourself:

■ **Slow it down with exercise.** Exercise slows the progress of atherosclerosis. It doesn't matter whether you go to an exercise class, take walks, or just work in the house or garden. Strive for 30 minutes or more of vigorous exercise just about every day, advises Dr. Cantwell.

■ **Control your problem areas.** If you can control your high blood pressure and cholesterol, you will help put the brakes on this condition, says Dr. Cantwell. He also notes that just being 20 percent overweight can trigger insulin resistance or diabetes, two key contributors to hardening of the arteries.

■ **Adjust your diet.** If you cut cholesterol and animal fats, you will also cut your risk, advises Frank Barry, M.D., a family practice physician in Colorado Springs and author of *Make the Change for a Healthy Heart.* You worsen the effects of insulin resistance and diabetes (both of which speed up hardening of the arteries) if you consume a lot of polyunsaturated oils, such as corn, safflower, and sunflower oils. Instead, mono-unsaturated fats, such as olive and canola oils, provide healthy alternatives.

■ **Take vitamin E.** Vitamin E spurs insulin activity and can prevent LDL cholesterol from being oxidized in the body, notes Dr. Barry. One study designed to find out how much vitamin E is necessary for this protection found that 400 international units of vitamin E per day is the minimum needed to prevent damage. It also found that 800 to 1,200 international units of vitamin E provided more protection. But talk with your doctor first, especially if you are already taking anticoagulant drugs, says Dr. Barry.

■ **Eat smaller meals.** Large meals raise insulin and blood sugar levels steeply, giving your system more problems to deal with, especially if your cells aren't taking in insulin and sugar as effectively as they used to. Smaller, more frequent meals will take off some of the pressure, says Dr. Barry.

Atrial Fibrillation

With atrial fibrillation, your heart loses its sense of rhythm—and your risk of stroke shoots up. According to the American Heart Association, this disorder is responsible for 75,000 strokes every year.

Symptoms of atrial fibrillation are subtle, including palpitations and shortness of breath. Often, you don't know that you have it until a routine physical picks up the irregular beat or an electrocardiogram maps it out.

This condition increases your risk of a stroke because blood tends to pool and be more likely to congeal. And atrial fibrillation usually goes along with other cardiovascular problems. You're at risk if you have had a stroke, heart attack, high blood pressure, congestive heart failure, hyperthyroidism, heart valve or rheumatic heart disease, or if you have abused alcohol.

Your doctor will probably prescribe an anticoagulant, followed by a regimen of medication to help your heart keep its steady beat.

Barrett's Esophagus

It seems pretty innocent at first—little benign tumors that develop on your esophagus, the pipe that moves food from mouth to stomach. The growths frequently start out as irritations caused by digestive juices that spurt upward from the stomach. Symptoms include heartburn and difficulty in swallowing.

But, as in the case of many cancers, harmless little lumps can turn malignant. Doctors once thought that this condition also increased your risk for colon cancer. But the good news is that a study performed in five French hospitals suggests that is not the case.

Chronic Infections

When your body's cells are damaged, repaired, then damaged again on a frequent basis, you're setting the stage for cancer, says Dr. Cantwell. Pay attention to skin sores, especially if they are exposed to the sun. Scar tissue, too, is more at risk.

"We know that chronic ulcerative colitis, an inflammatory disease of the colon, seems to be associated with increased risk of cancer. It is very likely that all of the body's tissues react the same way to chronic irritation," says Dr. Cantwell.

Colds and Respiratory Infections

In an English study of 96 older men and women, researchers found that the increased risk of winter colds may make blood more likely to clot in the arteries that supply the heart. That may be caused by increased levels of fibrinogen and factor VIIc, substances in the blood that lead to increased clotting.

Fibrinogen actually provides the scaffolding around which clots form, and it is linked to higher rates of heart disease. An Israeli study, for instance, followed more than 3,000 male heart patients for three years. The 111 men who died during the study all had higher levels of fibrinogen than did the survivors.

One theory is that respiratory infections trigger the body's infection-fighting mechanisms, which also speed up blood clotting. But the increase in winter strokes and heart attacks could also be due to seasonal variations in high blood pressure, weight gain, and lack of activity that occurs when the temperature drops.

One common bacterium, *Chlamydia pneumoniae,* may be tied to higher rates of heart disease. This bacterium causes upper and lower respiratory tract infections. It increases the concentration of fibrinogen and sialic acid in the blood, which is also associated with higher rates of heart disease. Furthermore, research shows that people with high levels of fibrinogen may have twice the amount of the harmful LDL cholesterol. Their levels of protective high-density lipoprotein (HDL) cholesterol tend to be lower than normal, too.

Still, experts aren't willing to put too much emphasis on colds and bacterial infections as risk factors for heart disease, cancer, and stroke. "It's much less significant than other factors, such as high blood pressure, cholesterol, and diabetes," believes Dr. Cantwell.

All the same, you can make changes in your lifestyle to keep fibrinogen levels down: Maintain a healthy weight and eat a diet low in saturated fat. Also, include vegetables, fruit, and fish in your diet, advises Dr. Cantwell.

Depression

You may already know that being the go-go-go type-A personality weighs heavily on your heart. But depression is actually worse for the heart, says Robert Carney, Ph.D., professor of medical psychology at Washington University School of Medicine in St. Louis. "Depression appears to be a risk factor for heart disease," he says. "It's more important than a type-A personality, but probably not as significant as high blood pressure and cholesterol." Still, he notes that depression is often treated long before patients show signs of heart disease. All the same, depressed people may have higher risk for heart trouble not because of their emotional states alone but because they're more likely to smoke and ignore doctors' recommendations.

Depression takes more than just a mental toll. If you're depressed, the nervous system becomes more active and the heart beats faster—and it is more likely to beat irregularly. "Any kind of chronic illness or problem affects the nervous system and adds to risk," says Dr. Carney.

Depression differs from your normal mood changes. You may be depressed if you experience some of these symptoms for two weeks or more:

Loss of interest in things you normally enjoy

Inability to concentrate

Trouble sleeping

Lack of appetite—you may lose five pounds or more

A hopeless and helpless feeling

Crying for no apparent reason

Sometimes depression itself can be fatal. If you have any symptoms that indicate you may be depressed, see your doctor immediately. Antidepressant medication can often reverse the dangerous effects of depression in short order.

There are ways you may be able to reverse short-term depression. Here's how:

■ **Do what's good for you.** Even though it's hard to stick to it when you are depressed, exercise and a healthy diet will help bring you out of the depths, advises Dr. Carney.

■ **Get emotional support.** People who are depressed feel isolated, as if they don't have anyone who cares for them. Ask for support from family and friends. "You need someone to put an arm around you and help you get through this," says Dr. Carney. "It's a lot easier if you ask for help and know that someone hears you, understands you, and is with you."

■ **Admit it to yourself.** Often, just acknowledging to yourself that you are depressed helps, particularly if your depression stems from a specific event, such as an illness. "This kind of depression can be treated quickly and effectively," says Dr. Carney. It may require short-term psychotherapy or antidepressants.

■ **Simplify your life.** If you are depressed, you may feel out of control or overwhelmed. "Focus on simple tasks and goals, things you can accomplish," advises Dr. Carney. "If you tell yourself that you have to stop smoking right now, you may not feel that you're in control enough to do so. You'll set yourself up for a failure and add to your depression." Instead, try to cut down. If you smoke 30 cigarettes a day, try to smoke only 25 a day. "That way, you can feel that you're making progress and setting goals that you can accomplish."

■ **Make a list.** Depression robs you of your concentration and makes it hard to remember things, says Dr. Carney. Keep a list of just a few tasks that you want to accomplish each day. Mark them off when you finish them. Don't overdo it—keep your list short and easy to manage. Tell yourself, "I may not be coping very well with this right now, but here are some things I can do to help myself. If I accomplish them, I'll feel more in control and less depressed."

■ **Look for your own basics in life.** When you're depressed, you may feel that life has no meaning. Make a list of your personal reasons for living—nothing fancy, just those things that you look forward to and that give you pleasure, says Dr. Carney. "For instance, that you can still enjoy your grandkids and you still play cards with friends." When you feel down, pull out your list and read it to yourself.

Diabetes and Insulin Resistance

Insulin resistance often leads to diabetes—and that's not all. "Insulin resistance and the abnormalities associated with it accelerate atherosclerosis, which leads to heart disease and stroke," says Gerald Reaven, M.D., a researcher at Stanford University. He estimates that insulin resistance affects 25 percent of all Americans.

Both insulin resistance and diabetes wage guerilla warfare on your circulatory system and significantly increase your risk of heart disease or stroke. These conditions also produce a domino effect in your body, making other systems go haywire.

Here's what happens: If you have insulin resistance, your system doesn't respond to the insulin your body produces. That's a problem because insulin is the substance that makes it possible for blood sugar to enter your cells and provide them with important nourishment. Think of insulin as the key that unlocks the door to your body's cells and allows nutrients to get in, says Dr. Reaven.

Don't Get X'd Out

Your children or grandchildren might be Generation X. But the X you really want to keep your eye on is *Syndrome X,* a cluster of medical conditions that dramatically increase your risk of heart disease and stroke.

Syndrome X is composed of several conditions, including high blood pressure, high triglyceride levels, low high-density lipoprotein (HDL) cholesterol levels, and premature coronary heart disease. Researchers see indications of this syndrome even in children, but it usually doesn't become a major problem until much later in life.

"All the components of Syndrome X are related to insulin resistance," says Gerald Reaven, M.D., the researcher at Stanford University who coined the term and has pioneered the research into Syndrome X. According to Dr. Reaven, when insulin cannot get into the cells, the body gets the wrong message and mistakenly thinks it needs to make more.

High blood levels of insulin lead to high levels of triglycerides, fats in the blood. This high triglyceride level is related to a low HDL cholesterol level—that is, the level of good cholesterol in the blood.

"You can make a big improvement with lifestyle changes, such as eating a healthy, low-fat diet and doing some aerobic exercise," says Dr. Reaven.

Your system is no slacker, so your pancreas gets the signal to work overtime to produce extra insulin because the amount it is producing is insufficient to do the job. Over time, your pancreas cannot keep up with the extra insulin production, and you end up with low insulin supplies. That's when insulin resistance turns into diabetes.

Though both insulin resistance and diabetes involve insulin, they are two different diseases affecting the body differently. First, let's look at the problems created by diabetes.

The lack of insulin means that blood sugar can't get into the cells where it is needed for energy, and it builds up in the blood. In type II diabetes, the most prevalent kind, some of this sugar gets into the cells by sheer force.

The blood sugar outside the cells exerts pressure—kicking the door down, so to speak, when the insulin key doesn't work. Having blood sugar levels that are either too high (hyperglycemia) or too low (hypoglycemia) is not good for your body.

As if that weren't enough, having diabetes seriously increases your risk of developing cardiovascular disease. According to the American Heart Association, approximately 80 percent of people with diabetes die of some type of heart or blood vessel disease. This is because diabetes increases triglyceride levels and lowers helpful HDL cholesterol levels. Diabetes is also the leading cause of blindness, kidney failure, and nerve damage.

Insulin resistance leads to its own share of problems. Several studies show that insulin resistance and high levels of insulin in the blood appear in as many as half of the patients with high blood pressure.

You'll want to alleviate insulin resistance because it changes the amount of LDL cholesterol in your blood, which is a risk factor in coronary heart disease. In this instance, the LDL cholesterol particles become smaller and denser and more easily oxidized, allowing them to grab on to artery walls and narrow them.

If you are insulin-resistant, you have more insulin floating around in your system trying to get that blood sugar into the cells. This is not good because insulin raises levels of triglycerides, those fats in the bloodstream that clog up the works. High levels of triglycerides are normally associated with low levels of HDL cholesterol. Also, high insulin levels and insulin resistance interfere with your body's system for breaking up clots in the bloodstream.

There are ways you can help your body use sugar and insulin more efficiently, reversing insulin resistance and preventing or minimizing diabetes:

■ **Get active.** People who exercise regularly can enhance how their bodies use insulin, which decreases their insulin resistance, says Dr. Reaven. In addition, physical activity can lower triglyceride and insulin levels, help lower blood pressure, and increase levels of "good" HDL cholesterol in the blood. The American Heart Association recommends that people try to get at least 30 to 60 minutes of aerobic exercise three to five times a week.

■ **Lose weight.** Being overweight is not the only factor that can lead to insulin resistance, but it is an important one. If you are overweight and subsequently lose weight, your body will improve its sensitivity to insulin, and you will become less insulin-resistant, says Dr. Reaven.

Where your body stores fat may be more important than how much your body stores. People who store fat in their upper body usually have more features of insulin resistance than those who store fat on their hips and thighs.

■ **Check your inheritance.** There is a genetic component to insulin resistance and diabetes. Your risk of developing these conditions is higher if you are of non-European ancestry. If that fits your family's description, be particularly careful to lower your risk, advises Dr. Reaven.

■ **Put out the cigarettes.** Another good reason to quit now: Smoking increases insulin resistance, forces triglyceride levels to go up, and makes HDL cholesterol levels go down, according to Dr. Reaven.

Hepatitis

This highly infectious disease comes in several forms. Two kinds, hepatitis B and C, are linked to liver cancer. You get type C from a blood transfusion or by sharing contaminated needles. Type B can get into your system through blood transfusion, sexual contact, or sharing contaminated needles or instruments.

High Blood Pressure

Many people think that high blood pressure is a natural part of getting older. But it doesn't have to be that way. When high blood pressure is lowered, you can cut your risk of heart disease and stroke in half or more, says Dr. Barry. That may seem hard to believe. After all, you can have high blood pressure and still feel great. But doctors don't call it "the silent killer" for nothing.

"When you blow up a balloon too much, you put too much pressure on a structure that's not built to take it. It pops," says Dr. Barry. "That's what high blood pressure does to your arteries."

The pressure rises when the muscles in your blood vessels constrict. Blood vessels narrow, and your heart works overtime, pumping more vigorously just to get enough oxygen and nutrients to your body's cells.

Because the blood is under more pressure, it travels more turbulently through your arteries. Imagine a wide river that suddenly narrows through a slender gorge. That wild river ride is similar to what happens in your arteries. And other things start to go wrong. The smooth walls

Low Stress Leads to Long Life

How do you lower stress? It depends on what motivates you, says Frank Barry, M.D., a family practice physician in Colorado Springs and author of *Make the Change for a Healthy Heart.* "Some people, in their heart of hearts, decide that it's easier to take a pill to reduce high blood pressure. Others prefer to make lifestyle changes."

Whatever your approach, you will feel less stress if you feel in control of your life, notes Dr. Barry. Get that control by establishing goals, writing them down, and working toward them, giving less attention to little things that aren't really important to you. Ask yourself, "What do I want to accomplish in life?" Here are a few techniques that many people find effective in relieving stress:

Relax and enjoy. Believe it or not, relaxation and enjoyment take some effort—or at least some calculation. "A lot of people realize that if they sit in a chair all day, they will make their health worse. But in the years of work, they have forgotten how to enjoy themselves," says Dr. Barry. "If you enjoy life and develop a sense of playfulness and humor, you'll be less prone to stress, anxiety disorders, and depression."

Make a study of what really relaxes you and what you really enjoy—the types of places (say, museums or parks) or activities (like cards, golf, or quilting). Then deliberately build those things into your day. Remind yourself that it is okay to have fun—you deserve it.

Lend a helping hand. You may get the greatest satisfaction from helping your children or grandchildren. But if you are considering providing financial assistance, think carefully: Will you find that satisfying or just stressful? "I've seen patients who have never had such joy as when they gave their grandchild a new car. In that case, money can be a stress reducer," says Dr. Barry.

Pay attention to changes. Stress increases with major life changes, such as adjusting to the first few months after retirement. "Your routine changes immediately, but your mind and body are still tuned to the habits that may have taken 65 years to form," says Dr. Barry. Often, just acknowledging that you are feeling stress helps to bring it down.

---

of your blood vessels get torn up and collect more debris, or plaque. The plaque builds up on your artery walls—and narrows them even more.

Under this extra pressure, the plaque may rupture. As it breaks loose, it turns into the stuff clots are made of, and your risk of heart attack and stroke rises.

Sometimes high blood pressure doesn't start in your arteries. If your kidneys don't work properly, they can produce hormones that tell the muscles in your blood vessels to tighten, constricting the arteries, and putting on the pressure. Stress can be another common cause of increased constriction of the blood vessels.

Here are lifestyle changes you can make that may help lower your blood pressure:

■ **Reduce personal stress.** Studies show that stress gets your heart pumping and your pressure rising, says Dr. Barry. As stress raises your heart rate and blood pressure, hormones may make the coronary arteries constrict, especially if they have been damaged by atherosclerosis (hardening of the arteries). The combination of

Low Stress Leads to Long Life...continued

Remember, less is more. Many older people feel the stress of a fixed income. "Take advantage of the burgeoning simplicity movement," says Dr. Barry. When you sit down and think about what makes you happy and what makes you worry, you may find that you don't need the second car, the cabin in the mountains, or the new furniture. You may find that what makes you happy are family and friends, and fewer material things. Letting go of what's not important helps cut costs and stop stress.

Get on with life. Especially when you retire, you may be tempted to live vicariously through your children and grandchildren. That always produces stress because it doesn't work. Instead, live your own life. Do volunteer work to establish a larger circle of friends and responsibilities. Take courses at your local college.

Change your inner environment. Biofeedback or meditation will relax you mentally and lower stress, says Dr. Barry. Try reducing the psychological stress that raises your blood pressure by repeating a sound, word, phrase, or muscle movement while you passively disregard other thoughts.

Say good-bye to beepers. A lot of people feel as though they are always on call, says Dr. Barry, thanks to pagers, cellular phones, and the like. Take a break from technology, perhaps spending a restful day with the phone unplugged. Get unbusy. Allow yourself time to do nothing.

Act like a B. People with type-A personalities suffer stress more often. Type A's are impatient, competitive, hostile, easily angered, and constantly struggling against the demands of real or imagined deadlines. (If you ever had to work for one, he/she probably gave you stress.) Type Bs, on the other hand, are more relaxed, accepting, and less impatient.

If you're a type A, practice being assertive but not hostile, advises John Cantwell, M.D., director of preventive medicine and cardiac rehabilitation at Georgia Baptist Hospital in Atlanta. You'll be more pleasant to be around—and you'll give your heart a break.

reduced blood supply and greater demand for blood can lead to a heart attack.

■ **Cut the salt.** As you get older, your system becomes more sensitive to salt and hangs on to it longer. The average American diet contains 3,500 to 5,000 milligrams of salt a day. Consuming 1,000 to 1,500 milligrams a day puts you in the low-salt and high-health range. So check those nutrition labels when you shop and look for no-salt or low-salt products, suggests Dr. Barry.

■ **Add potassium.** Low potassium intake can increase blood pressure, says Dr. Barry. Get more potassium by adding fresh fruit and vegetables, particularly bananas and potatoes, to your diet.

■ **Drop some pounds.** Being overweight can contribute to high blood pressure, says Dr. Cantwell, and a weight loss of just five to 10 pounds can actually make blood pressure medication unnecessary in some cases.

■ **Stay active.** Physical activity lowers high blood pressure. "If you're not doing anything, start to do something physical," says Dr. Barry. "Just accumulate 30 minutes of activity a day. This needn't be marathon running. You can walk, ride an exercise bicycle, work in the garden, or mow the lawn."

■ **Reduce dietary fat.** If you have been wondering why you've put on weight over the years, ponder this tidbit: 37 percent of most people's daily calories comes from fat. To lower high blood pressure (and get your cholesterol down), Dr. Barry suggests that you get 10 percent of your daily calories from fat, the amount recommended by Dean Ornish, M.D., to reverse heart disease. Make a habit of checking the labels on processed food—they will fill you in on the fat content.

■ **Increase antioxidant intake.** Some researchers suspect that high blood pressure is caused, in part, by a shortage of disease-fighting antioxidants in your system. Antioxidants prevent free radicals from blocking your body's production of nitric oxide and prostacyclin. These two compounds relax blood vessels to help keep blood pressure down.

You can get antioxidants through your diet by eating foods rich in beta-carotene and vitamins C and E, such as carrots, cantaloupe, broccoli, red bell peppers, and sweet potatoes. A multivitamin and a vitamin E supplement of 400 international units will also increase your intake, says Dr. Barry.

High Cholesterol

High cholesterol is the number-one risk factor for heart disease," says Dr. Barry. While HDL cholesterol protects you, LDL cholesterol and other fats do major damage to your arteries. Here's what happens:

The insides of your arteries start out with a smooth, elastic lining. Over time, it loses the elasticity and gets roughed up. The barrier between the cells in the lining breaks down. Fat cells get trapped within the lining and thicken artery walls. Microscopic fatty deposits even

form on the artery surface. The result: narrowed, plaque-filled arteries.

If these deposits break free, they can lodge in the blood's passageways, causing a heart attack or stroke. The good news is that one form of cholesterol, HDL, actually helps the body get rid of the harmful stuff before it can do damage.

Here is what you can do to keep cholesterol levels where they belong:

■ **Eat less fat.** Eat the standard American diet, and you take in gobs of fat, typically accounting for 37 percent of your calories. Your body makes a valiant effort to deal with the problem, but there is just too much. So it ends up as cholesterol. Reducing fat in your diet is the most important change that you can make because this may significantly lower cholesterol (especially harmful LDL) levels.

But not all dietary fats affect the body equally. Saturated fat, which you get in red meat and dairy products, is the real culprit. Eat less of foods that contain it, and you lower your total and LDL cholesterol levels, says Dr. Barry. Unfortunately, polyunsaturated fats (corn oil, for instance) are also problematic because they lower levels of the beneficial HDL.

If you need or crave fat, then lean toward monounsaturated fats instead (olive and canola oils), and you will reduce your LDL levels while raising HDL levels. But keep in mind that you should eat only moderate amounts of fat, even if it is monounsaturated.

The American Heart Association (AHA) recommends that you keep fat consumption to 30 percent or less of your daily calories. You will do your system even more favors if you get total fat intake below the AHA guidelines, to as low as 10 percent of calories, suggests Dr. Barry.

■ **Stop smoking.** No surprises here. Snuffing this habit tops doctors' lists, says Dr. Barry.

Are You Hot?

The standard tests that doctors use to tell whether you are an easily stressed "hot reactor" (and at greater risk for disease) are pretty simple, so take your pick, says Frank Barry, M.D., a family practice physician in Colorado Springs and author of *Make the Change for a Healthy Heart.* For the first two tests, you'll want to take a blood-pressure reading twice—once before the test and once during the test—for comparison.

Test 1: Chill out. In Test 1, put your hand into a bucket of cold water for one minute and have someone measure your blood pressure right after you have done it. If it goes up into the high range in response to physical stress, you are a hot reactor.

Test 2: Do some math. Test 2 is a little more cerebral. Start with the number 100 and mentally subtract 7, then continue to subtract 7s until you get to 2. In the midst of your figuring, have your blood pressure taken. "There's no exercise, no threat to your life, but a lot of people still feel mental stress and their blood pressures shoot up," says Dr. Barry.

Test 3: Talk to yourself. You can also test yourself without the shock of cold water or the mental anguish of math. Ask yourself: Are you working toward your own true goals or someone else's? If you are busy trying to keep up with the Joneses, "you're still in the rat race, even if you have retired. You're much more likely to feel the effects of stress regardless of whether you're a hot reactor," says Dr. Barry.

Nonsmokers have higher levels of the beneficial HDL cholesterol, 5 to 9 milligrams per deciliter (or mg/dL, as doctors measure cholesterol) above that of most smokers.

■ **Lose weight.** HDL—the "good" cholesterol—protects your heart, so you need as much of it as you can get. The problem is that if you gain weight, your HDL levels actually drop. A study showed that men's HDL cholesterol levels drop by 4 percent for every five pounds they gain. For women, it drops 2 percent. Lose the weight, and the HDL levels go back up.

■ **Raise a glass.** Studies show that very light drinking raises beneficial HDL cholesterol by up to 15 percent and lowers risk of heart attack. But more than two drinks a day for men, and more than one drink a day for women may cause more harm than good, says J. Michael Gaziano, M.D., director of cardiovascular epidemiology at Brigham and Women's Hospital in Boston.

■ **Add fiber to your diet.** Fiber can lower cholesterol levels, says Dr. Cantwell. Go for oats, oat bran, barley, legumes, prunes, apples, carrots, and grapefruit. If you like, add over-the-counter products that are rich in psyllium seeds, which are often sold as laxatives.

■ **Get enough vitamin E.** In a small study, researchers found that vitamin E supplements combined with a diet high in monounsaturated fat blocked LDL cholesterol and kept it from oxidizing. Some doctors recommend 400 international units of vitamin E a day for their patients who have coronary heart disease.

■ **Eat more soy.** Rather than a hamburger, reach for a soy or tofu burger. Soy protein is low in fat and rich in genistein. This substance has received a lot of attention because it may lower the risk of breast cancer, but researchers believe that it also decreases total cholesterol.

Stomach Ailments

Results from one study suggest that stomach cancer may be tied to a type of common bacteria, *Helicobacter pylori.* These little organisms produce chronic upset that may eventually allow cancerous cells to take over. In an American study, doctors found that half the people who visited their family doctors for stomach complaints had these bacteria to blame. Antibodies that your body produces to fight the bacterial infection may actually stimulate cancer cells in the stomach. Good news: The infection can be treated with antibiotics.

Stress

In the film *West Side Story,* members of the Jets, a New York street gang, urge each other to "stay cool." Researchers who study stress say the same thing, because stress can make you more vulnerable to heart disease, cancer, and stroke. Feeling stressed or overwhelmed raises your blood pressure and can even trigger heart arrhythmias. "We know that stress can contribute to increased cholesterol and hypertension," says Dr. Carney.

People who react strongly to stress are called "hot reactors" by cardiologists and psychologists. Their stress triggers an extra release in the flight-or-fight hormones that gave your Stone Age ancestors an edge over saber-toothed tigers. These hormones tell your heart to pump faster, which increases your blood pressure.

Stress also releases free fatty acids into your system, giving your body the energy boost it needs to react. But unless you're in serious danger, your body doesn't have a use for these compounds. Instead, they turn into artery-clogging cholesterol. Chronic stress may also decrease your body's immune response, leaving you more vulnerable to a cancer. Researchers at the National Institute of Mental Health in Bethesda, Maryland, found that stress activates hormones that allow viruses and cancerous cells to take hold.

If stress is a constant problem for you, see a psychologist or psychiatrist to learn ways you can keep it under control. Medications or short-term therapy can help lessen the effects of stress on your body.

Thyroid Imbalance

In a study of 2,000 men and women aged 60 and over, researchers found that a thyroid imbalance can interfere with the rhythm of your heart's beat. Those who had slightly overactive thyroids were most at risk, a condition called subclinical hyperthyroidism. If you have it, your thyroid releases a low level of thyrotropin, a pituitary hormone that controls the production of the thyroid hormone. Your doctor can prescribe medication to regulate hormone production.

Prescription for Preventing Disease

Cancer, heart disease, and stroke don't arrive out of nowhere. Lots of little problems pave the way for these major maladies. But all the little things you can do to assure your general good health will play important protective roles.

DO:

▶ **Keep cholesterol, blood sugar, blood pressure, and body weight within normal limits.**

▶ **Exercise regularly** to prevent the circulatory slowdowns that lead to heart disease and stroke.

▶ **Take vitamin E** at 400 international units daily to activate your insulin reserves and protect your cells from damage.

▶ **Eat small meals** to help your system take in insulin and sugar more efficiently.

DON'T:

▶ **Smoke.**

▶ **Let winter weather make you inactive.**

▶ **Stay in stressful situations** without getting help.

▶ **Get low on potassium.** You risk developing high blood pressure.

17

How Dangerous Is Sun Exposure?

I t's easy to get burned. Just stick an uncovered hand into a 550°F oven for a second or two. You'll quickly remember why you use potholders. The sun is 20 times hotter than a broiling oven. Sure, it's 93 million miles away, but in just 10 minutes it can toast you like a marshmallow over a campfire. And even after age 60, a sunburn—or even the lightest tan—can ignite cancer-causing skin damage. That's why doctors urge you to use sunscreen whenever you are out in the sun, and take other precautions, too.

"At this age, people want to live an active lifestyle. And I don't blame them. You don't have to live in a cave, but there are certain measures that you can take to protect yourself while you are enjoying the outdoors that will drastically reduce your risk of skin cancer," says Craig Eichler, M.D., a dermatologist at Cleveland Clinic Florida in Fort Lauderdale.

The Bronze Age Is Over

F or years, tans were in. Pale was out. But all that sun worshiping sparked an epidemic of skin cancer, Dr. Eichler says. Skin cancer is the most common type of cancer in the United States. In 1996, Americans over age 65 were expected to account for about half of the 838,000 new cases of skin cancer. In the same year, approximately 9,400 Americans—more than one every hour—were likely to die of some form of skin cancer, according to the American Cancer Society.

Almost all of this is unnecessary because without sun damage, cases of skin cancer—plus those nasty wrinkles and liver spots—would be virtually nonexistent, Dr. Eichler says.

Do You Need Sunscreen After Age 60?

A lot of my patients in this age range say, 'Well, I'm old and it doesn't matter how much sun I get anymore.' The point is that it does matter very much at that age," says Nancy Silvis, M.D., assistant professor of dermatology at the Arizona Cancer Center in Tucson.

Indoor Tanning Isn't a Bright Idea

The tropics beckon. Surf, sand, and lots of sun. You certainly don't want a nasty sunburn to spoil your fun. So before you leave home, you visit the neighborhood tanning parlor a few times to brown your skin a little.

A smart move?

"It may seem like a perfectly reasonable thought. The problem is that it doesn't work," says James Spencer, M.D., a dermatologist and director of Mohs Micrographic Surgery at the University of Miami School of Medicine. "The tan you get at a tanning parlor only provides an SPF [sun protection factor] of about four. So it won't protect you from burning, and tanning itself is a sign that the skin has already been damaged."

Most tanning parlors are unregulated and use UVA light in the mistaken belief that these rays are less harmful than other forms of radiation, Dr. Spencer says. In reality, UVA penetrates deep into the skin and can significantly increase the risk of melanoma and other skin cancers.

To get an idea of how sun damage accumulates, imagine sun exposure on a 100-point scale. When you're born, you have 0 points. When you reach 100 points, you get skin cancer, says Michael Kaminer, M.D., assistant professor of dermatology at Tufts University School of Medicine in Boston.

Every time you expose your unprotected skin to the sun, it damages your skin a bit more, and you add on points. One bad sunburn in your teens, for instance, might add 50 points to your lifetime total. Even tanning, which is really the skin's reaction to sun exposure, is a sign that harm has been done and more points are piling up. So if you are age 60 and your sun exposure score is 90, wearing sunscreen and taking other precautions may stop you from getting those last 10 points that would push you irreversibly toward skin cancer, according to Dr. Kaminer.

The problem is that you never really know where you are on that imaginary scale. You can look perfectly fine but could be getting close to topping 100 points and developing skin cancer. That's why it is important to start or continue taking sun precautions after age 60, Dr. Kaminer says.

How the Sun Does Its Damage

Sunlight contains two types of harmful ultraviolet rays: UVA, a long-wavelength ray that penetrates deep into the skin; and UVB, a medium-wavelength ray that is absorbed by the upper layers of the skin. Both scramble DNA, the genetic code that cells use to reproduce, and increase the likelihood that your skin will form abnormal cells. At the same time, these rays suppress the immune system so that your body will be less able to defend itself, says Kevin Cooper, M.D., chairman of the Department of Dermatology at Case Western Reserve University and University Hospitals of Cleveland.

Over years or decades, these skin changes can develop into one of three types of cancer:

1. *Basal cell carcinoma.* This is the most common type, and is also the least serious form of skin cancer. It rarely spreads to other organs.

2. *Squamous cell carcinoma.* It's a bit more aggressive than basal cell and is more likely to spread to the lymph nodes and other parts of the body.

(Both basal cell and squamous cell carcinomas are usually curable if removed early, but they can leave disfiguring scars.)

If You Live for a Tan...

Craig Eichler, M.D., a dermatologist at Cleveland Clinic Florida in Fort Lauderdale, says, "Some people tell me that they absolutely don't feel healthy unless they have a tan. For them, bronzers containing dihydroxyacetone (DHA) are worth trying. They are much better than they were years ago when they tended to give an orange-carrot-type look to the skin. Nowadays, these dyes are much more natural-looking and are a nice alternative for some people."

Bronzers contain chemical dyes that brown the skin without sun and are available over the counter at most drugstores and makeup counters. But remember, bronzers don't provide sunburn protection, so be sure to apply sunscreen as well.

3. *Melanoma:* The most tenacious and dangerous of all skin cancers, melanoma can quickly spread to the lungs, brain, and other vital organs if it isn't corralled early. It kills thousands of people every year. "Once melanoma spreads to a vital organ, it is resistant to radiation and chemotherapy. At that point, there is really nothing you can do. But if it is caught at the start, there is virtually a 100 percent cure rate," says James Spencer, M.D., a dermatologist and director of Mohs Micrographic Surgery at the University of Miami School of Medicine.

Lighten Your Risks

Most of the skin damage that leads to skin cancer occurs before age 20. But even if you have never taken any precautions when out in the sun, there are still plenty of reasons to start doing it now, Dr. Kaminer says.

Sun exposure can increase your risk of certain skin cancers after age 60, according to researchers at the British Columbia Cancer Agency in Vancouver. In a study of 586 men up to age 79, the researchers found that those who reported being outdoors 24 hours or more each week during the summer months were twice as likely to develop squamous cell carcinoma during the next 10 years than the men who got less sun exposure.

But taking preventive measures even at a late stage may help repair seriously damaged skin before it turns cancerous, Dr. Silvis says. For six months, Australian researchers tracked 588 people up to age 93 who had precancerous skin lesions called actinic keratosis. Those who began using sunscreen developed fewer new precancerous lesions and were 53 percent more likely to have existing actinic keratosis disappear.

"Studies like this have shown that patients over age 60 who use sunscreen are actually helping their skin recover," Dr. Silvis says. "But among patients who don't use any protection, the skin isn't doing the needed repair work because it is continually being damaged."

Here are a few ways to lower your chance of developing skin cancer, yet still enjoy the warmth of the sun:

■ **Make 15 your lucky number.** Use a sunscreen with a sun protection factor (SPF) of at least 15, Dr. Kaminer says. That means it will protect your skin from the sun for about 150 minutes, or 15 times longer than if you didn't wear it. Although sunscreens with SPFs up to 50 are available, a 15 should do the job. It will block out 93 percent of the sun's harmful rays. In comparison, an SPF of 35 only gives the skin about 4 percent more protection. (If you really want 100

You've Gotta Wear Shades

Sunscreens, hats, long pants, and shirts can protect 99.9 percent of your skin. But unless you don a pair of strong sunglasses, your eyelids are still vulnerable to the ravages of skin cancer.

"The eye is an easy pathway into the brain. That's why a tumor on the eyelid can be particularly dangerous," says René Rodriguez-Sains, M.D., chief of the Ocular Tumor and Orbital Clinic at Manhattan Eye, Ear, and Throat Hospital in New York City.

For optimal eye and eyelid protection, sunglasses should wrap around the face, fit snugly and comfortably as close to the forehead as possible, and absorb at least 99 percent of the sun's ultraviolet rays. Check the manufacturer's label.

When you are doing your monthly skin self-exam, don't forget to inspect your eyelids. See an ophthalmologist or dermatologist if you notice any lumps, growths, and discolorations, Dr. Rodriguez-Sains advises.

"Nine times out of 10, it will be nothing to worry about. It will probably just be the barnacles of life that go along with aging skin. But sometimes it may be a lesion that will need prompt attention," he says.

percent protection, choose a sunblock that contains either zinc oxide or titanium dioxide.)

■ **Establish a daily routine.** Sunscreen is easy to forget unless you make it a part of your morning ritual. After you bathe and before you dress for the day, apply sunscreen to every part of your skin that will be exposed to the sun, Dr. Cooper suggests. Allow at least 20 minutes for the lotion to soak into your skin before going out in the sun so that the sunscreen will stay on better once you swim or start sweating.

■ **Don't let the clouds fool you.** Wear sunscreen even on overcast days, since the sun's rays penetrate clouds and can still damage your skin, advises Dr. Eichler.

■ **Smear it on.** Many people, particularly in the over-60 age group, spread sunscreen on much too thinly, Dr. Kaminer says. Put at least one heaping teaspoon on your face and neck, another teaspoon on your chest, and yet another on your back. Then use a 1/2-teaspoon to cover both hands, another 1/2-teaspoon to cover both feet, a half- to a full teaspoon for each leg, and a 1/2-teaspoon for each arm and shoulder, he suggests. For men who have lots of body hair, more might be needed on their arms, chest, and legs because the sunscreen is absorbed by the hair before it reaches the skin.

■ **Do the hands, neck, and ears first.** "Three places where older people often forget to put sunscreen on are the neck, ears, and the back of their hands," Dr. Kaminer says. "So I tell my older patients to apply sunscreen to those areas first. It's important, especially on the back of the hands, because a lot of skin cancers develop there."

■ **Start all over again.** Reapply sunscreens at least every two hours to maintain maximum protection, Dr. Kaminer suggests. If you are swimming or perspiring heavily, you may need to do it every hour that you are in the sun. Some sunscreens are water-resistant or waterproof, but even these should be rubbed into your skin again every couple of hours, he says.

■ **No matter your color, beware.** People who have naturally dark skin pigment develop fewer skin cancers than fair-skinned

Don't Get Burned by Your Drugs

Medicines can do wonders for arthritis, high blood pressure, heart disease, and other ailments that are common after age 60. But when some drugs collide with the sun, your skin may pay a big price.

Certain oral drugs like antibiotics and diuretics can increase your sun sensitivity. That magnifies your chances of getting a cancer-promoting sunburn, says Nancy Silvis, M.D., assistant professor of dermatology at the Arizona Cancer Center in Tucson.

Ask your doctor or pharmacist if you should avoid the sun while taking any drug. Many common medications can increase your sun sensitivity:

Drug Class	Generic Name	Brand Name
Diuretics	Furosemide	Lasix
	Hydrochlorothiazide	HydroDIURIL
Sulfonylureas (for diabetes)	Chlorpropamide	Diabinese
	Tolbutamide	Tolbutamide
Antibiotics	Tetracycline	Achromycin V
	Doxycycline	Vibramycin
	Sulfamethoxazole	AZO Gantanol
	Nalidixic acid	NegGram
	Griseofulvin	Fulvicin
Nonsteroidal anti-inflammatory drugs	Naproxen	Aleve
	Piroxicam	Feldene
Antidepressants	Doxepin	Sinequan
	Imipramine	Tofranil
Anti-arrhythmic drugs (for irregular heartbeat)	Amiodarone	Cordarone
	Quinidine	Quinaglute

individuals, Dr. Spencer says, but it isn't perfect protection.

"African-Americans rarely develop skin cancers because their dark skin provides natural sun protection," he says. "Hispanics can and do develop skin cancers, so they should use sunscreen if they're going to be out in the sun for extensive periods, like fishing on a boat all day."

If you are African-American, keep an eye on the lighter portions of your skin, such as scars and the palms of your hands, which are often less resistant to sun damage, Dr. Spencer suggests. But no matter what color your skin, see your doctor if you develop any unusual spots or growths on your body.

■ **Check the weather.** Look for the UV Index in your local weather report, Dr. Silvis suggests. It is a forecast from the National Weather Service of how much ultraviolet light will reach the ground in your area at midday. It will help you decide when and for how long you may want to go out that day. The index ranges from 0 to 15.

Zero to 2 is minimal risk, meaning one hour of unprotected sun exposure may cause skin damage in sun-sensitive people.

■ **At high noon, take cover.** When the sun is directly overhead, its rays are traveling through less atmosphere than when it is on the horizon. That is why sunlight is considered more intense and damaging at midday than at sunrise or sunset, Dr. Eichler says.

"I suggest that my patients only go out in the sun when they cast a shadow that is longer than they are tall. It is an easy rule of thumb to remember, and it will protect you from the most damaging ultraviolet light," Dr. Eichler says.

■ **Wear a hat.** Hats are essential in the sun to cover your scalp and shade your neck and ears, particularly if you are over age 60, Dr. Kaminer says. Wear one that has at least a 3-inch brim all the way around the base.

■ **Reapply sunscreen under clothes.** Certainly, long-sleeve shirts and pants offer more protection from the sun than bare skin, Dr. Silvis says. But not much more—a dry T-shirt provides an SPF of 6 to 8, and only 2 to 3 when wet.

"Most people think that their clothing is enough to protect them from the sun," Dr. Spencer says. "But if you hold a white T-shirt up to the sun, you can see right through it. And if you can see through it, that means light is going through it." So be sure to regularly apply sunscreen every couple of hours underneath your clothes.

Some mail-order clothing manufacturers, such as Sun Precautions, however, make tightly woven clothing with an SPF of 30 even when wet. For a free catalog, write Sun Precautions, 2815 Wetmore Avenue, Everett, WA 98201. "Sun-protective clothing is an excellent option," Dr. Silvis says. "The clothing provides a broad range of protection from both UVA and UVB light."

■ **Soothe a burn.** If you do get a sunburn, only time will really help to relieve your symptoms, Dr. Spencer says. Your best bet? Take a 325-milligram aspirin every four to six hours and apply cool-water compresses to the burned area as needed. You also might try over-the-counter moisturizers like aloe vera to treat the burn.

■ **Examine your skin.** Conduct a self-exam of your skin once a month and see a dermatologist at least once a year for a professional evaluation. "It's so simple to do a head-to-toe. It doesn't take long, it doesn't hurt, and you can save yourself a lot of trouble," Dr. Spencer says. "Remember that most skin cancers are very easy to cure if they're detected early." Look for any new growths as well as changes in size, shape, color, texture, or thickness of existing moles, freckles, and birthmarks on all parts of your skin. If you do find a suspicious spot, have it checked promptly by a dermatologist.

Prescription for Being Safe in the Sun

Americans over age 65 account for about half of all new cases of skin cancer. Skin damage accumulates as you age. The more unprotected sun exposure you have, the greater your risk of skin cancer. But even after age 60, you can stop this process and reverse some skin damage if you begin taking precautions in the sun.

DO:

▶ **Use a sunscreen with an SPF of at least 15.** Apply it to your skin 20 minutes before sun exposure. Reapply every two hours when outdoors, even underneath clothing.

▶ **Look for the UV Index in your local newspaper.** It will help you decide when and for how long you may want to go out that day.

▶ **Wear a broad-brim hat and sunglasses in the sun.**

▶ **Conduct a self-examination of your skin once a month.** Look for any new growths or changes in moles, freckles, and birthmarks. See a dermatologist promptly if you discover any suspicious growths.

DON'T:

▶ **Let clouds fool you.** Sunlight penetrates clouds, so wear sunscreen even on overcast days.

▶ **Forget to apply sunscreen to your ears, neck, and back of the hands.** These spots are just as vulnerable to sun damage as other parts of your body.

18

Do You Need Hormone Replacement Therapy?

Sooner or later, every woman's menstrual cycle comes to an end. The transitional time (perimenopause) that leads to the cessation of periods and the complete end of them (menopause) can be an uncomfortable—even miserable—experience for many women. Hot flashes, night sweats, disturbed sleep, vaginal dryness, irritability, and difficulty concentrating are common, and these problems usually continue—to a varying degree—for several years. Most women reach menopause by their early 50s.

During the 1970s, doctors found that many patients could avoid the symptoms of menopause by using hormone replacement therapy (HRT). The therapy consists of taking drugs designed to replace the hormones that the body ceases to make. Many women welcomed HRT because it alleviated their often agonizing discomfort. What's more, HRT was hailed as a likely deterrent to heart disease and osteoporosis (a condition that causes thinning and weakening of the bones). A slightly elevated risk of breast cancer was suspected in connection with HRT, but many women were willing to run that risk in exchange for the symptomatic relief that HRT offered. In addition, for those who took HRT long term, studies suggested lower rates of heart disease and other serious medical conditions.

But, in 2002, a large government study on long-term use of combined HRT—a combination of estrogen and progesterone—was halted before its completion because women taking this type of HRT were found to be at higher, not lower, risk for heart attack, stroke, and blood clots, in addition to breast cancer. Another study showed that use of estrogen also increased the incidence of ovarian cancer. Even though the risks were small, the study results surprised the medical community and cast a pall over the routine use of HRT.

How Could Earlier Research Have Been So Wrong?

There are lessons here beyond HRT," says Timothy McCall, M.D., a Boston internist and author of *Examining Your Doctor: A Patient's Guide to Avoiding Harmful Medical Care*. "All scientific 'proof' is only tentative, subject to later revision as more data come in."

The studies on which prior recommendations for HRT were based didn't compare women who were chosen at random to receive either the treatment or a placebo, according to Dr. McCall. Instead, the early studies compared women who were using HRT by personal choice with other women who chose not to use HRT. As it turned out, the women who chose to use estrogen in the earlier tests tended to be in better health than those who did not, so their incidence of coronary disease and stroke were already lower. But randomized studies, such as the government study that was halted, provide more accurate information—any preexisting health factors are nearly equal between the groups.

"The decision to take HRT, as with many other medical choices, has always been complicated—and it still is, although opinion seems to be swinging against long-term use," says Dr. McCall. "There is a complex mix of purported benefits and side effects. Studies have flaws. Data are always incomplete. Marketing can influence doctors and patients." Clearly, as more new information comes along, you need to adjust your thoughts about using any other medical treatment that is under consideration.

Should You Give Up on HRT?

Don't be too quick to rule out HRT. "In the short term, taking hormones to relieve menopausal symptoms seems to be safe," says Steven R. Goldstein, M.D., professor of obstetrics and gynecology, New York University School of Medicine, in New York City.

"When taken for, say, a year or two, it may be worth the risk—depending on the severity of hot flashes and other symptoms and the degree of relief you get from alternative measures," Dr. McCall believes. That's because HRT is so effective at eliminating many of the uncomfortable symptoms of menopause. Of course, if you do

decide to take a short course of HRT, you must pay careful attention to your annual mammograms and get regular physical checkups—doing so will help you keep tabs on the increased risks of breast cancer, heart disease, and stroke. In addition, you should do all you can to lessen these risks by exercising, maintaining a healthy weight, and eating a low-fat diet that is rich in fiber.

A more complete randomized trial will be ready for publication in a few years. It should shed more light on the safety of HRT when taken over a longer period. Until then, consider how serious your menopausal symptoms are, and weigh them against your personal risk of developing breast cancer and heart disease. "If you are having menopausal symptoms that disrupt your life, you probably could take HRT safely for a few years to ease the transition," says Dr. Alexander J. Swistel, director of the Weill Cornell Breast Center and associate professor of surgery at New York Hospital–Cornell Medical Center, both in New York City.

What Happens When You Stop Taking HRT?

If you have been taking HRT for a few years and wish to stop, some or all of your menopausal symptoms may return. "Ask your doctor about gradually decreasing your HRT dosage," suggests Dr. Goldstein. The dosage can be tapered over several months to minimize the effects of withdrawal.

"I advise most women not to stop cold turkey," says Dr. McCall. Once you stop taking HRT, you will need to find another way to deal with the threat of osteoporosis. Supplementing with adequate calcium and vitamin D in addition to weight-bearing exercise and, in some cases, medication are things you should do to maintain your bone health. If you are at high risk for developing osteoporosis, Dr. McCall suggests that you talk with your physician about the advisability of using

Are Your Hormones in Balance?

If you're not feeling quite right, you may have too much estrogen (which increases your risk of breast cancer) and not enough progesterone (which helps you build new bone tissue). This imbalance in your system can be due to a number of factors, including the use of HRT or birth control pills; working night shifts under artificial lights; prolonged periods of stress; and eating too much sugar and starches, too few green leafy vegetables, or beef that has been injected with estrogen growth supplements.

"Every woman should get her estrogen and progesterone levels tested—and discuss the results with her doctor," says John R. Lee, M.D., a family physician in Sebastopol, California, and coauthor of *What Your Doctor May Not Tell You About Breast Cancer: How Hormone Balance Can Help Save Your Life*. Dr. Lee believes that a saliva test is more accurate than a blood test in measuring estrogen and progesterone levels. Contact the following sources for more information or to purchase a mail-order test (cost is approximately $50): Aeron Life Cycles Lab, 800-631-7900 or *www.aeron.com*; Great Smokies Diagnostic Laboratory, 800-522-4762 or *www.gsdl.com*; and ZRT Lab, 503-466-2445 or *www.salivatest.com*.

If the saliva test shows you have a low progesterone level: If testing reveals a progesterone/estrogen ratio below 200:1, Dr. Lee recommends rubbing your palms, chest, and neck with a topical progesterone cream, many of which are sold over the counter. Brands include Awakening Woman, Fem-Gest, Natra Gest, and Renewed Balance. They cost between $12 and $30. Use a quarter of a teaspoon once each day for three months, then have another saliva test to see if your ratio has improved.

If the saliva test shows you have a low estrogen level: If your level of estrogen is also low, Dr. Lee suggests that you ask your doctor about taking an oral estrogen such as Estradiol, starting with a dose of 0.25 mg. daily ($1/2$ a 0.5 mg. pill, the lowest dose currently available). And have another saliva test after three months to check your progress. Be careful to take no more than the minimum amount you need to return to balance, since an excess of estrogen increases the risk of developing breast cancer.

Warning: Be sure to speak with your physician about any progesterone/estrogen imbalance you may have before self-medicating with estrogen. Your doctor can thoroughly explain all the risks and benefits of this treatment.

one of the other drugs commonly prescribed to prevent or treat osteoporosis, such as alendronate sodium (Fosamax) and raloxifene (Evista).

Are There Other Treatments for Hot Flashes?

If you don't want to start taking HRT or are planning to taper off HRT, there are other ways to handle the challenges that menopause presents.

Warning: Do not take any medications or dietary supplements without first checking with your doctor. Some of them may interfere with other medications you are already taking.

There are several possible alternatives to HRT that can ease menopausal symptoms:

■ **Herbal remedies.** Black cohosh, licorice, red clover, and chasteberry are traditional treatments that have been used for decades to relieve menopausal discomfort. Check the recommended dosage on the labels of dietary supplements produced by reputable suppliers.

■ **Changes in diet.** Eating more soy-rich foods and ground flaxseed will help to compensate for the hormones that decrease during menopause. There are many ways to incorporate soy and flax into your meals. Start by sprinkling flaxseed over cereal or mixing it into a soy-milk smoothie.

■ **Prescription medications.** Estradiol and progesterone (the latter is available over the counter in a cream base) are identical to the hormones your body stops producing at menopause, according to Andrew L. Rubman, N.D., associate professor of clinical medicine, College of Naturopathic Medicine, University of Bridgeport, in Connecticut, and consultant to the North American Menopause Society, in Cleveland. Ask your doctor if they are suitable for you. (See the box on page 259 about how to keep your hormones in balance.)

"You may want to try the antiseizure medication called gabapentin [Neurontin]," suggests Thomas Guttso, Jr., M.D., a neurologist and senior instructor of neurology at the University of Rochester, in New York. "In one study, the intensity and frequency of hot flashes were cut in half in women who took 900 mg. of gabapentin daily. When the dose was increased to 2,700 mg. a day, hot flashes were diminished by two-thirds." There are, however, side effects to this medication. Approximately half the women in the trial experienced sleepiness, rashes, and swelling of their hands and feet. But the side effects may lessen the longer the medication is taken.

Prescription for Dealing with Menopause

Recent tests of hormone replacement therapy (HRT) indicate that it may be risky—even dangerous—to take, especially in regard to developing heart disease and breast cancer. You should take HRT only after thoroughly discussing your personal risk factors with your physician.

If you decide to take HRT to ease the symptoms of menopause:

DO:

▶ **Plan to take the prescribed medication for only a short period.**

▶ **Get regular mammograms** and any necessary tests to detect cardiovascular disease and cancer that could be related to HRT while using the therapy.

▶ **Taper off HRT medications slowly**—under the supervision of your doctor—when discontinuing use.

▶ **Find natural ways to cope with the possible return of menopausal symptoms** as you taper off the HRT regimen.

DON'T:

▶ **Take HRT unless you and your doctor agree that your personal medical history**—particularly how it relates to heart disease and cancer risk—indicates that the associated risks are acceptably low for you.

If you decide *not* to take HRT:

DO:

▶ **Ask your doctor if you need a prescription** for Evista, Fosamax, or another medication to replace the protection for your bones that HRT would give you.

▶ **Try traditional herbal remedies and dietary changes** to see if they help to alleviate your menopausal discomfort.

DON'T:

▶ **Try any alternatives to HRT** without discussing your plans with your doctor.

19

How Safe Is It to Shovel Snow?

Down comes the snow, out comes the shovel, and then comes the heart attack. It's a pattern that Stephen Hargarten, M.D., sees all too often. "After a heavy, wet snowfall, we'll get five to six times the number of heart attack cases that we would on any other typical winter day," says Dr. Hargarten, associate professor of emergency medicine at the Medical College of Wisconsin in Milwaukee.

At least 75,000 heart attacks occur each year during or shortly following strenuous physical exertion. About one in every three of those heart attacks are deadly, says Murray Mittleman, M.D., a researcher at the Institute for Prevention of Cardiovascular Disease at Beth Israel Deaconess Medical Center West in Boston. Many of these heart attacks and deaths occur among people over age 60 who have been shoveling snow.

It's More Than Just a Chore

A lot of people think, 'Oh, it's just snow. I can take care of this.' They think of it as just another domestic chore like mowing the lawn," Dr. Hargarten says. "But snow shoveling is a lot more strenuous an activity than power mowing. Shoveling causes changes in blood circulation that are a lot more stressful on the heart." Those changes in blood flow can be particularly risky for people over age 60 who are sedentary or who are unaware that they have heart disease. "As you move along in years, you tend to get less exercise, and activities like snow shoveling become more dangerous," Dr. Hargarten says.

A study of 10 sedentary men in Michigan, for instance, found that just two minutes of shoveling snow raised heart rates above the limit commonly recommended for safe exercise. If you are out of shape, the chances that you will have a heart attack in the hour following a physically draining task such as snow shoveling are 53 times greater than the chances for a person who is physically active on a regular basis, according to Dr. Mittleman.

"If you live in an area like Boston where snowfall is inevitable, it is important to get regular exercise throughout the year so that your cardiovascular system will be better prepared to handle the demands

Blowing Away Snow Isn't Necessarily Better

Snowblowers may make your work easier and put less stress on your heart rate and blood pressure. But even with power assistance, the demands of snow removal can still be too high for inactive people who have heart disease, says Barry Franklin, Ph.D., director of the Cardiac Rehabilitation and Exercise Laboratories at the Beaumont Hospital Rehabilitation and Health Center in Birmingham, Michigan. Plus, these devices may have limited value when the snowfall is extremely deep.

"In sedentary men, manual shoveling increases heart rates up to 175 beats a minute. But using a snowblower can elevate your heart rate to 120 beats a minute. If you have a heart condition, that could still be a real problem," Dr. Franklin says.

He suggests that, before you decide to clear any snow yourself—either by shoveling or using a snowblower—you ask your doctor if it is safe for you to do so.

of shoveling in the winter," Dr. Mittleman advises. If you've let yourself get out of shape, then you should make other arrangements for snow removal.

How Shoveling Strains Your Heart

When you shovel snow, you tend to hold your breath as you lift, Dr. Hargarten says. That increases pressure in your chest and reduces blood flow to your heart. At the same time, cold air constricts your blood vessels. All this raises your blood pressure and forces the heart to work even harder. If your heart arteries are damaged or partially blocked with plaque, these elements can combine to set you up for a heart attack. (Doctors are uncertain if physical exertion like snow shoveling also contributes to the onset of a stroke, Dr. Mittleman says.)

So is snow shoveling a good idea if you're older than 60? You can probably safely do it, Dr. Hargarten says, if all of the following four conditions are true for you:

1. *You exercise regularly.*

2. *You live a healthy lifestyle that includes low-fat eating.*

3. *You get regular physical exams.*

4. *You do not have any signs of heart disease, high blood pressure, or diabetes.*

Otherwise, it is smarter to get someone else to shovel snow for you.

If you are fit and really want to shovel, here is a checklist to consider:

■ **Get an annual checkup.** Before the first snow flurries begin to fall in your area, get a physical and ask your doctor if it's okay for you to shovel snow during the upcoming winter, Dr. Hargarten recommends.

■ **Let morning snow go.** If at all possible, avoid shoveling snow immediately after you awaken, Dr. Hargarten says. Most heart attacks occur early in the morning because blood is more prone to clotting after you have been asleep. Take your time getting around to shoveling. Stretch, take a warm shower. Allow yourself an hour or two before tackling this task.

■ **Lay off the smokes and java.** Avoid drinking caffeine or smoking tobacco for at least an hour before and after shoveling. Coffee and cigarettes can both elevate your blood pressure and pulse rate and increase the risk of a heart attack, Dr. Hargarten says. Smoking also elevates your carbon monoxide level, which further compromises the delivery of oxygen to the heart.

■ **Eat lightly.** Wolfing down a big meal may seem like a great way to rev yourself up for this exhausting chore, but you may be doing yourself more harm than good, says Barry Franklin, Ph.D., director of the Cardiac Rehabilitation and Exercise Laboratories at the Beaumont Hospital Rehabilitation and Health Center in Birmingham, Michigan. Eating draws blood into the stomach, which means that less blood is circulating to the rest of your body. So if you shovel after eating, you are more apt to strain the heart, he says. Consider waiting an hour or two after finishing a meal.

■ **Stretch out.** Before you begin shoveling, take five minutes to stretch and warm up your muscles, says John Emmett, Ph.D., an exercise physiologist and associate professor of physical education at Eastern Illinois University in Charleston. Stretching will help open up blood vessels and improve circulation to the heart. Try doing 20 to 25 knee bends and other stretching exercises or calisthenics before tackling the white stuff, he suggests. (To learn a warm-up routine, see "Warm Up for Comfort" on page 160.)

■ **Dress in layers.** Put on layers of clothes that can be easily removed so that you don't become overheated as you shovel, Dr. Mittleman suggests. As you work, your body will warm up. But you don't want to get too warm—if you get overheated, your blood vessels will dilate, blood will pool in your legs, and your blood pressure will drop. These conditions force your heart to pump harder, increasing your risk of a heart attack. If you start sweating or feeling warm, it's time to shed a layer of clothing, he says.

■ **Find the right tool.** The smaller and lighter the shovel blade, the lighter the load you will lift. And the lighter the load, the less strain you will put on your heart and back, says Dr. Emmett. Specially designed snow shovels that have a bend in the handle can lessen the strain on the body even more. These shovels are available at most hardware stores, he says.

Be sure that the shovel handle is the correct length so that you don't have to stoop too much, Dr. Emmett says. Here is one easy measurement: Grasp the handhold at the end of the shovel with one hand. Place your other hand about 18 inches from the point where the handle meets the blade. If your hands are a little more than a shoulder-width apart, you have the right size shovel for you.

■ **Work smart.** Start slowly and work your way up to a faster pace, Dr. Emmett says. During the first five minutes of shoveling, take half as many scoops as you will when you are going full speed.

When you lift the shovel, bend at the knees and lift with your legs. That will put less strain on your arms, back, and heart, Dr. Franklin says.

Try to keep the load as close to your body as possible. Avoid twisting and turning as you work. Instead, shovel in the direction that you want to toss the snow and throw it out straight from the shovel blade, Dr. Emmett suggests.

Don't work without pausing occasionally. Take a five-minute break from shoveling every 15 to 20 minutes.

■ **Watch for warning signs.** Immediately call for an ambulance or go to an emergency room if you feel very dizzy, light-headed, or short of breath or if you sense any tightness or burning in your chest, arms, or back, Dr. Mittleman says. "Don't worry about feeling embarrassed about coming into the emergency room for a suspected heart attack. It is better to be embarrassed and safe rather than be sick and dead," Dr. Hargarten says.

Prescription for Clearing Snow Safely

Heart attacks triggered by snow shoveling are quite common, particularly among people over age 60 who don't regularly exercise or who have heart disease. If you live a healthy lifestyle that includes regular physical activity, low-fat eating, and not smoking, you probably can safely shovel snow. If you don't, ask someone else to do it.

DO:

▶ **Get a physical** and ask for your doctor's consent before shoveling snow.

▶ **Dress in layers** to prevent overheating.

▶ **Stretch and warm up** before shoveling.

▶ **Work smart, not hard.** Use the right equipment, start slowly, and take frequent breaks.

▶ **Be on guard for the warning signs** of a heart attack, including tightness or pressure in your chest.

DON'T:

▶ **Smoke.**

▶ **Drink caffeinated beverages, such as coffee, or eat a meal** at least one hour before or after shoveling.

▶ **Shovel snow within one hour of waking in the morning.**

20

Healthy Living
After a Heart Attack

Okay, you've had a heart attack. Does that mean that you have to live the rest of your life in slow motion? Definitely not. For example, Dick Cheney has served as vice president of the United States after surviving several heart attacks. Other survivors have competed in marathon races.

"You can go on to a whole new, enjoyable life after a heart attack," says Andreas T. J. Wielgosz, M.D., Ph.D., head of the Division of Cardiology at Ottawa General Hospital in Canada. Researchers are finding that if you make certain lifestyle changes, they can help speed your recovery and even shield you from another attack.

And if you don't make these changes after a heart attack? Your risk of another attack skyrockets.

"If you've had a heart attack, your risk of a second one is three or four times greater than it is for someone who has never had an attack," says Daniel Levy, M.D., director of the Framingham Heart Study in Massachusetts, the nation's most important long-term study of heart disease. "You have to take aggressive steps to minimize your risk."

Changing Your Lifestyle Is Nothing New

At one time, heart attack survivors were urged to recuperate at health spas, with a regimen of relaxation, light exercise, and special diets—not too different from what contemporary cardiologists prescribe. But the patients in earlier times also underwent some treatments that by today's standards seem peculiar—long, hot baths in saltwater, for instance.

Today, when it comes to putting in time at a spa, researchers note that it could actually speed recovery. That's not surprising when you consider that life at the spa includes learning many elements that cardiologists believe are crucial if you want to avoid another heart attack:

The calm, ordered life that frees you from daily stresses.

A ready-made social support system, critical to prevention in today's world.

Regular exercise, also an essential part of a modern regimen for recovery.

If You Can Trim Even More Fat...

You'll get even greater results in lowering your heart attack risk if you switch to a diet with total fat levels at a super-low 10 percent of calories consumed, which is the level recommended by Dean Ornish, M.D. He has devised a widely known program for reversing heart disease. It's true that Dr. Ornish's programs are rigorous, but they are so successful that they are finding favor with some health insurance companies. The insurers reimburse subscribers for the cost of participating in the programs, which focus on making more extreme changes in lifestyle through diet, exercise, and meditation.

If you've had a heart attack, there are ways you can lower your risk of a recurrence:

Take Charge of Your Cholesterol

When you lower your cholesterol levels, you can stabilize or even reverse the atherosclerotic process," says Tom LaFontaine, Ph.D., manager of disease prevention and community wellness at Boone Hospital Center in Columbia, Missouri.

If you can lower your low-density lipoprotein (LDL) cholesterol count to 100 milligrams per deciliter (mg/dL) or less, keep your protective high-density lipoprotein (HDL) cholesterol above 35 mg/dL, and add exercise to the mix, something magical happens—you could help to reduce your risk for a second heart attack by 89 percent, according to Dr. LaFontaine.

"Cholesterol is a major risk factor for heart attacks. We've become much more aware in recent years of how important it is to lower cholesterol," says Dr. Levy. A good diet and exercise program can lower your cholesterol by 10 to 15 percent. If that's not enough, a combination of diet, exercise, and cholesterol-lowering drugs will usually do the trick.

That atherosclerotic process is a big part of what got your heart into trouble in the first place. Over the years, cholesterol in the blood found a home in your artery walls and really gummed up

the works. It built up thick deposits on your artery walls. Along the way, it turned into a hardened plaque that made your arteries stiffer and less flexible. It started to take up space that your blood needs to flow to your organs and tissue. Your narrowing arteries raised your blood pressure, leading to extra wear and tear on the artery walls.

And here's the worst part of the scenario—if the built-up plaque ruptures and breaks free, it can form a clot. Chances are, that's what caused your first heart attack. When blood flow to the heart is blocked, the heart muscle is denied the oxygen its cells need to stay alive and healthy. Beyond 20 to 30 minutes, the longer the heart muscle goes without oxygen, the more cells die, the more damage done to the muscle—and the slower your recovery.

Since you've already had a heart attack, it's a safe bet that some other arteries are filled with plaque and are now vulnerable to blockages. You need to get rid of that plaque—or at least stop its accumulation.

"You have to do everything you can to slow down the process that allows fats to oxidize and attach to your artery walls," says Dr. LaFontaine. "And it can be done. We're seeing that you can not only stabilize the plaque, but you can also change the way you live to make it less likely to rupture and cause clots." You should start to see lower levels of cholesterol in your blood

Be Careful in the Mediterranean

Monounsaturated fats, such as olive oil, are still high in calories. Dr. LaFontaine cautions that most of the studies showing the benefits of monounsaturated fat have centered on the Mediterranean diet. Although this approach to eating tends to be high in monounsaturated fats and low in other kinds, it is also loaded with fruits and vegetables, which protect against high cholesterol. So far, researchers haven't determined whether the heart-saving benefits of this diet come from the oil itself or the other food it flavors.

just a few weeks after you begin a cholesterol-lowering diet.

Regardless of your age or how much cholesterol has been setting up shop in your artery walls, bringing down cholesterol levels still lowers your risk. "In one study, the oldest adult in the project got the most benefit from lowering cholesterol," says Dr. LaFontaine.

Here's how to get your cholesterol down:

■ **Make a list.** After your heart attack, your dietitian probably prepared a list of menus and foods that you should eat to protect your heart. Make a list of what you are eating now and compare it with those recommendations. If you threw the list away when you started to feel better, ask your dietitian to review your current diet, suggests Dr. Wielgosz. As time passes, it is easy to fall back into old habits.

■ **Include your spouse.** If you've recently had a heart attack, you will probably meet with a dietitian or nutritionist who will help you plan a protective diet. Don't go alone—ask your spouse to go along with you, advises Dr. Levy. Your spouse needs to understands how important the new diet is to your future health. After all, both of you will probably end up eating the heart-protective diet that you are given. It will certainly be easier if both of you to stick to the plan.

■ **Cut down on fat.** Reduce your fat intake by a third, and you may help beat high cholesterol,

experts say. Look at product labels that show "calories from fat." Figure out the calorie and fat content of a day's worth of food. If you're consuming 2,000 calories a day, your fat content should total no more than 500 calories, or 25 percent of your total food intake. Make that figure—or a slightly lower one—your daily target, says Dr. LaFontaine.

Pay particular attention to the line on food labels that refers to artery-clogging saturated fat. Make sure that component adds up to less than 7 percent of total calories in the foods you eat each day.

■ **Count calories.** Just reaching for the low-fat products on grocery store shelves isn't enough by itself. You can select low-fat foods and still end up eating too many calories. Researchers from the National Center for Health Statistics note that in the 1970s, Americans took in about 36 percent of their daily calories from fat. In 1990, they took in only 34 percent of calories from fat. Sounds like an improvement, until you realize that total calorie consumption jumped and, therefore, the amount of the fat intake actually increased. Unfortunately, unburned calories get stored in the body as fat, increasing the problem.

■ **Decrease your dietary cholesterol.** When you read a package label, you'll see that many food products contain cholesterol, in addition to fat. Cholesterol is not as bad for your system as fat, but it still adds to the assortment of

Choose the Right Cardiologist and Hospital

Having the right cardiologist in your corner will go a long way toward avoiding a second heart attack, says Fredric J. Pashkow, M.D., medical director of the Cardiac Health Improvement and Rehabilitation Program at the Cleveland Clinic Foundation. Knowing that your doctor and recovery program are the best you can find provides important reassurance. And, if you do experience additional heart problems, you'll know that you will get up-to-date quality care.

Here are some pointers on how to choose wisely:

Check credentials. Call the local medical society or hospital physician referral service to get a guide to doctors in your area. You can find out about their education, training, and, sometimes, their specialities.

Look at the diplomas. Check to see if the cardiologist has degrees from top institutions. Quality education and training can make a difference.

Research the hospitals. Ask whether the hospitals that the cardiologist is affiliated with—the ones where you will end up—are accredited by the Joint Commission on Accreditation of Healthcare Organizations. That indicates that the hospital meets criteria for staffing and safety requirements. If possible, choose a cardiologist associated with a hospital that features a cardiac care center.

Visit the hospitals. Talk to friends who have been to the hospitals where your cardiologist works. If there is a regional or national heart health center in your area, ask your doctor whether you should go there. This is especially important if you have complex problems or advanced coronary disease.

---

harmful substances in the bloodstream. Look for products with low cholesterol. Try to consume less than 200 milligrams a day, suggests Fredric J. Pashkow, M.D., medical director of the Cardiac Health Improvement and Rehabilitation Program at the Cleveland Clinic Foundation.

■ **Eat more often.** Eat smaller meals more often, suggests Dr. Wielgosz. Emphasize fruits and vegetables. Your overall food consumption will probably drop, and your body will have an easier time burning the calories it takes in.

■ **Eat lean meats.** Buy "select" and "choice" cuts of meat because they are lower in fat than prime cuts, which are marbled with fat. Better yet, just generally cut down on the amount of meat you eat. Make portions smaller or, several days a week, prepare meatless entrées, suggests

Dr. LaFontaine. Instead of relying only on meat for your protein needs, look to beans, soy products, and vegetables. Not only will you take in less fat, but you'll consume more fiber, which also protects your heart.

■ **Pick the healthiest fats.** All fats are not created equal. "Substitute monounsaturated fats, such as olive oil or canola oil, for saturated or polyunsaturated fats," says Dr. LaFontaine. "Monounsaturated fats don't seem to contribute to fats in the bloodstream the way other fats do."

Use liquid fats for cooking. Keep away from oils like shortening that come in cans and are solid at room temperature. They're particularly high in the harmful kinds of fat.

Read the ingredients on every food label to make sure that oils appear far down on the

On Your Own? Work Out Anyway

Sure, it helps to have workout pals egging you on and charting your physical progress. But what if that's not possible? Here are some other strategies to increase your odds of sticking with an exercise program, suggested by Tom LaFontaine, Ph.D., manager of disease prevention and community wellness at Boone Hospital Center in Columbia, Missouri:

Make a display. Keep your exercise clothes and equipment where you can see them. They will provide constant reminders in case you start to lapse. Park your stuff by the front door, in the living room, in front of the TV, or in the den, at least until exercise becomes an ingrained habit.

Set a schedule. Exercise at the same time every day. You will be less likely to forget or become sidetracked. Exercise will become as much a part of your daily routine as brushing your teeth. Most heart attacks happen in the morning, but you can help condition your heart with light exercise, such as walking, during those early hours. Save the strenuous stuff until later in the day, says Andreas T. J. Wielgosz, M.D., Ph.D., head of the Division of Cardiology at Ottawa General Hospital in Canada.

Walk with energy. You'll probably include walking as a major component of your exercise program. Do it with vigor—the more energy you expend, the more benefit your cardiovascular system receives. Consult your doctor to find your optimal energy level, advises Dr. Wielgosz.

Tour the mall. Try getting your exercise by walking in an enclosed mall, especially if the weather is particularly hot or cold. You may find local mall-walking programs that welcome cardiac patients. "These organized exercise programs are particularly important because they also get people out in a group, helping to reduce social isolation, which is itself a major risk factor," says Dr. Wielgosz.

ingredients list, a sign that they played a small part in the food's production. Watch out for products that don't specify the type of oil they contain. They're probably high in the artery-clogging kind, says Dr. LaFontaine.

■ **Make substitutions.** Small changes can make big differences in getting cholesterol and fat levels down. For instance, instead of eating whole eggs, try egg whites or egg substitutes. And use fat-free salad dressing and fat-free margarine, says Dr. Pashkow.

Buy low-fat dairy products made from either skim or 1 percent low-fat milk. Try nonfat or low-fat yogurts. Choose cheeses that feature 3 grams of fat or less per ounce—and plan on eating a 1-ounce serving, suggests Dr. LaFontaine.

■ **Fortify with fiber.** When you eat a high-fiber diet, you're also picking foods that are generally low in cholesterol. Try to take in 25 to 35 grams of fiber a day. "You can get that by eating a lot of vegetable protein, consuming soy and other bean products, for example," says Dr. LaFontaine. "You can also get fiber in fruits, vegetables, and cereals. Evidence suggests that the fiber you get from cereal may be particularly important for protecting your heart."

■ **Step on the scales.** Every time you stand on the bathroom scale, you get an instant readout of your cholesterol risks. They go up as your weight goes up. "The best way to lower cholesterol is to burn off as many or more calories than you take in," says Dr. Wielgosz. What stays in the system can turn into fat and clog up your arteries.

■ **Ask for reminders.** Tell friends and family about the changes that you are making in your diet and how these changes can help keep you alive and healthy—with their support and encouragement. Ask them to remind you if you start to slip into your old eating patterns. Experts think that social support is one of the biggest motivators in keeping people on track.

■ **Call for help.** Your doctor or dietitian should be an important part of the support system that keeps you on the path to heart recovery. Choose a doctor who invites your calls, checks on your progress, and is interested in whether you are sticking to the lifestyle changes you've made to protect your heart. You'll get encouragement and psychological support just from knowing your doctor cares about how you are doing.

Get the Blood Pressure Down

Not that long ago, doctors thought that high blood pressure was okay as you got older. The theory was that you needed the extra pressure to keep the blood flowing. But study after study shows just how important it is that you get your blood pressure down into the normal range to lower your risk of a second heart attack. "Even if you're 80, your blood pressure can be similar to what it would be for someone 40 years old," says Dr. Pashkow.

Here's how to lower your high blood pressure:

■ **If you're carrying extra weight, lose it.** Not only will excess baggage make you more prone to high blood pressure, it will increase your risk of diabetes, which will raise your risk of a second heart attack even more, says Dr. LaFontaine.

■ **Again, add the fiber.** Fiber is one of those all-purpose substances. Not only does it lower your cholesterol, but it also helps reduce your blood pressure.

■ **Focus on fat.** Make sure that you're getting no more than 25 percent of your calories from fat—an eating approach that will lower both your cholesterol levels and your blood pressure, says Dr. LaFontaine.

■ **Cut the salt.** For the best heart protection, stay away from high-sodium foods, such as potato chips, anchovies, sauerkraut, pickles, and salami as well as other salty, highly processed products, advises Dr. Wielgosz. Your total daily sodium intake should be under 2,400 milligrams, according to the National Academy of Sciences. Your system may also be salt-sensitive, something that often contributes to high blood pressure. Talk with your doctor or dietitian about reducing your salt consumption.

■ **Check your supplements.** High blood pressure is linked to low levels of potassium, calcium, magnesium, and vitamin C. It's important to eat foods that are rich in these nutrients. Make sure that they are in your daily multivitamin. But don't consume more than the daily levels recommended by Jeffrey Blumberg, M.D., associate director and chief of the Antioxidants Research Laboratory at the U.S. Department of Agriculture Human Nutrition Research Center on Aging in Boston:

1,200–1,500 milligrams of calcium

400 milligrams of magnesium

3,500 milligrams of potassium

250–1,000 milligrams of vitamin C

Before you make any changes in your dietary supplements, discuss them with your doctor.

Dine Leisurely to Reduce Risk

Dr. Wielgosz speculates that enjoyment of eating may explain "the French paradox"—the fact that people in France eat a lot of fat but have fewer heart problems than Americans. "These people have more *joie de vivre* at the table," he says. "Their meals take longer. There is more socializing around the dinner table. People enjoy the moment and live in the moment."

Stop the Stress

Stress has been identified as an important risk factor for heart attacks. Researchers found that the way someone responds to mental stress gives as clear a picture of heart attack risk as does the traditional exercise stress test. This finding underscores just how important a stressful environment may be in heart attack risk.

"While you can't eliminate stress a lot of the time, you can change how you cope with it. That may be an important factor in reducing your risk for a second heart attack," Dr. Wielgosz says.

Here's how you can manage stress:

■ **Take time out.** During the day spend a few minutes for quiet reflection, contemplation, or isolation from daily life. In your office, bedroom, or outdoors, tune out stress-provoking pressures and thoughts. Focus on pleasant reflections. Many people relax by repeating a single word or a prayer over and over again.

■ **Walk the dog.** Fido may not be up for a brisk, nonstop, 20-minute walk, the kind of intense aerobic workout that benefits the heart. But even leisurely dog-walking will help reduce stress. You'll benefit from the repetitive action of your muscles as you walk. You'll enjoy the scenery. But most important, you'll have social interaction with another being, says Dr. Wielgosz.

■ **Find a hobby.** "An amazing number of cardiac patients can't name anything that they do

to relax and unwind," Dr. Wielgosz says. "They don't have a hobby or other activity that's unrelated to the demands of their daily life. Think about what you might get pleasure and satisfaction from." A hobby can refresh you and help clear out stress. He suggests that you write down a list of things that you enjoy. Knitting? Reading? Card games? Volleyball? Dancing lessons? Pottery? Continuing education courses? Find a way to make these activities a regular part of your life.

■ **Enjoy the moment.** Practice getting enjoyment out of routine activities, such as preparing a meal. "It's easy to see everything you do as one more thing to be checked off on the agenda," says Dr. Wielgosz. "But you end up not enjoying anything, whether it's watching your grandchild in a school recital or eating dinner."

Get Moving

You'll need a two-part program that combines strength training and aerobic exercise to help optimize your recovery from a heart attack, says Dr. LaFontaine. Strength training builds a larger musculature, which burns more calories and helps to keep weight down—important for lowering risk. Aerobic exercise builds up your cardiovascular system and reduces the levels of atherosclerosis that contributed to your first attack.

"If you've had a heart attack or have coronary artery disease, you have to do more exercise, not

Symptoms May Be Different the Second Time

When you are over age 60, the symptoms of a heart attack are often different than they are in younger people. Instead of the classic crushing, heavy feeling in the middle of the chest, you may get a cluster of subtle symptoms. They might not seem serious individually, but you should call your doctor if you experience several of these minor symptoms together.

Equally important, "Don't put off making the call," says Andreas T. J. Wielgosz, M.D., Ph.D., head of the Division of Cardiology at Ottawa General Hospital in Canada. If you experience a second heart attack or stroke, you need to get treatment as quickly as possible to minimize the impact. Every second counts. The longer your heart or brain goes without oxygen, the more tissue is damaged.

Watch for these symptoms as they occur together or separately:

- A heavy fullness or pressure in the center of your chest that radiates to your left arm or shoulder
- Weakness or lethargy
- Nausea
- Clammy perspiration
- Shortness of breath
- Pain traveling down the left or right arm
- Back pain or deep aching in the left or right biceps or forearm
- A feeling of doom, as though something awful is about to happen
- Angina that continues for more than 15 to 20 minutes
- Dizziness
- Confusion
- Pain in the neck, jaw, or shoulder
- Indigestion
- Difficulty breathing

less," says Dr. LaFontaine. "Of course, you have to work up to it gradually."

"If your cardiologist didn't automatically refer you to a cardiac rehabilitation exercise program after you left the hospital and didn't recommend exercise, call him or her for a referral," adds Dr. Pashkow. "Even if your heart is severely damaged and you don't think that you can tolerate exercise, you should get into a program."

Cardiologists sometimes assume that older patients may be too physically frail or won't par-

ticipate in an exercise program. But it can mean the difference between life and death for you. "Researchers in Finland did a 15-year follow-up study and found that people who participated in a cardiac rehabilitation exercise program and risk factor-reduction program had a significantly lower risk of death," says Dr. LaFontaine.

Here's how exercise can help you:

■ **Exercise burns away plaque.** As you burn off calories, levels of beneficial HDL

273

What About Sex?

Six weeks after a heart attack, you have probably regained most of your strength. But how to judge if you are ready for sex? "If you can climb three or four flights of stairs without panting and puffing, you can have normal sex," says Tom LaFontaine, Ph.D., manager of disease prevention and community wellness at Boone Hospital Center in Columbia, Missouri.

If your heart attack resulted in severe damage to your heart, and your exercise tolerance is quite low, you may need to adjust your sexual activities, perhaps playing a more passive role or taking medication before you have sex. Your heart rate and blood pressure do go up during sex, but this generally happens only for about 30 seconds during orgasm.

There is an important caveat, and a great reason (if you need one) for staying with one partner: Researchers found that heart rate escalates far more with new partners or extramarital encounters. "Those levels could, theoretically, be dangerous," says Dr. LaFontaine.

cholesterol go up. That's the stuff that helps keep your arteries clean and helps stop plaque from building up. The effort that you expend through exercise also helps lower triglycerides, the harmful fats in the blood.

■ **Exercise improves your metabolism.** Dr. Pashkow says that, as you get older, your metabolism shifts into lower gear. "That seems to accompany a drop in the beneficial HDL cholesterol," he says. Higher metabolic rates are tied to higher levels of protective HDL cholesterol.

Improving your metabolism also helps fight off diabetes. As you age, some of your systems may not work as well as they used to. You don't metabolize carbohydrates as efficiently, which can lead to insulin insufficiencies and diabetes, a major risk factor for heart problems, says Dr. Pashkow. "When you change your metabolism, you also make it easier for your body to use carbohydrates over the next 24 hours," he says.

The Catch: How Much Exercise?

Yes, exercise will help your heart get healthy. But to get the job done, you'll have to put the pump to work for two to five hours a week. "Studies show that people with coronary artery disease

show the most benefit from this amount of exercise," says Dr. LaFontaine. "That's the threshold at which their atherosclerosis stabilizes or even regresses. If you do less exercise, the atherosclerosis continues and more plaque builds up in the arteries." Several short daily bursts of activity (10 to 15 minutes in length) seem to help prevent cardiac problems in the first place, but Dr. LaFontaine believes this isn't enough to reverse risk if you've already had a heart attack.

And what if you have been inactive for a long period of time? You won't have the capacity to exercise as strenuously as you need to. You won't burn calories at as high a rate as someone with more exercise tolerance. This means that you will have to exercise for even longer periods, although at a more moderate level, to get similar results. Dr. LaFontaine recommends that you talk with your doctor about the exercise level that is appropriate for you. It's important to make sure that you are not overdoing it.

Once you have determined the level of exercise you can handle, here's how to get the most out of your workout:

■ **Get attention.** When you start an exercise program, you may be going against a lifetime of habits. You'll have the most success in sticking with your efforts if your cardiologist provides extensive follow-up and support. If this kind of follow-up isn't a routine part of your cardiologist's program, ask for it.

"We get patients in four times a year just to monitor their progress because it helps them stay on track," says Dr. LaFontaine. "We ask them about their exercise and diets, check their symptoms, and look for improvement." This follow-up procedure is particularly important once you recover from the heart attack and start to feel fine. It will be tempting to go back to your old habits. "In the early months, people have a lot of incentive to stay with the program. They see the heart attack as a wake-up call to make lifestyle changes. But it is easy to revert to former habits when everything seems back to normal," he says.

■ **Get rhythm.** You can get your aerobic workout through walking, bicycling, working out on ski machines, or using other exercise equipment. "What makes exercise aerobic is that it's rhythmical, can be sustained for 30 minutes, and burns about 300 calories in a session," says Dr. LaFontaine.

■ **Build slowly.** "At first, do what you can handle," says Dr. Pashkow. "You may not be able to work up to 45 minutes of aerobic activity five times a week—what I recommend for people who have had a heart attack. If you can just do 10 minutes, start there."

Regardless of how long you exercise, make it fairly intense, says Dr. Pashkow. "The exercise stress test that you had in the hospital and in follow-up visits will let you know what you can safely handle. The kind of exercise that helps prevent another heart attack is different from just strolling in the mall and window shopping."

■ **Choose your rehab center with care.** Sticking with an exercise routine will be a lot easier if you get support from your rehabilitation group or exercise program as well as friends and family. "It's probably as hard to stay with exercise as it is to stop smoking," says Dr. Pashkow. After a year, you have a one-in-three chance of returning to inactivity. After four years of regular exercise, your chances of becoming sedentary are about one in 13.

So if you have a choice of rehabilitation centers, pick one that will help you stay with the program. "We know that can make a big difference. We put a lot of effort into getting to know the patients, having special events and dinners with them, and recognizing their birthdays," says Dr. LaFontaine.

■ **Extend your exercise after rehab.** Your in-hospital program is classified as a Phase 1 program, and the 8- to 12-week program conducted at the hospital or in another institution is the Phase 2 program. The ideal program goes to a Phase 3, and even a Phase 4 cardiac rehabilitation program, also called a maintenance program. If your local hospitals don't offer a rehabilitation exercise program beyond the standard 8- to 12-week Phase 2 regimen, discuss other programs with your doctor.

Phase 3 programs are usually supervised and may be geared for people who have had heart attacks or coronary procedures. They may be offered through a community center. They aren't generally covered by insurance, but the costs tend to be very low, says Dr. Pashkow.

In a Phase 4 program, you can exercise on your own, perhaps at home, or better yet, in an unsupervised group. Your options for finding a Phase 4 program may be the local YMCA or a community center program designed for the general public rather than cardiac patients. But you can ask your cardiologist to discuss your

Always Be Prepared for Another Attack

You're doing all you can to prevent another heart attack. But just in case it does happen, prepare your own plan of attack to minimize the damage and risk, advise many medical experts. Here is how to do it:

1. Choose a hospital. Look for a hospital with a strong cardiology department in case of future heart problems or an emergency, says Fredric J. Pashkow, M.D., medical director of the Cardiac Health Improvement and Rehabilitation Program at the Cleveland Clinic Foundation. Find out whether the physicians in the cardiology department are board certified, an indication that the doctor has completed a specified course of training in this field.

2. Compile the data. Prepare a list of instructions for the hospital staff and include the following information, advises Dr. Pashkow:

- Information about any clot busters administered to you during your first heart attack. (If you received streptokinase, administering it again may produce an allergic reaction.)
- Your doctor's telephone number and those of close friends and relatives. (Ask hospital personnel to call them as soon as you're admitted.)
- Any history of bleeding.
- Name of a cardiac surgeon recommended by your doctor.
- A copy of your current electrocardiogram (EKG), the readout of your heartbeat. (If you've had one heart attack, your current EKG may look abnormal. A copy of it will help the hospital staff determine if you've had another attack.)

3. Get an assistant. Have your spouse, family member, or close friend learn cardiopulmonary resuscitation (CPR), suggests Daniel Levy, M.D., director of the Framingham Heart Study in Massachusetts. "Many people who have a heart attack live in enormous fear that they'll have a recurrence, and so do their spouses," he says. Having friends or family members who know how to administer CPR provides reassurance. CPR should be administered if someone is not breathing and has no heartbeat.

Contact your local office of the American Heart Association to find out how to get CPR training. You might also want to become certified in Basic Life Support, available through local community centers or adult education programs, adds Dr. Pashkow.

exercise treatment with the class leaders. They can work together to set up target goals and monitor your progress through periodic telephone calls, says Dr. Pashkow. That way, it can become a low-cost program tailored just for you. The follow-up involvement from your cardiologist and class leader will also provide an important psychological incentive for you to keep at it.

■ **Find safety in numbers.** Regardless of where you are in the recovery process, you're better off exercising with a group. "Group exercise sessions give you social interaction—as important for recovery from a heart attack as the exercise itself," says Dr. Pashkow. This can help you ward off the feelings of social isolation and depression that often come after a heart attack. Those feelings dramatically increase your risk of another attack, he says.

■ **Go high-tech.** If you live in a rural area or if it is hard for you to get to group exercise sessions, look for a cardiac center that has developed "transtelephonic" programs. In these programs,

Be Prepared for Another Attack...continued

4. Check the exterior of your house. Now, before you have a second heart attack, says Dr. Pashkow, make sure that your house number is clearly visible and that your exterior lights work. If you have an episode at night, turn on the outside lights to help the ambulance driver locate the right house.

5. Plan how to work fast. The time between the attack and your arrival at the hospital determines the amount of damage to your heart. That's because the longer your heart goes without oxygen, the more cells die, explains Dr. Pashkow. Some medications that actually stop a heart attack, such as clot busters, are best given within a few hours of the attack. Ask your doctor for a prescription, and keep it readily available.

    If you suspect a heart attack is occurring: Call 911 immediately. Tell the dispatcher you may be having a heart attack. Many communities have ambulances that carry advanced cardiac life support technicians and equipment.

    Never try to drive yourself to the hospital, advises Andreas T. J. Wielgosz, M.D., Ph.D., head of the Division of Cardiology at Ottawa General Hospital in Canada. If it is a heart attack, your heart could develop an irregular rhythm and you could pass out behind the wheel—even if you're only experiencing a cluster of subtle symptoms, such as clammy perspiration and shortness of breath.

6. At the hospital, go to the front of the line. Explain that you may be having a heart attack. Remember, it is important for you to get treatment as quickly as possible. Prompt attention and medications can actually stop a heart attack and allow the blood to get to your heart. If you're asked to wait, be assertive and make sure that everyone understands that you need immediate treatment, says Dr. Pashkow. Ask to see a triage nurse, the person who decides the order of patients to be treated.

several patients exercise at home, in their physician's office, or in a medical clinic. Regardless of where they are, a telephone link allows their cardiologist to monitor their activities with an electrocardiogram readout. Four to six people can exercise together, even though they are in different settings. Participants can also communicate with each other during exercise. Such communication is important to provide the social support that helps them stay with the exercise program and keeps them healthier in general, says Dr. LaFontaine.

    ■ **Spread the word.** Tell your loved ones and friends that you are starting an exercise program to help your heart. Ask them to remind you to exercise if you lapse, says Dr. LaFontaine. Ask them to ask you about your progress. Let them know that their support is important to your success. Not only will their support help you stay with your exercise regimen, it will also reinforce your sense of being related to friends and family, which will help you fight off the depression that often follows a heart attack.

Tell Tobacco Good-Bye

If you smoke, this habit played a big part in your first heart attack. If you have continued to smoke, you will just have to snuff out the habit. "Studies show that even in people age 75 and over, quitting smoking reduces the chance of recurrent cardiac problems," explains Dr. LaFontaine. "That's the most important thing that you can do to prevent future attacks."

Dr. Wielgosz says, "If you continue to smoke, you will have a sevenfold increase in risk for a second heart attack and a threefold increase in the risk of dying within the first year after the attack."

Here are some suggestions for getting over the habit:

■ **Keep trying.** "We know that smokers go through phases to quit. And often it takes many attempts. So, if you have tried and tried but haven't been able to quit, don't be discouraged—it's part of the normal process," says Dr. Wielgosz.

■ **Take the three-pronged attack.** You are most likely to stop smoking if you take the three-pronged approach, consisting of:

1. *Counseling*

2. *Group therapy*

3. *Wearing the nicotine patch*

Dr. Wielgosz recommends looking for a cardiac rehabilitation program that puts all these pieces in place to help you quit. Your health insurance may cover the costs.

■ **Think long-term.** Cardiologists agree that you can claim to have kicked the habit only if it has been a year or more since your last puff. Even then, there is a 50-50 chance that you will fall back into your old ways. Minimize the risk by joining a heart attack survivors' discussion group, says Dr. Wielgosz. You'll get important psychological support from other heart attack survivors.

■ **If you start smoking again or feel the urge:** Call your cardiologist immediately. Ask for a referral to a smoking-cessation group for support (possibly covered by insurance) and jump-start the quitting process without delay.

Evaluate Your State of Mind

Researchers believe that your mental outlook can make a big difference in whether you experience a second heart attack. "Depression and social isolation put you at greater risk for a second heart attack than even smoking," says Dr. Wielgosz. "If you fall into that category, you have the highest mortality rate after a heart attack."

In fact, people with heart disease who become depressed are four to six times more likely to die than those who don't, regardless of other risk factors, says Robert Carney, Ph.D., professor of medical psychology at Washington University School of Medicine in St. Louis. He says that if you are depressed, you'll have a more difficult time following your doctor's instructions and staying on medication that you need. And you'll be more likely to smoke. Most important, researchers believe that depression affects your autonomic nervous system, which regulates heartbeat and heart rhythm.

People who have had a heart attack tend to go through bouts of depression. But if your depression lasts longer than a week, contact your cardiologist—you may need help to break free, says Dr. Carney. Let your cardiologist know if you experience some of these symptoms:

Depressed mood

Loss of interest in things that you normally enjoy

Problems concentrating

Feelings of hopelessness or helplessness

Appetite and weight loss

Sleep problems

Crying for no apparent reason

The good news is that, by working with your doctor, there is a lot you can do to end the isolation and depression you are feeling.

Get Connected

A lot of people are more isolated than they realize. Ask yourself: If your car was broken down, would someone drive you to the doctor? If the answer is "no," you need to work on making friends. And that takes practice. "Studies show that people who belong to groups and have social interaction are less likely to have a second heart attack," says Dr. Pashkow.

Here are some ways to make friends and stay connected:

■ **Find a confidante.** Having one close friend makes a difference. You need someone with whom you feel comfortable sharing your worries and feelings. "Heart patients who have someone that they can confide in generally do better than those who don't," says Martin Sullivan, M.D., a cardiologist at the Duke University Center for Living in Durham, North Carolina. It could be your spouse. Or it may be someone else you can talk to. You may find people with whom you have something in common by following the rest of these suggestions.

■ **Get family support.** "People who are depressed feel isolated," says Dr. Carney. "They worry that they don't have anyone who cares for them. They often ask after a heart attack, 'Is there a future for me?'" Discuss your feelings with family members and friends. Their emotional support is critical. You will all benefit—you won't feel quite so isolated, and they will understand your needs better.

■ **Join something.** Start by getting out. Get involved in a religious group, a social/hobby club, or neighborhood activities.

■ **Give advice.** Be part of the community, helping others as you help yourself. Do volunteer work, perhaps as a senior business consultant or in a partner program in which you work with disadvantaged young people, such as Big Brothers and Big Sisters. You will benefit your community and lower your risk of another heart attack because you will feel part of a social network.

■ **Connect with survivors.** Join a focused support group for heart attack survivors. These groups often engage in community activities. They may do fund-raising for nonprofit heart associations. Groups often sponsor educational sessions, meet with nutritionists and exercise specialists, or just discuss their health problems with people who have had similar experiences, says Dr. Wielgosz.

Usually, group members talk about their heart attack experiences and their concerns for the future. Cardiac rehabilitation programs often include programs of this type.

"Group sessions are very important in our program," says Dr. LaFontaine. "After an attack, patients are scared, nervous, depressed, and anxious. It helps them to interact with other people, to know that other people have the same worries and concerns. Once they get better and find that they can exercise and carry on life normally, they can bring that information back to the support group to help other people who have recently had a heart attack. It benefits everyone." These groups also provide an important sense of community.

Seek Out Professional Help

Researchers at the University of Montreal in Canada found that people who have become depressed and/or angry following a heart attack are much more likely to die within one year than people who aren't. If you do become depressed despite your best efforts, getting some good counseling can ease your mood and literally save your life.

Here are some ways to find the help you need:

■ **Make an appointment.** Talk to a counselor, a social worker, or a religious advisor. Talk about your feelings and worries. Even if this activity seems foreign to you, remember that you are helping your heart by doing it.

■ **Get a follow-up.** Your cardiologist or cardiac rehabilitation program can help you combat depression, says Dr. Wielgosz. A Canadian study showed that even simple follow-ups make a significant difference. For instance, patients showed more improvement if a nurse made a follow-up call to check on their progress and, if necessary, referred them to a doctor. If your program or doctor doesn't do such follow-ups, ask for it, or look for an alternative program, suggests Dr. Pashkow.

■ **List your medical questions.** Next time you visit your doctor, ask questions. You will feel more in control of your fate, which helps reduce depression and isolation. You will also get used to interacting with people who you don't know very well. "Many elderly patients, especially women, don't ask questions," says Dr. Wielgosz. The more you ask, the easier it will be to talk in other settings and become involved.

Dr. Pashkow suggests that, before your next appointment, you should write down the questions that you want to discuss with your doctor. Ask a spouse or other family member to go over them with you to help clarify the issues that are important to you. Take the list to your appointment—and go over each point with your doctor.

■ **Stay informed.** Subscribe to one of the quality newsletters, such as the *Harvard Heart Letter*, that keeps heart patients up to date on research and relevant issues, says Dr. Pashkow. Learning this kind of information will also help you feel in control.

Change Your Outlook

Expect that you will have to behave differently from the way you have always behaved if you are to strengthen your defenses against a killer depression.

Consider the following methods that may help you to overcome a tendency toward depression:

■ **Put things in perspective.** Emotions play an important role in heart attack risk. Teach yourself to spot and defuse anger and hostility, emotions that could pave the way for a second heart attack. When you are feeling upset or worried, just stop, step back, and try to analyze the emotion. Ask yourself if what is bothering you is really important, says Dr. Sullivan.

If, for instance, you get cut off in traffic, is it worth getting angry? Did the incident really slow you down? Is your anger at another driver worth an increased risk of a heart attack? With time, putting your emotions into perspective will become second nature, and you will learn to control heart-threatening feelings.

■ **Redefine yourself.** A lot of people define themselves by what they can do: their jobs, their physical activity, or their health. A heart attack can lower your self-esteem, says Dr. Sullivan. "It can take away a layer of who you are, especially if you define yourself by the things you can't do right after a heart attack." Determine other ways of defining yourself. For example, even though you've had a heart attack, you are still just as important to family and friends.

■ **Use existing resources.** If you're just recovering from a heart attack and have physical limitations, use the resources already in place in your community. Take advantage of programs that offer senior transportation or home delivery of meals—at least until you feel better.

A lot of cardiac patients don't like to feel dependent, but these organizations also help you feel like a part of the community, which speeds recovery and lowers your risk. Remember that the whole community benefits, because staying healthy is a lot less costly. "You're doing everyone a favor by taking advantage of resources and staying involved in the community," says Dr. Pashkow.

■ **Consider adopting a pet.** At Brooklyn College of the City University of New York, researchers found that cardiac patients who owned pets had better survival rates than those who didn't. Pet owners were less anxious, less depressed, and less angry. Dog owners fared the best in the study, but Dr. Pashkow notes that you should benefit from any pet to whom you are strongly attached. It will provide you with crucial support and interaction. "Pets depend on you, and that gives your life a purpose and gratification that can sustain you," says Dr. Wielgosz.

Prescription for Preventing Another Heart Attack

Get back on track for a healthy, active life by making the lifestyle changes that both help your heart recover and protect it from another attack. If you don't, your risk of another attack soars.

DO:

▶ **Become a label reader in the grocery store.** Choose low-fat, low-cholesterol, and low-calorie products.

▶ **Increase your consumption of breads, cereals, pasta, grains, fruits, and vegetables.**

▶ **Choose a doctor and a cardiac rehabilitation program** that provide you with encouragement and follow-up.

▶ **Reduce stress.** Make time every day for quiet reflection, contemplation, and hobbies.

▶ **Get two to five hours of aerobic exercise a week.**

DON'T:

▶ **Smoke.**

▶ **Let small things stress you out.**

▶ **Live in isolation.** Get involved in a religious group, social/hobby club, or neighborhood activities. Help others by doing volunteer work. Join a focused support group for heart attack survivors.

21

Healthy Living After Cancer

The fear that cancer will return dances a ceaseless jig in your mind. Sure, you're scared. Yes, you're nervous. But never forget that you are in remission.

"Every time you go to bed think, 'I'm in remission.' Every morning when you wake up think, 'I'm in remission.' Always, always think about remission instead of recurrence. Thank God every day that you are in remission. Embrace that feeling and hang on to it as tightly as you can," said one breast cancer survivor in her seventies—who had been in remission for more than 25 years.

Increase the Odds You'll Stay in Remission

People shouldn't just sit around waiting to die. Sure, you have a chance of recurrence. But assuming you didn't come in with a cancer that was in an advanced stage to begin with, then chances are you're going to be cured or survive for many years," says Hugh Shingleton, M.D., the American Cancer Society's national vice president for cancer detection and treatment. "So you should keep on practicing good health habits."

Although no direct evidence exists that lifestyle changes can reduce the risk of recurrence, some doctors suspect that the same measures recommended for preventing an initial cancer—a low-fat and high-fiber diet, regular exercise, weight control, optimism, spirituality, not smoking, and avoiding nitrites and excessive alcohol consumption—can help fend off a return of the disease.

"These preventive steps, which are beneficial to the general public, may be of heightened importance for someone who has already had a cancer," says Wendy Schlessel Harpham, M.D., attending physician at Presbyterian Hospital of Dallas, herself a cancer survivor, and author of *After Cancer: A Guide to Your New Life.* "All people are at risk for developing the same cancer again. Many survivors are at an increased risk for developing another type of cancer just because of the original type of cancer they had. Some treatments themselves increase the risk of developing cancer. Taking these preventive steps can reduce survivors' overall risk of future cancers."

Another Reason to Quit Smoking

Patients who are cured of lung cancer are more prone to develop new cancers of the lung, throat, or mouth. That's because lung cancer is difficult to detect early and cure. And smoking—the number-one cause of lung cancer—damages numerous cells in the respiratory tract and makes them more susceptible to cancer, according to Dr. Engstrom. Five years after recovering from lung cancer, the risk of recurrence is about 15 percent and doubles to 30 percent within a decade.

Often the Odds Are with You

For certain cancers that are detected and treated early, a cure is likely, and the odds of a recurrence are small, Dr. Shingleton says.

Take breast, colon, and prostate cancer, for instance. These three cancers are among the most common in men and women over age 60 and account for about 44 percent of all cancers. For women, the risk of renewed breast cancer rises by about 1 percent each year after treatment. So after 10 years, there is about a 10 percent chance of cancer developing in the other breast, says Charles Taylor, M.D., director of medical oncology at the Arizona Cancer Center in Tucson. In the colon, there is a 10 to 15 percent risk of a second new cancer occurring in the remaining bowel.

Prostate cancer seldom recurs if the tumor is confined to the prostate and the organ can be surgically removed, says Paul Engstrom, M.D., a medical oncologist and senior vice president of population science at Fox Chase Cancer Center in Philadelphia. As with all cancers, there is a small chance that some prostate cancer cells will elude detection and spread to other organs even after the prostate has been removed. But if caught early, there is less than a one-in-10 chance that prostate cancer will revive in some other part of the body in the next five years.

Living with Uncertainty

Yet, even with these favorable statistics, doctors can't guarantee that your cancer will never recur. Why? Sometimes, radiation or chemotherapy doesn't destroy all the cancer cells in a person's body. These microscopic cells, which often are undetectable, begin to grow, and eventually a tumor takes hold in another spot, says Peter Greenwald, M.D., head of cancer prevention and control at the National Cancer Institute in Bethesda, Maryland.

In other cases, it is possible for cells at several sites in the same organ to be damaged by carcinogens like cigarette smoke. These damaged cells can develop into cancer at different rates. So even while you're being treated for one tumor, it is possible that a second or even third cancer may be slowly developing within the same organ, says Dr. Greenwald.

If a cancer does recur, it is usually more difficult to fight than the initial cancer, according to Dr. Engstrom. That's because the remaining cancer cells often are more resistant to treatment than those destroyed the first time around. "Unless all of the factors, such as smoking, that may have contributed to that cancer developing in first place are reversed, the risk of it happening again is still high," Dr. Harpham says.

That is why lifestyle changes—such as improving your diet and getting regular exercise like walking 30 minutes a day, three to five times a week—are so important after cancer. These and other preventive steps bolster the immune system and increase its ability to seek out and destroy any stray cancer cells, according to Dr.

How I Did It: A Super Bowl Coach Wins the Big One

There is only one recurrence that Marv Levy would welcome in his life.

"A chance to go back to the Super Bowl and win," says Levy, who retired as the winningest coach of the National Football League's Buffalo Bills and now is a member of the Pro Football Hall of Fame. But even though he might never get that opportunity, Levy has already won the biggest challenge of his life. In 1995, he survived prostate cancer.

"I think I was doing all the right things before I got prostate cancer. I was exercising. I was eating a very low-fat, high-fiber diet. So I don't know what else I could have done to prevent it. I was just fortunate that it was detected early during an annual physical," Levy says.

He opted for surgical removal of the prostate. Like many other men, Levy feared impotence and incontinence, but neither of these two possible side effects of the surgery affected him. After surgery, his faith in his lifestyle has remained strong.

"I got back into living a healthy life very quickly after my surgery," Levy says. "I work out, I run, I lift weights at least twice a week, I eat correctly, and I make sure that I get the proper amount of rest. I think all of that helped me come back very quickly." He also went back to coaching for two more years before beginning a career as a sports columnist and TV analyst.

Still, anxiety about a recurrence does rumble through Levy's mind every once in awhile like a blitzing linebacker. "Those concerns exist, but I can't live in fear," he says. "One thing that helped was that I did quite a bit of studying about prostate cancer once I discovered that I had it. That was very reassuring to me because I found out about treatments and ways to live with it even if it does spread. So education always helps.

"I also talked with a lot of people who have been through similar experiences. And I found that to be very helpful."

He also advises diving back into your regular routine.

"As quickly as possible, I'd say return to as vigorous a life as you can," Levy says. "You don't have to become a workout nut. But don't make yourself an invalid mentally just because you've had cancer. Don't ever let this disease make you feel old."

Harpham. "If your immune system is in good shape and you are well nourished, I do think that helps the body keep a cancer in check," he says.

Making Your Remission Last

Your battle against recurrence begins in the doctor's office, since early detection is your first line of defense. Your doctor will determine the best follow-up plan for you. "In a sense, follow-up is further assurance for both you and your doctor that everything is okay," Dr. Shingleton says.

In general, most oncologists like to see patients every three months during the first year of remission, every four months in the second year, and then every six months until year five. After that, your doctor will probably want to examine you annually, says David Bouda, M.D., assistant professor of oncology at the University of Nebraska College of Medicine in Omaha.

Here are a few tips to make your follow-up sessions more fruitful:

■ **Chart your progress.** Keep a record of your medications, side effects, and symptoms, Dr. Shingleton advises. Take it with you every time you see your oncologist. It will help you plan the next step in your recovery.

Supplement Wisely to Prevent Recurrence

After cancer diagnosis and treatment, the use of vitamin supplements, along with diet modifications and lifestyle changes, can reinforce your body's natural defenses and help prevent a recurrence, says Kedar N. Prasad, Ph.D., director of the Center for Vitamins and Cancer Research at the University of Colorado Health Sciences Center in Denver, and author of *Vitamins in Cancer Prevention and Treatment*. "Taking these supplements may boost your immune system so it can seek out and destroy any undetected cancer cells that remain in your body." Here is the combination of oral supplements he recommends:

Beta-carotene: 15 milligrams (mg.) a day.

Vitamin A: 5,000 international units (IU) a day, divided into two doses, taken once in the morning and once in the evening. Most vitamin A supplements come in a 10,000 IU dose, so quarter the tablet (equivalent to 2,500 IU) to get your 5,000 IU a day.

Vitamin C: Up to 2,000 mg. a day, divided into at least two doses, in the form of calcium ascorbate. *Note:* Amounts of vitamin C over 1,200 mg. a day may cause diarrhea in some people.

Vitamin E: 400 IU per day, divided into two doses, taken in the morning and evening. Each dose should contain 100 IU of alpha-tocopheryl-succinate and 100 IU of alpha-tocopherol.

B vitamins: Take a multiple vitamin that contains two to five times the Daily Value for thiamin, riboflavin, and vitamins B_6 and B_{12}.

Selenium: 100 micrograms (mcg.) a day, divided into two doses, once in the morning and once in the evening. Levels above this should only be taken under medical supervision. Selenium must be taken in the form of organic selenium. Inorganic selenium, such as sodium selenite, is poorly absorbed by the small intestine.

■ **Express yourself.** Before each appointment, make a list of questions that you may have about your follow-up treatment. Then discuss these concerns with your oncologist, says Dr. Bouda.

"You need to be open about your feelings. Some people never discuss anything with their doctors, so the doctors don't have a clue that there are any concerns," Dr. Bouda says. "Your doctor isn't a mind reader. You need to talk with your physician regularly and give him a fair chance to address your concerns."

If the doctor doesn't seem interested in your problems, find another oncologist. "The doctor–patient relationship is a partnership. If your doctor isn't your partner, fire him," says Dr. Bouda.

■ **Don't panic over tests.** Blood tests such as prostate-specific antigen (PSA), which measures cancer activity in the prostate, can provide doctors with valuable clues about the status of your remission. But don't panic if a single test is elevated. Some tests have a wide range of normal readings, while others may be prone to imprecise results, Dr. Bouda explains.

"People who focus on the outcome of every test tend to be fixated on recurrence," says Dr. Bouda. "They're often paralyzed to the point that they can't enjoy life." If you're like that, you may be better off not getting tested, because any fluctuation is going to drive you nuts, he adds.

In fact, doctors may be able to detect some forms of recurrent cancer just as well without complex tests. Researchers, for instance, have found that doctors who used sophisticated medical testing detected breast cancer recurrence only four weeks earlier than doctors who relied solely on physical exams, Dr. Bouda says. The earlier detection by testing made no difference in overall survival rates.

Dr. Bouda suggests that you ask your doctor what a test really means. How reliable is it? What does it actually measure? How concerned should you be if it isn't normal? Is it really necessary?

"If it's a simple, specific test, it should be done. But ordering too many tests just causes unnecessary anxiety," Dr. Bouda says.

■ **Suspend alternative treatments.** Or at least let your doctor know if you are using any alternative treatments like homeopathy, ayurveda, or vitamin and mineral therapy, Dr. Bouda says. And be sure to discontinue them before your appointments. These treatments may interfere with traditional medication and testing.

Saw palmetto, for instance, an herbal treatment used by some men to prevent swelling of the prostate, may decrease PSA test readings. That can mislead you and your doctor into thinking that your prostate cancer is under control, says E. David Crawford, M.D., chairman of the Division of Urology at the University of Colorado Health Sciences Center in Denver.

"If you're doing something that is off the mainstream, you probably shouldn't take any alternative therapy for at least 24 hours before or after your conventional treatment," Dr. Bouda recommends.

■ **Know the warning signs.** Ask your doctor to explain the most important signs and symptoms of a possible recurrence, Dr. Harpham says. If you have any concerns about a symptom, don't hesitate to contact your doctor and make an appointment.

"After surviving cancer, particularly soon afterward, it is very normal to be a bit alarmist about changes or symptoms," says Dr. Harpham.

"But you owe it to yourself and your doctor to go in with your concern and get it checked out. If it turns out to be nothing, what have you lost? But if it does turn out to be something, you have maximized your health."

Diet: Get Back to the Pyramid

No particular diet or foods have been proven to suppress the recurrence of cancer, says Carolyn Clifford, Ph.D., chief of the diet and cancer branch at the National Cancer Institute in Bethesda, Maryland. But several ongoing studies sponsored by the Institute are attempting to determine if eating a low-fat, high-fiber diet will help to lower recurrence rates of breast, lung, and neck cancer.

Although the results of these long-term studies are several years away, following the U.S. Department of Agriculture's food pyramid recommendations after you have dealt with cancer is probably prudent.

"The feeling is, it is best to follow these guidelines to reduce the risk of recurrence as much as possible," says Christine Polisena, R.D., an oncology dietitian at the Cleveland Clinic Foundation. "For someone who has successfully gotten through cancer treatment, the recommendations I would give are to maintain your desirable body weight, watch your fat consumption, increase your fiber intake, try to eat more fruits and vegetables, and limit nitrate-cured foods and alcohol consumption."

Here are a few specific tips regarding diet that are especially important after recovering from cancer:

■ **Eat more lean meat.** "When some people are recovering from cancer, they'll think now is the time to become a vegetarian. But that's not necessarily true," says Cheryl Ritenbaugh, Ph.D., head of nutrition research at the Arizona Cancer Center in Tucson. "Many people lose muscle

How I Did It: A Survivor Helps Others

Terri S. still cries a lot.

"Crying is a blessing," she says. "If I couldn't cry, I couldn't have gotten through all of this."

"All of this" began when she was diagnosed with breast cancer and underwent a radical mastectomy and radiation treatment. More than a quarter-century later, she's still in remission.

"The prognosis was really grim. But from the beginning I told myself, 'You're not going to think about dying,' " she says. "I've known so many people who from the minute they knew they had cancer told themselves that they were going to die. And many did. I simply didn't want to think like that. I focused on living."

Once she recovered, she became a volunteer at the cancer center, visiting new patients and running errands for families. "Volunteering is healing. If you can help patients get through their trauma and their anger, that certainly helps you, too," Terri says. "The possibility of recurrence does pop into the back of my mind every once in awhile, particularly when someone comes in with a recurrence after 20 years. But I just focus on helping others, and any fear or anxiety that I may have about my cancer coming back just fades away."

Instead, she reserves her tears for others. "I hurt when someone doesn't make it. And I cry whenever I hurt. That's when I feel angry about cancer," she says.

"But I'm happy because I've had 25 years that I wouldn't have had," Terri says. "I thank God for every day that I've had. I love every day that I'm alive, whether it's good, bad, or indifferent."

mass rapidly while fighting the disease, so getting enough lean meat and other forms of protein onto your plate is important at that point."

To help your body rebuild muscle, eat three servings—a total of 5 to 7 ounces a day—of fish, poultry, and lean meat for at least four months after your treatment ends, Dr. Ritenbaugh suggests. "You don't need to go overboard on meat. You don't need to eat a 16-ounce steak," she says.

■ **Hold down the fat.** In laboratory experiments, excessive amounts of dietary fat fueled the growth of certain types of tumors like prostate cancer, says William R. Fair, M.D., chief of urologic surgery and chairman of urologic oncology at Memorial Sloan-Kettering Cancer Center in New York City. Reducing dietary fat also may slow recurrence.

Try to limit yourself to 20 percent of calories from fat daily, Dr. Fair recommends. If you eat 2,000 calories a day, for instance, that means you can consume about 400 calories—44 grams—from fat. Look for total fat grams on food labels.

■ **Stoke up on fruits and vegetables.** Try eating at least five servings each day of fruits and vegetables like apples, oranges, carrots, and broccoli. Not only are these foods an excellent source of fiber, they contain important antioxidants and cancer-preventing nutrients, according to Polisena.

Fruits and vegetables are good sources of fiber, which speeds food through your body so that fewer carcinogens can be absorbed by your digestive tract, Dr. Bouda explains.

■ **Cut out nitrites.** Limit or avoid nitrate-cured, salt-cured, or smoke-cured foods like ham, sausage, or bacon, Polisena says. These foods have been linked to stomach cancer.

■ **Lighten up on liquor.** Alcohol may promote the recurrence of cancers of the neck, mouth, and esophagus. Limit your consumption each day to no more than one 12-ounce beer, one 4-ounce glass of wine, or one cocktail containing an ounce of liquor, Polisena recommends.

Look to the Future

When she was diagnosed with lymphoma in 1990, Dr. Harpham didn't know what to do about her magazine subscriptions.

"I always used to renew my magazines and medical journals for several years at a time," she says. "When I first got sick, I questioned whether it was worthwhile renewing any of them. Then when I felt a little more secure, I renewed them for a year. Now I renew them for three to five years at a time. Instead of making me feel vulnerable, these subscriptions empower me, because I plan on being here to use them."

The lesson? Hang on to hope and cling to the future as you move into remission, she says. Not only can that improve the quality of your life and lessen your fears of recurrence, it may actually boost your immune system's ability to wipe out any emerging cancers, Dr. Bouda says.

"Try to figure out some way to think positively every day, despite having had cancer," Dr. Bouda advises.

Here are some suggestions for retaining a positive frame of mind:

■ **Seek support.** Cancer support groups can breed optimism. You'll probably meet many long-term survivors who can inspire you and offer lots of empowering self-help tips. "A doctor may just tell you what the textbook says," Dr. Bouda says. "Someone at a support group meeting may tell you, 'Yeah, I tried what my doctor suggested, and it never worked. But I tried this instead, and I haven't had a problem since.'"

Most cancer treatment centers or hospitals can provide you with a list of support groups in your area.

■ **Look to your past.** You have lived for more than 60 years and probably have coped with many stressful and tragic situations before. Evaluate those experiences and try to identify what helped you survive those emotional upheavals, suggests Joan Hermann, director of social work services at Fox Chase Cancer Center in Philadelphia. Did it help to jot down your feelings? Talk to close friends? Pray? Whatever it was, it probably will help you deal with your fears and anxieties now.

"Older people often handle cancer and its aftermath better than younger men and women because of their wisdom and experience," Hermann says. "An older person tends to think, 'This is how I dealt with another tragedy in my life, and I can get through this situation in the same way.' A younger person simply doesn't have that experience to fall back on."

■ **Tame your wild imagination.** It's easy to imagine the worst. But if you learn to control your imagination, it can actually help calm your fears and strengthen your body's natural defenses, says Gloria Malone, Ph.D., a Phoenix psychologist who counsels many older people who have cancer. "It's like a remote control on your television. With a little practice, you can literally learn to turn off an unwanted thought," she says.

To do it, you might begin by imagining yourself in a very relaxed place in nature like a meadow filled with wildflowers or a lush tropical beach. See it, feel it, smell it, sense it. Practice that for a minute or two, 20 to 30 times a day, until visualizing your special place becomes almost automatic, Dr. Malone says. Then when fear or any other unwanted thought pops into your mind, imagine reaching for a remote control. Press the "on/off" button and—zap—turn off the unwanted thought or fear. Take a deep breath, then press the button again and visualize yourself calm and relaxed in your special place in nature.

■ **Treat yourself.** Plan to do something special for yourself each day. It doesn't have to be time-consuming or costly. List two dozen nurturing activities like watching a sunrise, playing with your grandchildren, or reading from an inspirational book. Then pick one activity each day and do it, advises Dr. Malone.

"Doing something to nurture yourself every day will help you feel less angry or deprived," Dr. Malone says. "It will help you focus on the positive aspects of your life instead of negative thoughts about recurrence."

■ **Find hope.** Look for touchstones and other special items that make you feel hopeful about the future. Souvenirs from a memorable vacation, inspirational posters, and meaningful pictures from your life can help. "I have a poster in my kitchen that reads, 'Keep on hoping, keep on wishing, keep on believing.' It would be easy to say that poster is childish and silly," Dr. Harpham says. "Well, you know what? This physician and mother derives benefit from looking at that poster. It is one more thing that helps me believe that I can get well again—and stay well."

Prescription for Preventing a Cancer Recurrence

Fear of a recurrence is a common emotion after surviving cancer. Although your doctors can't guarantee that you won't get cancer again, the odds of a complete cure for many forms of this disease are getting better every day, particularly if you adopt a healthy lifestyle.

DO:

▶ **Focus on remission rather than recurrence.** Rejoice every day that you are cancer-free.

▶ **Know the warning signs and symptoms of a recurrence.** Like your initial cancer, early treatment of a recurrence increases your chances of recovery.

▶ **Consume no more than 20 percent of daily calories from fat.** If you eat 2,000 calories a day, that means you can have about 44 grams of fat daily.

▶ **Eat plenty of fruits and vegetables** that are rich in antioxidants and other cancer-suppressing nutrients. Try to eat at least five servings of foods like oranges and broccoli daily.

DON'T:

▶ **Get hung up on test results.** Small fluctuations in a single test don't necessarily mean your cancer has returned.

▶ **Take alternative treatments within 24 hours** of a conventional cancer treatment or test. Some alternative medicines can interfere with more traditional treatments.

▶ **Overindulge.** Excessive alcohol consumption can promote head, neck, and other cancers. Limit yourself to one drink a day or less.

▶ **Eat bacon and other nitrate-laden foods.** Salt-cured, smoke-cured foods like ham or bacon might reignite cancer. If you can't completely give up these foods, limit your intake.

22

Healthy Living After a Stroke

A s he walks, his right foot slowly rises about two inches in the air before it mechanically plunges to the ground, as if it were attached to a puppeteer's string. Often, he still says "water" when he really means something else like "hand," "chair," or "tree." But John C. is happy. "I feel great. I'm not sick anymore," he says.

Indeed, John, who was nearly 60 when he had a massive stroke, came a long way in the first year after it happened. With the help of therapists, he regained the use of his paralyzed right arm and leg. His speech, which was once limited to "One, two, three, water," returned to complete, understandable sentences after months of rehabilitation. He recovered so well that he is now a volunteer—transporting patients in wheelchairs—at the center where he was treated.

But as healthy as he seems, John still is at high risk for another stroke. "He doesn't worry about it, but I do because I know the statistics," says John's wife, Mary. In fact, people over age 60 who have had a stroke are 10 times more likely to have another one. Up to one in three will have another stroke within five years of the first one.

But even if you've had a stroke, this doesn't have to be your fate. "Changing your lifestyle now can make a dramatic difference," says Lawrence M. Brass, M.D., professor of neurology and co-director of the Yale Cerebrovascular Center at Yale University School of Medicine. "In some cases, lowering blood pressure, quitting smoking, and making other lifestyle changes can reduce your risk of subsequent stroke by more than 50 percent."

Anatomy of a Stroke

W hen you were going through stroke rehabilitation, you probably noticed a lot of people your age working through similar problems. There are reasons for that.

Every minute, someone in the United States has a stroke. Of those, two of every three strokes—more than 350,000 a year—occur in people over age 65. And after age 55, the risk of stroke doubles with each passing decade you live.

Stroke becomes more common with age, in part, because it is provoked by many of the same habits—smoking, sedentary living, high-fat eating—that, when done over many years, tend to trigger heart attacks. In fact, most strokes are caused by the same mechanism that causes a heart attack, according to Arthur Ancowitz, M.D., author of *The Stroke Book* and founder of the Stroke Foundation in New York City.

These "brain attacks," or ischemic strokes, occur when a blood vessel gets blocked and blood flow to a part of the brain ceases, causing death of brain tissue. A less common type of stroke, called a hemorrhagic stroke, happens when a weakened blood vessel bursts and causes bleeding in the brain. This kind of stroke, which killed President Franklin Roosevelt, is often more debilitating than an ischemic stroke, says Michael Schneck, M.D., assistant professor of neurological sciences at Rush-Presbyterian-St. Luke's Medical Center in Chicago.

Aftermath of a Stroke

Even a small stroke, if it occurs in a vital part of the brain, can cause extensive damage that may rob you of speech, vision, or movement, Dr. Schneck says. But at least 1/3 of all strokes are mild, meaning the person may have little or no disability. Another 1/3 of stroke survivors are completely debilitated, requiring special care. The remaining 1/3 are somewhere in between— for example, they may have extreme weakness in one or more limbs. Those who have moderate effects are often functionally independent in their daily activities, although they may or may not be able to return to work.

But no matter how severe the initial damage, most stroke survivors do get better, says Richard C. Senelick, M.D., neurologist, medical director of HealthSouth Rehabilitation Institute of San Antonio, Texas, and co-author of *Living with Stroke*.

And regardless of type, "Most effects of stroke can improve with therapy," notes Dr. Schneck.

Some early improvement probably occurs as swelling surrounding the damaged area of the brain slowly diminishes in the first few weeks after the stroke, says Carlos Kase, M.D., professor of neurology at Boston University School of Medicine. It's also possible that in the months following the stroke, other parts of the brain compensate for some of the functions of the damaged area, he says.

Still, it may take up to a year before a survivor regains many of the capabilities that he had prior to the stroke, Dr. Schneck says. "The first six months of rehabilitation are the hardest. Don't let yourself give up."

Preventing Another One

Now that you feel better, you certainly don't want it to happen again. Depending on the type of stroke you had, your doctor may prescribe an anticoagulant drug like anisindione (Miradon) or antiplatelet drugs like ticlopidine (Ticlid) or aspirin.

Your doctor also might recommend surgery (carotid endarterectomy) to unclog your carotid arteries. In this procedure, a surgeon makes a 3-inch incision in your neck and cleans plaque from one or both of the carotids—two major arteries that supply blood to the brain.

Although surgery can't reverse the damage already done by stroke, says Dr. Ancowitz, this procedure can help prevent a recurrent or even an initial attack in those at high risk. Among people who have had a previous stroke, this surgery reduces the risk of recurrence in the following two years from 27 percent to 8 percent, according to Richard Libman, M.D., assistant professor of neurology at the Albert Einstein College of Medicine of Yeshiva University in New York City.

Take Stroke Signs Seriously

Strokes can fool you. The warning signs of a recurrent stroke, such as blurred vision, dizziness, and an unsteady gait, can be subtle, says Michael Schneck, M.D., assistant professor of neurological sciences at Rush-Presbyterian-St. Luke's Medical Center in Chicago.

A symptom like numbness in the hands will last only a few minutes, for instance, then suddenly disappear. But don't be deceived.

"If there is even the slightest chance that you're having symptoms of a stroke, don't wait to see your doctor. All that does is delay treatment. Go to a hospital emergency room immediately, then have someone notify your doctor of the situation," advises Richard Libman, M.D., assistant professor of neurology at Albert Einstein College of Medicine of Yeshiva University in New York City.

Since a stroke can impair your judgment and ability to communicate, it's important that people in your life be aware of a stroke's warning signs, says Harold P. Adams, Jr., M.D., director of the Division of Cerebrovascular Diseases at the University of Iowa in Iowa City. They can help you get immediate medical help if you become incapacitated.

It's also important to remember that a stroke can occur in any area of the brain, affecting different parts of the body. If you've already had a stroke, a subsequent stroke can have completely different warning signs than your first one.

Here are some of the key warning signs of any impending stroke:

- Sudden weakness or numbness of the face, arm, or leg
- Sudden dimness or loss of vision, particularly in one eye
- Double vision
- Any sudden unexplained drowsiness, nausea, or vomiting
- Sudden difficulty speaking, finding words, or understanding speech
- Sudden severe headache with no known cause
- Unexplained dizziness, unsteadiness, or sudden falls, especially with any of these other symptoms
- Difficulty swallowing
- Memory loss
- Loss of consciousness

But even if you take medication or have surgery, it is still important to take command of your own health after a stroke. Granted, some risk factors for stroke are out of your control. Among these are family history of stroke, age, gender (men are slightly more prone to strokes than women), and race (African-Americans are almost twice as likely to have a stroke than people of European heritage). But many other factors, such as high blood pressure, high cholesterol levels, diabetes, a smoking habit, being overweight, a sedentary lifestyle, and excessive alcohol consumption, can and should be tamed.

"If a person has a stroke and doesn't stop smoking or change his diet or get his blood pressure under control, then his chances of having a second stroke in the next year are overwhelming," Dr. Ancowitz says. "Without those changes, all

Make "I Can" Your Motto

If you've had a stroke, it's easy to give in. If you're a caregiver, it's easy to overprotect. Resist these temptations.

People who have had strokes often can do much more than many caregivers suspect, says Michael Schneck, M.D., assistant professor of neurological sciences at Rush-Presbyterian-St. Luke's Medical Center in Chicago.

"Whenever possible, I advise caregivers to err on the side of independence," Dr. Schneck says. "Let the person who has had the stroke do as much as they want to, and then some. Don't let the survivor be an invalid."

With adaptive equipment and techniques, many people who have had strokes can master skills like driving, gardening, woodworking, and other activities, says Caryn Abel, a recreation therapist at the Kessler Institute for Rehabilitation in West Orange, New Jersey. If you have a hobby or vocation that you would like to try, first clear it with your doctor, then ask your recreation therapist how you might do it, Abel suggests.

It is also important that the stroke survivor be allowed to reassume his/her role within the family, says Wayne Sotile, Ph.D., director of psychological services for the Wake Forest University Cardiac Rehabilitation Program in Winston-Salem, North Carolina, and author of *Heart Illness and Intimacy.*

"If the person with a stroke becomes a spectator instead of a participant in life, that can be devastating emotionally," Dr. Sotile says. "Allow the stroke survivor to be as much of a person as he can."

So if the stroke survivor loves to cook, for example, but no longer has full use of his arms, he can still be helpful in the kitchen by sharing his expertise with others, Dr. Sotile suggests. That will help to relieve depression and boost self-esteem.

---

the ingredients that caused stroke number one will still be there to provoke stroke number two."

Banish High Blood Pressure

Uncontrolled high blood pressure is a major cause of stroke. And treatment is crucial," says Sidney C. Smith, Jr., M.D., professor and chief of the Division of Cardiology at the University of North Carolina at Chapel Hill and past president of the American Heart Association.

In fact, after a four-year study of 662 men and women in their sixties and seventies who had strokes, researchers at Allegheny University in Philadelphia concluded that those people who didn't correct their high blood pressure were substantially more likely to have a recurrent stroke, says Milton Alter, M.D., Ph.D., clinical professor of neurology at Allegheny University Hospitals, a neuroepidemiologist, and co-author of the study.

That's because high blood pressure—which is a reading consistently higher than 140/90 millimeters of mercury (mmHg)—strains your arteries, especially in the brain. This makes them more susceptible to clotting or rupture, Dr. Ancowitz says.

There are many ways to combat high blood pressure. Here are some suggestions:

■ **Shed pounds.** If you lose excess weight, you'll be less likely to have high blood pressure, Dr. Ancowitz says.

Caregivers: You Deserve a Break Today

Caregiving is a grind that can wear down even the best of us. In fact, up to half of all long-term caregivers will seek help for a stress-related disorder. Often, the exhausting routine of this ceaseless job creates more stress for the caregiver than the illness itself does for the person who is ill, says Wayne Sotile, Ph.D., director of psychological services for the Wake Forest University Cardiac Rehabilitation Program in Winston-Salem, North Carolina, and author of *Heart Illness and Intimacy.*

"It's important for caregivers to realize that this isn't a sprint. It's a marathon, so you have to pace yourself," Dr. Sotile says. "The best gift you can give to people that you care for is taking time to care for yourself both mentally and physically."

Here are some ways to lessen the strain of caregiving:

Reach out for help. Don't be afraid to ask family members, friends, and neighbors to take some of the load off your shoulders, suggests Pam Erickson, R.N., private care manager for Eldercare Advisors in Denver. Make a list of people who are willing to care for your loved one when you need a break. Call upon those who have said, "If there's anything I can do, just ask." Even if the respite person will just cook a meal, do laundry, or do other chores for you once a week, accept it. It will ease your burden and allow you to have more quality time for yourself. If friends or family aren't available, consider home health care or nursing services listed in the Yellow Pages. Rates range from $10 to $18 an hour.

Get away from it all. Take 30 minutes daily to do something that you enjoy, like gardening or reading. At least once a week, get outside the home, advises Dr. Sotile. Go to a movie, walk around a park, or play bridge with friends for a couple of hours. Not only will these activities boost your morale but also, when you come home, you may have new experiences and stories to share with your less-mobile loved one.

■ **Curtail cocktails.** Limiting your daily consumption of alcohol to no more than two 12-ounce beers, two 4-ounce glasses of wine, or two cocktails containing 1 ounce of alcohol also can slash your chances of having a stroke, Dr. Ancowitz says. Women are advised to drink half these amounts (or less).

■ **Stay physically active.** "Exercise is extremely important after you've had a stroke for many reasons. Not only will it help lower blood pressure and protect against the development of cardiovascular disease, but it will help you maintain muscle tone that is so vital during rehabilitation," explains Dr. Ancowitz.

Regular exercise dilates blood vessels so that blood pressure falls and stays down when you're not exercising. Sweating also may coax sodium out of your bloodstream and help lower blood pressure, Dr. Ancowitz says. Plus, developing more muscle strength through exercise will make daily tasks that much easier to perform.

Ask your doctor or physical therapist about the types of exercise that are best for you. But in general, Dr. Ancowitz suggests that you try to get some type of moderately intense aerobic exercise for at least 30 minutes daily.

"If you can walk, do that. If you can't walk, then try upper-body exercises like swinging your arms over your head. Just do as much as you can," Dr. Ancowitz recommends.

■ **Stoke up on calcium.** If you're not getting enough calcium in your diet, not only will

Caregivers: You Deserve a Break Today...continued

Vent your feelings. At times, every caregiver feels frustrated, angry, guilty, lonely, and overwhelmed. Form a telephone network of caregivers who are facing similar problems so that you can share your ups and downs, Dr. Sotile suggests. The National Stroke Association (9707 E. Easter Lane, Englewood, CO 80112; 800-STROKES) can provide a list of stroke support groups in your area with interested members.

If you're having a particularly bad day, don't try to hide it from the person you're caring for, Dr. Sotile says. "Holding in your feelings and letting interpersonal tension accumulate isn't healthy for either you or the stroke survivor. Sometimes, you need to proclaim to the person you're caring for: 'I really need your help, love, and care today as much as you need mine.' "

Set limits. People who have had strokes have mood swings, frustrations, and bad days, too. But that doesn't mean they have a right to take it out on you.

"Ask yourself how you would react to this behavior if the stroke had not occurred," Dr. Sotile says. "If your loved one came home from work and started calling you names, you probably wouldn't tolerate it. So take off those kid gloves. Say, 'Listen, I love you, I care about you, and I know you're scared. But you can't treat me like this and get away with it. It's important to me that I am respected and loved. We can't let a stroke ruin what we have built between us.' You simply can't let yourself be violated, or else you're going to end up resentful, and that doesn't help anyone in this situation."

Get counseling. If mood swings and other emotional outbursts persist for more than six months for either the patient or anyone in a caregiving position, seek counseling, advises Dr. Sotile. The emotional effects of dealing with serious illness can be far-reaching, he says, so it is important for each family member to examine his feelings and seek help if needed.

you be at greater risk of developing osteoporosis, but also you may be more likely to have high blood pressure. "Individuals that fail to meet the Daily Value for calcium are more likely to develop hypertension," says David McCarron, M.D., professor of medicine and head of the Division of Hypertension at Oregon Health Sciences University in Portland.

Edith Howard Hogan, R.D., a spokesperson for the American Dietetic Association in Washington, D.C., recommends consuming 1,500 milligrams of calcium daily. A 1-ounce piece of Swiss cheese, about the size of a domino, has 270 milligrams of calcium and only 7 grams of fat. One cup of low-fat yogurt, 8 ounces of skim milk, or canned sardines or salmon packed with bones are also good sources. If you don't think you're getting enough calcium from your diet alone, ask your doctor about taking a supplement to boost your intake, says Hogan.

■ **Substitute herbs for salt.** Instead of reaching for the salt, which can raise blood pressure, add herbs and spices like ginger, oregano, garlic, or onion powder to your foods, Dr. Ancowitz suggests. Not only will that add aroma and zest to your meal, but it will also reduce your salt consumption and may lower your risk of a recurrent stroke.

■ **Try the dilution solution.** In many cases, you can do a lot to shave the sodium content of a favorite food or ingredient, Hogan says. If, for example, you buy a sodium-rich spaghetti sauce, try adding a can of no-sodium-added stewed tomatoes to the mixture. That will dilute the sodium in the sauce with little effect on the flavor.

■ **Be wary of salt substitutes.** Many salt substitutes contain potassium in the form of potassium chloride, which can help lower blood pressure in healthy people. But some men and women over age 60 who have weakened kidneys may not be able to rapidly excrete potassium from their bodies, says Thomas Pickering, M.D., professor of medicine at New York Hospital-Cornell Medical Center in New York City and author of *Good News about High Blood Pressure.* Also, excessive amounts of potassium in the blood can cause abnormal heart rhythms. Before using a salt substitute, he suggests that you check with your doctor.

Really Quit Smoking This Time

Smoking elevates blood pressure, speeds up the narrowing of artery walls, and forces the heart to work harder. Overall, smoking at least doubles your chances of having another stroke.

"If you want to increase your risk of a recurrent stroke and take the chance of being further debilitated, then you should continue to smoke," Dr. Libman says. "Smoking is the most modifiable risk factor for stroke. You have complete control over whether you do it."

Of course, there are many ways to quit. Deep breathing, for instance, helps many people learn to relax without cigarettes and can help them resist cravings, experts say. Mitchell Nides, Ph.D., a psychologist specializing in smoking cessation at the University of California, Los Angeles, explains that long, deep breaths mimic the sensation of smoking and can be reassuring and satisfying to someone who is trying to quit. "Deep breathing may be one of the best ways to cope with an urge to smoke," he says.

Try the following deep-breathing exercise whenever you feel the urge to smoke:

1. Take a deep, slow breath through your nose or through pursed lips as if smoking a cigarette. But instead of smoke, feel the fresh air filling your lungs.

2. Hold the breath for a count of three.

3. Exhale slowly, letting all of the air out of your lungs. As you exhale, feel the muscles in your neck and shoulders relax.

4. Repeat this exercise two or three times.

You also may want to consider the suggestions in Chapter 10 for how you can stop smoking.

Sex: Love Conquers All

Intimacy hasn't been forgotten at Jim and Cathy's home in Iowa.

"We're keeping on pace with the national record for sex in a month by a stroke survivor," Jim says, laughing. "I'm holding up my end."

Jim survived a paralyzing stroke in his fifties. His wife Cathy, a nurse, says, "I don't think you should ever give intimacy up because of a disability. You find what is the best way for you to fulfill your intimacy. We have managed to do that. We're probably as sexually active as some of the younger couples in our neighborhood."

Cathy discounts the aftereffects of her husband's stroke on their sex life. "I don't see Jim's disability," she says. "I don't look at him like I'm longing for something that isn't there. He is who he is, and I am who I am."

Many stroke survivors and their spouses fear that sexual activity will trigger another stroke. In reality, although blood pressure and heart rate do increase during sex, the increase probably isn't enough to be concerned about, according to Roger Crenshaw, M.D., a psychiatrist and sex therapist in private practice in San Diego. "The sexual part of the brain doesn't dissolve during a stroke," he says. "Just because there has been a muscular difficulty doesn't mean that the person can't desire and enjoy sexual activity."

How I Did It: Regaining an Active Life

Jim K. has a message for everyone who's had a stroke: Life goes on. "A stroke isn't the end of the world. You just change your routine, switch to another track, and proceed onward. You can still have the same enjoyment of life. I used to love golf. But since my stroke, I've found lots of other things to do," he says.

Jim has lived with complete paralysis of his left arm and leg since he suffered a stroke in his fifties. He can stand and walk with the aid of a leg brace.

"I was at least 30 pounds overweight, I had high cholesterol, my blood pressure was running high, I drank more than I should, and I was working in a high-pressure job," he says. "But for some reason, I didn't think it would happen to me."

After rehabilitation, he went back to work, but made little effort to change his lifestyle. His job continued to wear him down. His daily routine still included two or three drinks after work. In addition, he and his wife, Cathy, continued eating a high-fat diet that included lots of fried foods. Then, in his sixties, Jim had a massive heart attack that forced him to retire.

But this time, the lesson was learned. Now he adheres to a low-fat diet, walks as much as possible, limits himself to one beer a day, and lives at a slower pace.

"I think one of the things that saved me from another stroke is that I got away from the pressures. That's very important. I'm just more relaxed. I'm not living my life full-speed ahead anymore."

But Jim remains active. He uses a power mower to cut the grass on the couple's 4-acre lot, enjoys building doll furniture and wooden storage trunks for his grandchildren, and serves on his community's cemetery board. "I don't understand people who sit around and feel sad about what life has dealt them," he says. "I just don't have any room for that in my life."

Still, there are times when anxiety does overwhelm him. "It's unrealistic to believe that a fear of recurrence isn't going to be in the back of your mind occasionally," he says. "I just do everything I can, including prayer, to prevent a stroke from happening again."

In fact, intimacy of all kinds, including hugging and kissing, can boost self-esteem and relieve depression, says Dr. Senelick. The better your primary intimate relationship is after a stroke, he says, the better the odds that you'll have a more complete recovery.

"It's a huge boost to your self-esteem if your partner finds you attractive," says Domeena Renshaw, M.D., director of the Sexual Dysfunction Clinic at Loyola University of Chicago Stritch School of Medicine. "And yes, it's still possible to be a very good lover even if you've had a stroke."

Ask your doctor if and when you can resume sexual relations, Dr. Crenshaw recommends. Like all aspects of stroke rehabilitation, regaining intimacy may require some adaptation and experimentation.

Here are some suggestions for renewing sexual intimacy after a stroke:

■ **Take it slow.** Once you and your partner decide to resume sexual relations, put intercourse out of your mind for a couple of weeks. Instead, focus on other pleasures of intimacy like kissing, touching, and hugging, suggests Dr. Renshaw, author of *Seven Weeks to Better Sex*. Gradually building up to renewed sexual relations will boost your self-esteem and self-confidence, reduce performance anxiety, and foster feelings of mutual trust.

Empowering Ways to Help Your Caregiver

Jim K. wrote these 10 commitments after he suffered a paralyzing stroke. Even after his recovery, they have helped him maintain an understanding and fulfilling relationship with his wife and caregiver, Cathy. Originally published by the National Stroke Association, the commitments are as follows:

1. Don't ask my caregiver for anything that I can do for myself.
2. Make sure that I thank my caregiver each time he/she provides assistance to me.
3. Make sure that when my caregiver suggests we go out to eat, shopping, and so forth, I make every effort to go.
4. I will do my best not to complain about my stroke or handicap and my limitations.
5. I will try my utmost, on my own, to improve my skills, so as to improve the quality of my life and my caregiver's quality of life.
6. Encourage my caregiver to do things on his/her own, always giving my caregiver some space.
7. I will try to never feel sorry for myself, and I will do my best to keep my sense of humor.
8. I enjoy telling my caregiver that he/she looks nice, and to me he/she is always attractive.
9. I will not live in the past but live for today and the future, learning to live with my new lifestyle, my handicap.
10. I tell my caregiver I love him/her, because I do.

"Love play that avoids the genitals can strengthen the relationship between a couple in this situation," she says. "It lets the person who had the stroke know that his partner really loves him in many ways. And that ultimately makes sex much easier."

■ **Play it again, Sam.** Setting the right mood is also important, particularly after a life-changing event like a stroke, Dr. Renshaw says. Take time to reminisce about past romantic moments in your relationship. Play a favorite love song on the stereo. Take a moment to gaze at a sunset or full moon together, and realize that the romance you had before the stroke can continue.

■ **Stay in sight.** Many people who experience a stroke lose vision in one eye. If this is the case, ask your spouse to move so that you can see him or her better, or tilt your head to the side so that your partner remains in your line of sight when you're making love, Dr. Renshaw suggests.

■ **Go with your strength.** Lie on the side of your body that is weaker so that your strong hand is free to caress your spouse's body. This position will also allow you to thrust by using your strong leg to push off against the foot of the bed or a wall, Dr. Renshaw recommends.

■ **Keep laughing.** Sex at any age or with any physical problem is better if you don't take it too seriously. Have fun, be frivolous, use your imagination, Dr. Renshaw says. Remember that you're not at a stockholders meeting—you're with someone you love. Enjoy it.

■ **Check out your drugs.** If you have difficulty getting aroused or maintaining arousal, ask your doctor about it. Some medications prescribed for high blood pressure or depression, for instance, can interfere with your sexual abilities, says Dr. Renshaw. But under no circumstances should you discontinue taking a drug without your doctor's consent. Instead, discuss a switch.

■ **Give yourself time.** After six months, if you are not back into the same sexual routine that you were prior to the stroke, consider seeing a sex therapist who has experience in dealing with stroke survivors, advises Dr. Crenshaw.

"It usually isn't protracted therapy—just six to eight sessions that will help the couple deal with their specific concerns," Dr. Crenshaw says.

Rehabilitation Is a Lifetime Job

Although rehabilitation may not lower your risk of having another stroke, it can vastly improve the quality of your life and keep you more active. Dr. Senelick says that exercise, along with other lifestyle changes like quitting smoking, can lessen your risk factors—such as hypertension, diabetes, or obesity—as well as reduce your chances of having another stroke.

That's why it is important to keep the muscles in the affected area of your body well toned even after your rehabilitation ends, says Matthew Lee, M.D., medical director of the Rusk Institute of Rehabilitation Medicine at New York University Medical Center in New York City, and co-author of *Recovering at Home After a Stroke*.

"If you don't do the exercises given to you, if you don't maintain the flexibility you've gained during rehabilitation, you're going to lose it.

Your movements are going to get tighter, and eventually you may not be able to put on a shirt or pair of pants again. What's going to be affected is your quality of life," says Dr. Lee.

Maintenance Exercises

In addition to walking, strength training, or any other regular exercise you can perform, the daily arm and leg toning regimen on the following pages is suggested by Regina Kelly, a physical therapist at the Kessler Institute for Rehabilitation in West Orange, New Jersey.

Wear comfortable, loose-fitting clothing and do these exercises slowly and smoothly. Count out loud during your workout, says Kelly. Saying numbers aloud will require you to breathe normally, while helping to keep track of your reps.

1. Do one set (10 repetitions) of each exercise.

2. Rest for 1 minute, or until you feel able to continue.

3. Do two more sets of 10 repetitions with rest periods in between.

4. Switch sides where appropriate.

5. Repeat the cycle.

Caution: If your stroke happened recently, be sure to check with your doctor before starting any exercise program.

Another Difference Between Men and Women

Unusual stroke symptoms are more likely to occur in women, according to Lewis B. Morgenstern, M.D., director of the Stroke Program, University of Michigan Health System, Ann Arbor. In both women and men, symptoms of stroke include sudden onset of weakness on one side of the body, difficulty speaking, and/or vision problems. But one study shows that 28 percent of women and 19 percent of men eventually diagnosed with stroke initially complained of face and limb pain, nausea, chest pain, shortness of breath, palpitations—even hiccups.

The reason for this is believed to be a biological difference in the brains of women and men, which may explain the greater prevalence of atypical stroke symptoms in women.

Bottom Line Health

UPPER-BODY EXERCISES

Making Fists: Curl your fingers, beginning at the tips, and make a fist. Uncurl your fingers, completely straightening and spreading them. You can work both hands at once or alternate sides.

Wrist Flexions: To strengthen your wrists, sit in a chair and rest the forearm of your left hand on a table next to you, with your wrist extending over the edge, palm down. Bending at the wrist, raise the hand up and down, leaving your forearm on the table. Do three sets of 10, rest, then turn your palm up and repeat. Switch arms.

Sitting Push-ups: To strengthen your triceps muscle, sit on a firm surface like the edge of a bed and lean to one side. Support your weight with your bent elbow and forearm. Now push up so that your weight is on your hand and your arm is straight. Slowly lower yourself again and repeat for three sets of 10. Switch sides.

Elbow Extensions: Lie on your back on a firm bed. Touch your left hand to the opposite shoulder. Your elbow should be pointing toward the ceiling. Raise your hand slowly toward the ceiling until your arm is straight. Then lower your hand to the starting position. Do three sets of 10 with rest periods in between. Repeat with your other arm.

Biceps Curls: This exercise can be done lying down, sitting, or standing. Begin with your arms straight and at your sides. Bend your left elbow, bringing your left hand toward your left shoulder. Straighten your arm and repeat for three sets of 10. Rest, then switch sides.

Shoulder Squeezes: To improve your posture and strengthen your back muscles, stand or sit straight and tall. Tuck your chin in and relax your arms. Pull your shoulders back and squeeze your shoulder blades together. Try to get your elbows as close together as possible behind your back. If you're sitting, you can bend your elbows slightly as you draw your arms back. Otherwise, try to keep your arms straight. Relax and repeat for three sets of 10.

LOWER-BODY EXERCISES

Heel Slides: On a firm bed, lie on your back with your legs straight. Bend your left leg at the hip and knee, sliding your heel up toward your buttocks with your foot flat on the bed. Your knee should eventually point toward the ceiling. Hold for a count of five, then return to the starting position. Do three sets of 10 with rest periods in between. Repeat with your other leg.

Leg Slides: On a firm bed, lie on your back with your legs straight, and slide your left leg out to the side. Keep the leg straight and toes pointed up. Don't lift the leg, just slide it. (As you get stronger, you can try lifting your leg up slightly as you swing it out.) Return to the starting position and repeat. Do three sets of 10 with each leg.

More Leg Work: Lie on your back on a firm bed with knees bent and feet flat. Keeping your knees bent, slowly lower your left knee out to the side as far as possible. Return to the starting position. Repeat for three sets of 10. Rest, then switch legs.

Bottom Lifts: To strengthen your buttocks, lie on your back on a firm bed with your legs together and your knees bent and pointing toward the ceiling. Your feet should be flat on the bed and your arms by your sides. Using your arms for leverage, if necessary, lift your bottom as high as possible. Don't forget to breathe regularly. Slowly lower your bottom, then repeat for three sets of 10.

Knee Extensions: Lie on your back with a pillow or large towel rolled under your knees. Slowly lift one foot up a couple of inches. The back of your knee should remain on the pillow and your leg should become as straight as possible. Slowly lower and repeat for three sets of 10. Rest, then switch legs.

Prescription for Preventing Another Stroke

With therapy, many people can regain use of the arms, legs, and speech after a stroke. Strokes are often provoked by many of the same lifelong habits—smoking, sedentary living, high-fat eating—that trigger heart attacks. But modifications in lifestyle can diminish your chances of having a recurrence.

DO:

▶ **Exercise.** Walking and other activities will help lower blood pressure, a major risk factor for stroke.

▶ **Season foods with herbs and spices instead of salt.** Excess sodium can drive up blood pressure in some people who are salt-sensitive.

▶ **Quit smoking.** Lighting up doubles your chances of having another stroke.

▶ **Continue practicing the exercises** your physical therapist or doctor has recommended for you.

DON'T:

▶ **Drink too much alcohol.** In excess, alcohol increases your risk of stroke. Limit yourself to no more than two drinks a day.

▶ **Reach for salt substitutes.** Many are made with potassium chloride, which can cause irregular heart rhythms and other problems in some people over age 60.

▶ **Shy away from intimacy.** Sex can boost your self-esteem. It is unlikely to cause a stroke.

▶ **Give up.**

Index

Page numbers in **bold** indicate a table or box. Page numbers *italicized* indicate an illustration.